Cardio-oncology Related to Heart Failure

Editors

DANIEL J. LENIHAN
DOUGLAS B. SAWYER

HEART FAILURE CLINICS

www.heartfailure.theclinics.com

Founding Editor
JAGAT NARULA

April 2017 • Volume 13 • Number 2

ELSEVIER

1600 John F. Kennedy Boulevard • Suite 1800 • Philadelphia, Pennsylvania, 19103-2899

http://www.theclinics.com

HEART FAILURE CLINICS Volume 13, Number 2
April 2017 ISSN 1551-7136, ISBN-13: 978-0-323-52408-7

Editor: Stacy Eastman
Developmental Editor: Alison Swety

Heart Failure Clinics (ISSN 1551-7136) is published quarterly by Elsevier Inc., 360 Park Avenue South, New York, NY 10010-1710. Months of publication are January, April, July, and October. Business and editorial offices: 1600 John F. Kennedy Boulevard, Suite 1800, Philadelphia, PA 19103-2899. Periodicals postage paid at New York, NY, and additional mailing offices. Subscription prices are USD 247.00 per year for US individuals, USD 448.00 per year for US institutions, USD 100.00 per year for US students and residents, USD 288.00 per year for Canadian individuals, USD 519.00 per year for Canadian institutions, USD 309.00 per year for international individuals, USD 519.00 per year for international institutions, and USD 100.00 per year for Canadian and foreign students/residents. To receive student and resident rate, orders must be accompanied by name of affiliated institution, date of term, and the *signature* of program/residency coordinator on institution letterhead. Orders will be billed at individual rate until proof of status is received. Foreign air speed delivery is included in all *Clinics* subscription prices. All prices are subject to change without notice. **POSTMASTER:** Send address changes to *Heart Failure Clinics*, Elsevier Health Sciences Division, Subscription Customer Service, 3251 Riverport Lane, Maryland Heights, MO 63043. **Customer Service: 1-800-654-2452 (US and Canada). From outside of the US and Canada, call 314-447-8871. Fax: 314-447-8029. For print support, E-mail:** JournalsCustomerService-usa@elsevier.com. **For online support, E-mail:** JournalsOnlineSupport-usa@elsevier.com.

Reprints. For copies of 100 or more of articles in this publication, please contact the Commercial Reprints Department, Elsevier Inc., 360 Park Avenue South, New York, NY 10010-1710. Tel.: 212-633-3874; Fax: 212-633-3820; E-mail: reprints@elsevier.com.

Heart Failure Clinics is covered in *MEDLINE/PubMed (Index Medicus)*.

Contributors

EDITORS

DANIEL J. LENIHAN, MD, FACC
Professor of Cardiovascular Medicine, Director of Clinical Research, Vanderbilt University Medical Center, Nashville, Tennessee

DOUGLAS B. SAWYER, MD, PhD
Chief of Cardiovascular Services, Maine Medical Center Cardiovascular Institute, Portland, Maine

AUTHORS

SADEER G. AL-KINDI, MD
Onco-Cardiology Program, Advanced Heart Failure & Transplantation Center, Harrington Heart & Vascular Institute, University Hospitals Cleveland Medical Center, Case Western Reserve University School of Medicine, Cleveland, Ohio

SARO H. ARMENIAN, DO, MPH
Division of Outcomes Research, Department of Population Sciences, Comprehensive Cancer Center, City of Hope, Duarte, California

ANA BARAC, MD, PhD
Associate Professor of Medicine and Oncology, Georgetown University, Washington, DC

CHRISTOPHER M. BIANCO, DO
Onco-Cardiology Program, Advanced Heart Failure & Transplantation Center, Harrington Heart & Vascular Institute, University Hospitals Cleveland Medical Center, Case Western Reserve University School of Medicine, Cleveland, Ohio

ANNE BLAES, MD, MS
Division of Hematology and Oncology, University of Minnesota, Minneapolis, Minnesota

WILLIAM L. BORDER, MBChB, MPH
Department of Pediatrics, Sibley Heart Center Cardiology, Division of Pediatric Cardiology, Department of Pediatrics, Emory University School of Medicine, Atlanta, Georgia

JOSEPH CARVER, MD, FACC
Abramson Cancer Center, University of Pennsylvania, Philadelphia, Pennsylvania

ERIC J. CHOW, MD, MPH
Clinical Research Division, Fred Hutchinson Cancer Research Center, University of Washington, Seattle, Washington

ROBERT F. CORNELL, MD, MS
Division of Hematology and Oncology, Department of Internal Medicine, Vanderbilt University School of Medicine, Nashville, Tennessee

JOSE EMANUEL FINET, MD
Assistant Professor of Clinical Medicine, Krannert Institute of Cardiology, Indiana University, Staff Physician, Cardio-Oncology and Advanced Heart Failure and Transplant Cardiology, IU Health Academic Health Center, Indianapolis, Indiana

SANJEEV A. FRANCIS, MD, FACC
Director of Education and Director of Cardiovascular Disease Fellowship Program, Division of Cardiovascular Medicine, Maine Medical Center, Portland, Maine

STACEY GOODMAN, MD
Division of Hematology and Oncology,
Department of Internal Medicine, Vanderbilt
University School of Medicine, Nashville,
Tennessee

JOERG HERRMANN, MD
Department of Cardiovascular Diseases, Mayo
Clinic, Rochester, Minnesota

BORAH J. HONG, MD
Division of Pediatric Cardiology, Department
of Pediatrics, Seattle Children's Hospital,
University of Washington School of
Medicine, University of Washington,
Seattle, Washington

VARUN JAIN, MD
MedStar Washington Hospital Center,
Washington, DC

MICHELLE N. JOHNSON, MD, MPH, FACC
Memorial Sloan-Kettering Cancer Center, New
York, New York

BENJAMIN KENIGSBERG, MD
MedStar Washington Hospital Center,
Georgetown University Hospital,
Washington, DC

MICHEL G. KHOURI, MD
Division of Cardiology, Department of
Medicine, Duke University, Durham, North
Carolina

YONG-HYUN KIM, MD
Department of Cardiovascular Medicine,
Kaufman Center for Heart Failure, Heart and
Vascular Institute, Cleveland Clinic, Cleveland,
Ohio; Cardiovascular Medicine, Korea
University College of Medicine, Korea
University Medical Center Ansan Hospital,
Ansan, Korea

JENNIFER KIRSOP, BS
Department of Cellular and Molecular
Medicine, Lerner Research Institute, Cleveland
Clinic, Cleveland, Ohio

RYAN J. KOENE, MD
Division of Cardiology, University of Minnesota,
Minneapolis, Minnesota

SUMA KONETY, MD, MS
Division of Cardiology, University of Minnesota,
Minneapolis, Minnesota

GEORGIOS KOULAOUZIDIS, MD
NIHR Cardiovascular Biomedical Research
Unit, Royal Brompton Hospital, London, United
Kingdom

DANIEL J. LENIHAN, MD, FACC
Professor of Cardiovascular Medicine, Director
of Clinical Research, Vanderbilt University
Medical Center, Nashville, Tennessee

AMIR LERMAN, MD
Department of Cardiovascular Diseases, Mayo
Clinic, Rochester, Minnesota

GRACE LIN, MD
Department of Cardiovascular Diseases, Mayo
Clinic, Rochester, Minnesota

ALEXANDER R. LYON, MD, PhD
NIHR Cardiovascular Biomedical Research
Unit, Royal Brompton Hospital, Imperial
College London, London, United Kingdom

ANANT MANDAWAT, MD
Division of Cardiovascular Medicine, Duke
University School of Medicine, Durham, North
Carolina

SHARON MULVAGH, MD
Department of Cardiovascular Diseases, Mayo
Clinic, Rochester, Minnesota

GUILHERME H. OLIVEIRA, MD
Chief of Heart Failure Section and Director of
Onco-Cardiology Center, Onco-Cardiology
Program, Advanced Heart Failure &
Transplantation Center, Harrington Heart &
Vascular Institute, Associate Professor of
Medicine, University Hospitals Cleveland
Medical Center, Case Western Reserve
University School of Medicine, Cleveland, Ohio

JAE YOON PARK, MD
Department of Cardiovascular Diseases, Mayo
Clinic, Rochester, Minnesota

NAVEEN PEREIRA, MD
Department of Cardiovascular Diseases, Mayo
Clinic, Rochester, Minnesota

ANNA PRIZMENT, PhD
School of Public Health, University of
Minnesota, Minneapolis, Minnesota

ALEXANDRA J. RITTS, MD
Department of Internal Medicine, Vanderbilt University School of Medicine, Nashville, Tennessee

MARTIN RODRIGUEZ-PORCEL, MD
Department of Cardiovascular Diseases, Mayo Clinic, Rochester, Minnesota

KIRSTEN ROSE-FELKER, MD
Department of Pediatrics, Sibley Heart Center Cardiology, Division of Pediatric Cardiology, Department of Pediatrics, Emory University School of Medicine, Atlanta, Georgia

THOMAS D. RYAN, MD, PhD
The Heart Institute, Cincinnati Children's Hospital Medical Center, Cincinnati, Ohio

JAI SINGH, MD
Division of Cardiovascular Medicine, Department of Internal Medicine, Vanderbilt University School of Medicine, Nashville, Tennessee

DAVID SNIPELISKY, MD
Department of Cardiovascular Diseases, Mayo Clinic, Rochester, Minnesota

RICHARD STEINGART, MD, FACC
Memorial Sloan-Kettering Cancer Center, New York, New York

KRIS SWIGER, MD
Division of Cardiovascular Medicine, Department of Internal Medicine, Vanderbilt University School of Medicine, Nashville, Tennessee

WAI HONG WILSON TANG, MD
Department of Cardiovascular Medicine, Kaufman Center for Heart Failure, Heart and Vascular Institute, Cleveland Clinic, Department of Cellular and Molecular Medicine, Lerner Research Institute, Cleveland Clinic, Center for Clinical Genomics, Cleveland Clinic, Cleveland, Ohio

HECTOR R. VILLARRAGA, MD
Department of Cardiovascular Diseases, Mayo Clinic, Rochester, Minnesota

ANDREW E. WILLIAMS, PhD
Division of Health Services Research, Center for Outcomes Research and Evaluation, Maine Medical Center Research Institute, Portland, Maine

Contents

and mortality with cardiovascular disease as a leading cause of death. Heightened awareness in providers with increased surveillance and improvement in cardiovascular imaging modalities have led to earlier detection of cardiac dysfunction, but the outcomes remain poor once this has dysfunction developed. A great deal of work remains to be done to refine screening and identify high-risk patients more precisely, and to develop more evidence-based strategies for effective primary and secondary cardioprotection and treatment.

End-stage heart failure in cancer survivors may result from cardiotoxic chemotherapy and/or chest radiation and require advanced therapies, including left ventricular assist devices (LVADs) and transplantation. Traditionally, such therapies have been underutilized in cancer survivors owing to lack of experience and perceived risk of cancer recurrence. Recent data from large registries, however, have shown excellent outcomes of LVADs and transplantation in cancer survivors, albeit subject to careful selection and special considerations. This article summarizes all aspects of advanced heart failure therapies in patients with cancer therapy–related cardiac dysfunction and underscores the need for careful selection of these candidates.

Hematopoietic cell transplantation (HCT) has been used for curative intent in patients with hematologic and nonhematologic malignancies, resulting in an increasing number of HCT survivors. These survivors are at risk for serious and life-threatening complications, including cardiovascular disease (CVD). This article provides an overview of CVD in HCT survivors, describing the pathophysiology of disease, with a special emphasis on therapeutic exposures and comorbidities unique to this population. This article also discusses novel screening and prevention strategies that have shown promise in non-HCT cancer populations, emphasizing opportunities for collaboration between cardiologists and hematologists to improve the cardiovascular health of HCT survivors.

Cardiovascular demands to the care of cancer patients are common and important given the implications for morbidity and mortality. As a consequence, interactions with cardiovascular disease specialists have intensified to the point of the development of a new discipline termed *cardio-oncology*. As an additional consequence, so-called cardio-oncology clinics have emerged, in most cases staffed by cardiologists with an interest in the field. This article addresses this gap and summarizes key points in the development of a cardio-oncology clinic.

Management of cardiovascular disease in patients with cancer and cancer survivors requires particular clinical expertise and skills that are central to cardio-oncology.

The areas of knowledge required include specific cardiovascular complications directly related to oncologic therapies and the impact of cancer and its therapies on existing or potential cardiovascular comorbidities. Many cancer therapeutics have potential cardiotoxicity. The conversion of many cancers to chronic conditions, rather than fatal diseases, has produced a population of patients with cancer at high risk for cardiovascular diseases that require specialized knowledge of treating physicians. Thus, there is a compelling need for enhanced cardio-oncology training.

There is a growing body of evidence that suggests cancer and cardiovascular disease have a shared biological mechanism. Although there are several shared risk factors for both diseases, including advancing age, gender, obesity, diabetes, physical activity, tobacco use, and diet, inflammation and biomarkers, such as insulinlike growth factor 1, leptin, estrogen, and adiponectin, may also play a role in the biology of these diseases. This article provides an overview of the shared biological mechanism between cancer and cardiovascular disease.

Chemotherapy-related cardiac dysfunction (CRCD) has challenged clinicians to hesitate in using cardiotoxic agents such as anthracycline and several protein kinase inhibitors. As early detection of CRCD and timely cessation of cardiotoxic agents became a strategy to avoid CRCD, cardiac troponin and natriuretic peptide are measured to monitor cardiotoxicity; however, there are inconsistencies in their predictability of CRCD. Alternative biomarkers have been researched extensively for potential use as more sensitive and accurate biomarkers. The mechanisms of CRCD and previous studies on traditional and novel biomarkers for CRCD are examined to enlighten future direction of investigation in this combined biology.

Despite its challenges, a "big data" approach offers a unique opportunity within the field of cardio-oncology. A pharmacovigilant approach using large data sets can help characterize cardiovascular toxicities of the rapidly expanding armamentarium of targeted therapies. Creating a broad coalition of data sharing can provide insights into the incidence of cardiotoxicity and stimulate research into the underlying mechanisms. Population health necessitates the use of big data and can help inform public health interventions to prevent both cancer and cardiovascular disease. As a relatively new discipline, cardio-oncology is poised to take advantage of big data.

Cardiac amyloidosis is a complex and vexing clinical condition that requires a high degree of suspicion for the diagnosis with a substantial amount of discipline to discern the extent of disease and the best available therapy. There is a complex interplay between multiple organ systems, and the clinical presentation may involve a myriad of confusing clinical symptoms. The diagnosis of cardiac amyloidosis can be confirmed with a combination of physical findings, cardiac biomarkers, noninvasive testing, and, if necessary, myocardial biopsy. Genetic testing is critical to establish the type of amyloidosis.

HEART FAILURE CLINICS

ISSUE OF RELATED INTEREST

Magnetic Resonance Imaging Clinics, February 2015 (Vol. 23, Issue 1)
Updates in Cardiac MRI
Karen G. Ordovas, *Editor*
Available at: http://www.mri.theclinics.com

THE CLINICS ARE AVAILABLE ONLINE!
Access your subscription at:
www.theclinics.com

Preface

Cardio-Oncology—A Rapidly Evolving and Expanding Field of Medicine

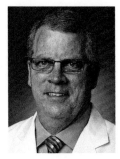 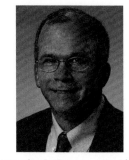

Daniel J. Lenihan, MD, FACC   Douglas B. Sawyer, MD, PhD

Editors

We are excited to share with you this series of articles by experts in the rapidly evolving field of cardio-oncology. In 2011, we guest edited a *Heart Failure Clinics* issue devoted to this topic. The editors asked us to revisit this in order to keep up with this important field of cardiovascular medicine with special relevance to heart failure. In this update, a compendium of topics of practical relevance is covered, which we consider valuable additions to the literature.

It has become increasingly clear that there are common risk factors for cancer and heart failure that hold special relevance to understanding and mitigating risk as well as detection of both of these diseases. Epidemiologic and clinical databases are helping to recognize and highlight the magnitude of these problems and opportunities. Rapid advances in the care of heart failure need careful consideration in the specific group of patients who experience heart failure as a complication of or concomitant with cancer treatment. These include the polypharmacy of heart failure medical therapy as well as application of advanced treatment options.

We are at an interesting juncture. The promise of the molecular revolution of medicine is coming to fruition. And yet there is incomplete understanding of how the common biology of tumors and normal tissue limit the precision of "precision medicine." As new therapies emerge through clinical trials, approval for use may occur with incomplete recognition of the potential adverse effects as well as strategies to reduce risk for these and/or treat them. With widespread availability of technical information, patients with newly diagnosed cancer are often aware of the potential adverse effects of new cancer therapies, often before their health care providers.

Recognizing the rapid expansion in this field, and in response to patient requests, a number of medical centers and clinical practices are moving to offer specialized cardio-oncology clinics for appropriate patients. For most patients, this specialized expertise is likely to improve patient experience as well as outcomes. Perhaps specialized training in this field, cardio-oncology fellowship training, should be considered to address this need.

Daniel J. Lenihan, MD, FACC
Vanderbilt University Medical Center
1215 21st Avenue South, Suite 5209
Nashville, TN, 37232, USA

Douglas B. Sawyer, MD, PhD
Maine Medical Center Cardiovascular Institute
22 Bramhall Street
Portland, ME 04102, USA

E-mail addresses:
daniel.lenihan@vanderbilt.edu (D.J. Lenihan)
dsawyer@mmc.org (D.B. Sawyer)

Heart Failure Clin 13 (2017) xiii
http://dx.doi.org/10.1016/j.hfc.2017.01.001
1551-7136/17/© 2017 Published by Elsevier Inc.

Management of Heart Failure in Cancer Patients and Cancer Survivors

 CrossMark

Jose Emanuel Finet, MD

KEYWORDS

- Heart failure • Cancer • Cardiotoxicity • Cardioprotection • Anthracyclines • Trastuzumab
- Cardio-oncology • Myocardial dysfunction

KEY POINTS

- Patients at high risk of cancer therapeutics–related cardiac dysfunction (either high-risk patients because of their inherent cardiovascular risk factor burden, or planned cardiotoxic cancer therapeutics) should be referred to a cardio-oncology specialist for prevention, surveillance, early management, and recovery of cardiomyopathy.
- Baseline and serial echocardiographic evaluation of systolic and diastolic left ventricular function should be performed in all patients undergoing anthracyclines and/or ERBB2 inhibitors, irrespective of baseline cardiovascular risk, with the exception of asymptomatic patients with metastatic disease.
- If left ventricular ejection fraction declines to less than 40%, cardiotoxic chemotherapy should be stopped; alternative cancer therapies should be discussed, standard heart failure therapies should be implemented, and other causes of left ventricular dysfunction should be excluded.
- Patients with cancer who develop left ventricular dysfunction should be aggressively treated with standard heart failure guideline–directed medical therapies, just as any other patient with heart failure, especially if the neoplasia allows a long-term survival.
- Cancer survivors exposed to high cumulative anthracycline doses and/or chest radiotherapy should be offered lifelong cardiac surveillance.

DEFINITION, CLASSIFICATION, AND EPIDEMIOLOGY OF HEART FAILURE

Heart failure (HF) is currently defined as a complex clinical syndrome that results from any structural or functional impairment of ventricular filling or ejection of blood.[1] This condition can be classified by stages of disease progression (A–D), severity of symptoms (New York Heart Association [NYHA] class I–IV), degree of left ventricular (LV) systolic dysfunction (HF with preserved ejection fraction [HFpEF] or HF with reduced ejection fraction [HFrEF]), and need for either standard or advanced HF therapies (Table 1).[1–3]

This syndrome is characterized by pulmonary and/or splanchnic congestion, and/or peripheral edema; impaired end-organ perfusion is the hallmark of advanced HF.[1] A list of typical clinical features of this syndrome is provided in Table 2. It is most commonly caused by LV diastolic or systolic dysfunction; however, disorders of the other cardiac chambers, pericardium, heart valves, and great vessels can also elicit an HF syndrome.

It is estimated that 20% of the US population greater than or equal to 40 years of age will develop HF in their lifetime.[4] As with cancer, the

Disclosures: The author has nothing to disclose.
Krannert Institute of Cardiology, Indiana University, IU Health Methodist Hospital, 1801 North Senate Boulevard, MPC-2, Suite 2000, Indianapolis, IN 46202, USA
E-mail address: jefinet@iu.edu

Heart Failure Clin 13 (2017) 253–288
http://dx.doi.org/10.1016/j.hfc.2016.12.004
1551-7136/17/© 2016 Elsevier Inc. All rights reserved.

Table 1
American College of Cardiology Foundation/American Heart Association heart failure classifications

Stages		Definition	LVEF	NYHA Class
A: At Risk of HF				
B: Asymptomatic LV dysfunction				I: No physical activity limitation
C: Prior or current symptomatic HF	HFpEF	Diastolic HF	LVEF ≥50%	I: No physical activity limitation
		Borderline HF	LVEF 41%–49%	
		Improved HF	LVEF >40%	II: Slight physical activity limitation
	HFrEF	Systolic HF	LVEF ≤40%	III: Marked physical activity limitation IV: Unable to perform physical activity
D: Refractory HF		Advanced HF	LVEF <30%	III: Marked physical activity limitation IV: Unable to perform physical activity
INTERMACS Profile[2]				**UNOS Status[3]**
7: Advanced NYHA III				2
6: Exertion limited				
5: Exertion intolerant				
4: Resting symptoms on home oral therapy				
3: Stable but inotrope dependent				1B
2: Progressive decline on inotropes				1A
1: Critical cardiogenic shock				

Abbreviations: AHA, American Heart Association; INTERMACS, Interagency Registry for Mechanically Assisted Circulator Support; LVEF, left ventricular ejection fraction; UNOS, United Network of Organ Sharing.
Data from Refs.[1–3]

incidence of HF proportionally increases with age[5]; 5.7 million adults have HF currently in the United States, and it is projected to affect 46% of the population by 2030,[6] and cost $69.7 billion.[7]

HF is involved in 1 every 9 deaths in the United States.[6] Although stable in recent years,[8] the mortality in the HF population has progressively declined since 1979[9] because of the implementation of evidence-based approaches to prevent and treat this condition.[10] Nonetheless, the 5-year mortality risk of the overall HF population is still more than 50%, increasing proportionally with age.[8,9]

In the general population, LV diastolic dysfunction has a prevalence of 21%, whereas 6% of the population has systolic dysfunction.[11] Even when asymptomatic, both systolic and diastolic LV dysfunction have an increased risk of developing HF and all-cause death.[12] Approximately half of patients who seek attention for HF symptoms have a normal or near-normal LV ejection fraction (LVEF)[13]; the prevalence of HFpEF is higher in older patients, especially in women with hypertension, obesity, and anemia.[6,14] The long-term survival of patients with HFpEF in the community is lower than that of patients with HFrEF,[15] mostly driven by noncardiovascular causes[16]; however, in most clinical studies, HFrEF carries a worse prognosis.[17]

Coronary artery disease, hypertension, diabetes mellitus, age, tobacco smoking, and obesity continue to be the leading risk factors for HF.[6] Age, tobacco smoking, diabetes mellitus, and obesity are also cancer risk factors.[18,19] Recently identified shared pathophysiologic mechanisms,[20] and similar long-term survival and prognosis,[21] seem to relate both conditions more than was previously thought. In addition, certain cancer therapies have been recognized to cause or exacerbate HF; among these, anthracycline agents have historically been the most notorious.[22–24]

HEART FAILURE IN CANCER PATIENTS AND CANCER SURVIVORS

The number of cancer survivors continues to increase annually, because of both advances in early detection and treatment, and the aging and growth of the population.[25] It is projected that there will be more than 20 million cancer survivors by 2026.[25] This increase in cancer survivorship has brought forth a concomitant increase in morbidity and mortality from other conditions related to the adverse effects of cancer treatments.[26] Cardiovascular diseases, and

Table 2
Heart failure syndrome

	Signs	Symptoms	Biomarkers
Congestion	Peripheral edema Jugular venous distention S3 gallop Tachypnea Lung rales Pleural effusion Hypoxemia Regurgitant murmurs Hepatojugular reflex Hepatomegaly Splenomegaly Ascites	Dyspnea on exertion Orthopnea Paroxysmal nocturnal dyspnea Dyspnea at rest Frothy cough Early satiety Nausea and vomiting Oliguria Angina	Labs: BNP/NT-proBNP, Troponin, ALT/AST, lactate, LDH, and Cr elevation ECG: LV strain, ST depression, sinus tachycardia, PACs, PVCs CXR: Pulmonary edema, pleural effusion, cardiomegaly
Hypoperfusion	Tachycardia Hypotension Cool and pale skin Liver injury Kidney injury Myocardial injury Altered mental status	Fatigue Confusion Oliguria Angina Nausea and vomiting	Echo: RV and LV systolic dysfunction, diastolic LV dysfuntion, cardiomegaly, LVH, LAE, MR, TR

in particular LV dysfunction and HF, are among the most significant.[23,27,28] For example, adult cancer survivors are at increased risk of ischemic heart disease and HF.[28] Pediatric cancer survivors also have a 15-fold increased lifetime risk of asymptomatic LV dysfunction and HF,[29] and a 5-year HF incidence of 17% in those adult patients receiving CHOP (cyclophosphamide, doxorubicin, vincristine, and prednisolone) and Rituximab + CHOP chemotherapy regimens.[30] Recent data suggest that the highest incidence of anthracycline-induced cardiomyopathy (AIC) occurs during the first year after the completion of chemotherapy.[31] This condition has historically carried an increased risk of mortality compared with idiopathic nonischemic cardiomyopathy[32]; however, modern evidence-based HF therapies seem to have improved its prognosis.[33]

Heart Failure Related to Chemotherapy

The American Heart Association (AHA) recently released a scientific statement enumerating and describing drugs that may cause or exacerbate HF according to currently available clinical data.[22] Several chemotherapy agents were included in this list, each with its incidence and magnitude of cardiotoxic effect, and the weight of supporting evidence.[22] Correspondingly, the European Society of Cardiology (ESC) just published a comprehensive position paper containing a similar list, along with evidence-based guidelines

for the evaluation and management of cardiovascular toxicity caused by chemotherapy and other cancer therapies.[23]

The referenced cardiotoxic chemotherapy agents cause or exacerbate HF either by causing direct myocardial injury (anthracyclines, antimetabolites, alkylating agents, interleukin-2), by exacerbating hypertension (vascular endothelial growth factor [VEGF] inhibitors), by impairing myocardial stress response (ERBB2 inhibitors), by facilitating arrhythmias (some BCR-ABL inhibitors), or by other cardiotoxic mechanisms that are still not well understood.[22] Patients with cancer and cancer survivors exposed to these agents are at increased risk of developing HF.[23,34]

Table 3 lists the cardiotoxic chemotherapy agents recently acknowledged by the AHA and ESC to cause or exacerbate HF, including their incidence and magnitude of LV dysfunction effect, mechanism of action, common cancer uses and chemotherapy regimens, and other clinically relevant cardiovascular toxicities.[22,23,35–41]

Heart Failure Related to Radiotherapy

The true incidence of radiation-induced cardiotoxicity is difficult to evaluate because of the long delay between exposure and manifestation of heart disease, the consequential reporting bias, and the frequent concomitant use of cardiotoxic chemotherapy, in particular anthracyclines.[23] Nonetheless, it is estimated that cancer survivors who received chest radiation have an 4.9-fold

Table 3
Chemotherapy agents that cause or exacerbate heart failure (American Heart Association/European Society of Cardiology 2016)

Chemotherapy Family	Chemotherapy Agent	Incidence and Magnitude of Cardiac Dysfunction	Cancers Uses and Chemotherapy Regimens	Mechanism of Action	Other Cardiovascular Toxicities
Anthracyclines	Doxorubicin	3%–26% (major)	Breast cancer [AC (CA), CAF (FAC), ACT (TAC), CMF] Non-Hodgkin lymphoma [CHOP, R-CHOP, EPOCH, R-EPOCH, hyper-CVAD-R, BACOD, m-BEACOD, CHOEP, CVAD, MACOP-B, ProMACE-MOPP, ProMACE-CytaBOM, CODOX-M, CODOX-M/IVAC] Burkitt lymphoma [CODOX-M, CODOX-M/IVAC, hyper-CVAD] Mantle Cell lymphoma [R-hyper-CVAD, VcR-CAP] Hodgkin lymphoma [ABVD, BEACOPP, Stanford V, VABCD, VAMP, ChlVPP/EVA, GVD, VAPEC-B] Waldenström macroglobulinemia [R-CHOP] Acute lymphocytic leukemia [CALGB 8811, CALGB 9111, hyper-CVAD, VAD/CVAD] Small cell lung cancer [CAV] Multiple Myeloma [DT-PACE, VAD, hyper-CVAD, VAMP, VD-PACE, VTD-PACE, PAD] Gastric cancer [FAM, FAMTX] Bladder cancer [MVAC] Wilms' Tumor [DD-4A, Regimen I, VAD] Bone Sarcoma [VAC/IE] Soft Tissue Sarcoma [MAID, AD, AIM, VAC/IE, VAIA, VIDE, VAI] Thymoma [CAP, ADOC] Neuroblastoma [A3, CAV-P/VP, CE-CAdO, New A1] Hepatoblastoma [IPA, PA-CI] Endometrial cancer [AP, APT]	Anthracyclines bind directly to DNA (intercalation) and also inhibit DNA repair (via topoisomerase II inhibition) resulting in blockade of DNA and RNA synthesis and fragmentation of DNA. It is active throughout the cell cycle (cell cycle nonspecific). Doxorubicin is also a p53 inhibitor and powerful iron chelator; the iron-doxorubicin complex binds to DNA and cell membranes, producing free radicals that cleave the DNA and cell membranes	Acute myocarditis, atrioventricular block, bradycardia, bundle branch block, extrasystoles (atrial or ventricular), nonspecific ST or T wave changes on ECG, sinus tachycardia, supraventricular tachycardia, ventricular tachycardia

Daunorubicin	2.8%–3.7% (major)	Acute Myelocytic Leukemia [7 + 3 (DA/DAC), DAT (TAD)] Acute lymphocytic leukemia [hyper-CVAD] Kaposi sarcoma Non-Hodgkin lymphoma [EPOCH, R-EPOCH]
Idarubicin	5%–18% (major)	Acute Promyelocytic Leukemia [APL] Acute Myelocytic Leukemia [7 + 3 (IA/IAC), 5 + 2, FLAG-Ida]
Epirubicin	1%–11% (major)	Breast cancer [EC, FEC] Soft Tissue Sarcoma [EI] Bone sarcoma [IPE] Gastric cancer [ECF, EOX] Esophageal cancer [ECF, EOX]
Mitoxantrone	2.6% (major)	Non-Hodgkin lymphoma [FCM (FMC), R-FCM, FM, R-FM] Hodgkin lymphoma [MINE-ESHAP, VIM-D] Prostate cancer [MP] Breast cancer [MMM] Acute Promyelocytic Leukemia [APL] Acute Myelocytic Leukemia [5 + 2, 7 + 3, CLAG-M, MEC-G, FLAG-Mito]

(continued on next page)

Table 3
(continued)

Chemotherapy Family	Chemotherapy Agent	Incidence and Magnitude of Cardiac Dysfunction	Cancers Uses and Chemotherapy Regimens	Mechanism of Action	Other Cardiovascular Toxicities
Alkylating agents	Cyclophosphamide	7%–28% (major)	*Breast cancer [AC (CA), CAF, CMF, CT (TC), EC, FEC, ACT (TAC)]* Non-Hodgkin lymphoma [CHOP, R-CHOP, R-CVP (COP), CVAD, EPOCH, R-EPOCH, PEP-C, hyper-CVAD-R, BACOD, m-BEACOD, CHOEP, CEPP, FCM (FMC), R-FCM, MACOP-B, ProMACE-MOPP, ProMACE-CytaBOM] Mantle cell lymphoma [PEP-C, R-hyper-CVAD, VcR-CAP, FC] Follicular lymphoma [R-CVP, FCR] Burkitt lymphoma [CODOX-M, CODOX-M/IVAC, hyper-CVAD] Hodgkin lymphoma [BEACOPP, C-MOPP/ABV Hybrid, VAPEC-B] Waldenström macroglobulinemia [R-CHOP] Acute lymphocytic leukemia [CVAD, hyper-CVAD, CALGB 8811, FC, R-FC, R-PC] Small cell lung cancer [CAV] Lymphoma [CBV] AL Amyloidosis [CTD, CYBORD, RdC] Multiple Myeloma [CYBORD, DCEP, DT-PACE, hyper-CVAD, VBCMP, C-VAMP, VD-PACE, VTD-PACE, CRd] Gastric cancer [ECF] Esophageal cancer [ECF] Soft Tissue Sarcoma [VAC] Wilms' Tumor [Regimen I] Gestational Trophoblastic Tumor [EMA/CO, MAC] Neuroblastoma [A3, CAV-P/VP, CE-CAdO, CT, New A1]*	Alkylating agents prevent cell division by cross-linking DNA strands and binding with nucleic acids and other intracellular structures, inhibiting protein synthesis and DNA synthesis, resulting in cell death. It is active throughout the cell cycle (cell cycle nonspecific). Cyclophosphamide also possesses potent immunosuppressive activity	Atrial ectopy, atrial fibrillation, atrial flutter, bradycardia, capillary leak syndrome, cardiac arrest, cardiogenic shock, hemopericardium, hemorrhagic myocarditis

Ifosfamide	0.5%–17% (moderate)	Bone Sarcoma [CT, VACIIE]
		Brain Tumor [COPE]
		Ovarian cancer [VAC]
		Thymoma [CAP, ADOC]
		Hodgkin lymphoma [DICE, ICE, IGEV, MINE-ECHAP, VIM-D, R-ICE, MINE, R-MINE]
		Non-Hodgkin lymphoma [R-ICE]
		Burkitt lymphoma [CODOX-M/IVAC]
		Neuroblastoma [DICE, ICE, R-ICE]
		Small cell lung cancer [PEI]
		Penile cancer [TIP]
		Testicular cancer [TIP, VIP, VIP-16, VeIP]
		Hepatoblastoma [IPA]
		Bone Sarcoma [PEI, EI, VACIEI]
		Soft Tissue Sarcoma [MAID, AIM, EI, VACIIE, VAIA, VIDE]
Mitomycin	10% (moderate)	Gastric cancer [FAM]
		Anal cancer [FM]
		Pancreatic cancer
		Lung cancer [MVP]
		Mesothelioma [MVP]
		Bladder cancer
		Breast cancer [MMM]

(continued on next page)

Table 3
(continued)

Chemotherapy Family	Chemotherapy Agent	Incidence and Magnitude of Cardiac Dysfunction	Cancers Uses and Chemotherapy Regimens	Mechanism of Action	Other Cardiovascular Toxicities
Antimetabolites	Fluorouracil	2%–20% (major)	Breast cancer [CAF (FAC), FEC, VIFUP] Anal cancer [FM] Gastric cancer [FAM, FAMTX, CF, ECF] Esophageal cancer [PF, FLOX, ECF] Colorectal cancer [FL (Mayo), FOLFIRI, FOLFOX, IFL, FLOX] Cervical cancer [PF] Bladder cancer [PF] Head and Neck cancer Pancreatic cancer [FOLFIRINOX, FOLFOX, FL, FLI]	Fluorouracil is a fluorinated pyrimidine antimetabolite that inhibits thymidylate synthetase, blocking the methylation of deoxyuridylic acid to thymidylic acid, interfering with DNA and, to a lesser degree, RNA synthesis. Fluorouracil seems to be phase specific for the G1 and S phases of the cell cycle. Capecitabine is a prodrug of fluorouracil	Angina pectoris, vasospasm, myocardial infarction, nonspecific ECG changes, ventricular ectopy, atrial fibrillation, bradycardia, collapse, pericardial effusion, cerebrovascular accident, local thrombophlebitis
	Capecitabine	2%–7% (moderate)	Colorectal cancer [CAPOX (XELOX)] Breast cancer Billiary cancer [CAPOX (XELOX)] Esophageal cancer [EOX] Pancreatic cancer [CAPOX (XELOX), GTX] Gastric cancer [EOX]		
Anti-ERBB2 monoclonal antibodies	Trastuzumab	1.7%–20.1% (major)	Breast cancer (ERBB2+) [TCH] Gastric cancer (ERBB2+)	Trastuzumab binds to ERBB2 (HER-2), mediating antibody-dependent cellular cytotoxicity of cells that overexpress HER-2 protein. Pertuzumab binds to a different ERBB2 (HER2) epitope than trastuzumab	Peripheral edema, HF, tachycardia, hypertension, arrhythmias
	Pertuzumab	0.7%–1.2% (major)	Breast cancer (ERBB2+)		

Drug class	Drug	Incidence (severity)	Cancer indications	Mechanism	Cardiovascular effects
Anti-VEGF monoclonal antibody	Bevacizumab	1.6%–4% (major)	*Non-Small cell lung cancer* *Cervical cancer* *Ovarian cancer* *Breast cancer* *Endometrial cancer* *Renal Cell cancer* *Glioblastoma* *Soft Tissue Sarcoma* *Colorectal cancer*	Bevacizumab binds to and neutralizes VEGF-A, preventing its association with the endothelial receptors VEGFR1 and VEGFR2, inhibiting angiogenesis, and thus retarding the growth of all tissues (including metastatic tissue)	Hypertension, venous thromboembolism, peripheral edema, hypotension, arterial thrombosis, deep vein thrombosis, syncope, intra-abdominal thrombosis, LV dysfunction, pulmonary embolism
Multitargeted (VEGFR) tyrosine kinase inhibitors	Sunitinib	2.7%–19% (major)	*Renal Cell cancer* *Soft Tissue Sarcoma* *GIST*	Inhibits multiple receptor tyrosine kinases (VEGFRs; PDGFRα/β; FLT3; CSF-1R; RET), preventing tumor growth and angiogenesis.	hypertension, peripheral edema, chest pain, venous thrombosis, pulmonary embolism
	Pazopanib	7%–11% (major)	*Renal cell cancer* *Soft tissue sarcoma* *Thyroid cancer*	Inhibits multiple receptor tyrosine kinases (VEGFRs; FPDGFRα/β; LT3; CSF-1R; RET; FGFR-1/3; cKIT; IL-2R; Lck; c-Fms), preventing tumor growth and angiogenesis	Hypertension, bradycardia, peripheral edema, HF, chest pain, venous thrombosis, ischemia, myocardial infarction, prolonged QT interval on ECG
	Sorafenib	4%–8% (Minor)	*Renal cell cancer* *Hepatocellular cancer* *Soft tissue sarcoma* *GIST* *Thyroid cancer*	Inhibits multiple receptor tyrosine kinases (VEGFRs; PDGFRβ; FLT3; RET; cKIT; RET/PTC; CRAF; BRAF), preventing tumor growth and angiogenesis	Hypertension

(continued on next page)

Table 3
(continued)

Chemotherapy Family	Chemotherapy Agent	Incidence and Magnitude of Cardiac Dysfunction	Cancers Uses and Chemotherapy Regimens	Mechanism of Action	Other Cardiovascular Toxicities
Multitargeted (BCR-ABL) tyrosine kinase inhibitors	Imatinib	0.2%–2.7% (moderate)	*Acute lymphocytic leukemia* *Acute myelocytic leukemia* *GIST*	Inhibits multiple receptor tyrosine kinases (Bcr-Abl; PDGFRβ; SCF; cKIT), inducing apoptosis	Edema (anasarca, ascites, pericardial and pleural effusion, peripheral edema, pulmonary edema, and superficial edema), hypotension, chest pain, hypertension, HF
	Dasatinib	2%–4% (moderate)	*Acute lymphocytic leukemia* *Chronic myelocytic leukemia* *GIST*	Inhibits multiple receptor tyrosine kinases (Bcr-Abl; PDGFRβ; SRC; LKC; YES; FYN; cKIT; EPHA2), inducing apoptosis. Targets most imatinib-resistant BCR-ABL mutations (except the T315I and F317V mutants)	Peripheral edema, HF, pericardial effusion, prolonged QT interval on ECG, pulmonary hypertension, arrhythmias, angina, hypertension, tachycardia
	Nilotinib	1% (minor)	*Chronic myelocytic leukemia* *GIST*	Inhibits multiple receptor tyrosine kinases (Bcr-Abl; PDGFRβ; cKIT), inducing apoptosis. Targets most imatinib-resistant BCR-ABL mutations	Peripheral edema, hypertension, peripheral arterial disease, cerebral ischemia, pericardial effusion, angina pectoris, cardiac arrhythmia (including AV block, atrial fibrillation, bradycardia, cardiac flutter, extrasystoles, and tachycardia), prolonged QT interval on ECG

ERBB1/2 tyrosine kinase inhibitor	Lapatinib	0.2%–1.5% (major)	Breast cancer (ERBB2+)	Inhibits of EGFR (ERBB1) and HER2 (ERBB2), regulating cellular proliferation and survival in tumors expressing ERBB1 and ERBB2	Peripheral edema, HF, tachycardia, hypertension, arrhythmias
Proteasome inhibitors	Carfilzomib	11%–25% (major)	Multiple myeloma	Carfilzomib inhibits the 20S proteasome, leading to cell cycle arrest and apoptosis	Hypertension, chest pain, peripheral edema, HF, hypotension, myocardial infarction, pulmonary embolism, venous thrombosis
	Bortezomib	2%–5% (moderate)	AL Amyloidosis [CYBORD] Follicular lymphoma Mantle Cell lymphoma [VcR-CAP] Waldenström macroglobulinemia Multiple Myeloma [CYBORD, RVD, VD-PACE, PAD, VTD-PACE]	Bortezomib inhibits the 26S proteasome, leading to cell cycle arrest, and apoptosis	Hypotension, acute pulmonary edema, HF, cardiogenic shock, atrial fibrillation, angina pectoris, atrial flutter, atrioventricular block, bradycardia, cerebrovascular accident, deep venous thrombosis, peripheral embolism, hemorrhagic stroke, myocardial infarction, pericardial effusion, pericarditis, peripheral edema, portal vein thrombosis, pulmonary embolism, sinoatrial arrest, torsades de pointes, transient ischemic attacks, ventricular tachycardia

(continued on next page)

Table 3
(continued)

Chemotherapy Family	Chemotherapy Agent	Incidence and Magnitude of Cardiac Dysfunction	Cancers Uses and Chemotherapy Regimens	Mechanism of Action	Other Cardiovascular Toxicities
Antimicrotubule agents	Paclitaxel	<1% (moderate)	*Breast cancer [ACT (TAC), TCH]* *Bladder cancer [PCG]* *Cervical cancer* *Endometrial cancer* *Esophageal cancer* *Gastric cancer* *Head and neck cancer* *Non-Small cell lung cancer* *Small cell lung cancer* *Testicular cancer [TIP]* *Soft tissue sarcoma* *Thymoma/thymic carcinoma* *Penile cancer* *Ovarian cancer*	Inhibits microtubule disassembly, interfering with the late G2 mitotic phase, and inhibits cell replication. In addition, it can distort mitotic spindles, resulting in the breakage of chromosomes	Abnormal ECG, edema, hypotension, bradycardia, tachycardia, hypertension, rhythm abnormalities, syncope, venous thrombosis
	Docetaxel	2.3%–13% (moderate)	*Breast cancer [CT (TC), ACT (TAC)]* *Bladder cancer* *Bone Sarcoma* *Esophageal cancer* *Gastric cancer* *Head and Neck cancer* *Non-Small cell lung cancer* *Small cell lung cancer* *Ovarian cancer* *Pancreatic cancer [GTX]* *Prostate cancer* *Soft tissue sarcoma* *Uterine sarcoma*	Inhibits microtubule disassembly, interfering with the M mitotic phase, and inhibits cell replication	Hypotension

Immunomodulators	Interleukin-2	25% (major)	*Melanoma [CVD-Interleukin-Interferon]* *Neuroblastoma* *Renal cell cancer*	Promotes proliferation, differentiation, and recruitment of T and B cells, NK cells, thymocytes, LAK cells, and TIL cells, causing subsequent interactions between the immune system and malignant cells	Hypotension, peripheral edema, supraventricular tachycardia, HF, arrhythmia, cardiac arrest, myocardial infarction, ventricular tachycardia
	Interferon	25% (major)	*Melanoma [CVD-Interleukin-Interferon]* *Renal cell cancer*	Inhibits cellular growth, alters cellular differentiation and cell surface antigen expression, interferes with oncogene expression, increases phagocytic activity of macrophages, and augments cytotoxicity of lymphocytes	Chest pain, edema, hypertension
	Thalidomide	15% (minor)	*AL Amyloidosis [CTD]* *Waldenström macroglobulinemia* *Multiple Myeloma [DT-PACE, ThalfDex, TD-PACE]*	Thalidomide increases natural killer cell number and levels of interleukin-2 and interferon gamma. Also inhibits angiogenesis, increases cell-mediated cytotoxic effects, and alters expression of cellular adhesion molecules	Edema, thrombosis/ embolism, hypotension
	Lenalidomide	20% (major)	*Mantle cell lymphoma* *Multiple Myeloma [CRd, BLD]* *Chronic lymphocytic leukemia* *Myelodysplastic syndrome* *AL amyloidosis* *Renal cell cancer* *Non-Hodgkin lymphoma*	Inhibits secretion of proinflammatory cytokines; enhances cell-mediated immunity by stimulating proliferation of anti-CD3 stimulated T cells	Peripheral edema, deep vein thrombosis, hypotension, hypertension, chest pain, atrial fibrillation, myocardial infarction, pulmonary embolism,

(continued on next page)

Table 3
(continued)

Chemotherapy Family	Chemotherapy Agent	Incidence and Magnitude of Cardiac Dysfunction	Cancers Uses and Chemotherapy Regimens	Mechanism of Action	Other Cardiovascular Toxicities
				(resulting in increased IL-2 and interferon gamma secretion); inhibits trophic signals to angiogenic factors in cells	syncope, stroke, angina pectoris, bradycardia, HF, cardiac arrest, cardiogenic shock, increased cardiac enzyme levels, supraventricular arrhythmias
mTOR inhibitors	Everolimus	<1% (minor)	*Breast cancer Renal cell cancer Astrocytoma PNET*	Reduces protein synthesis and cell proliferation by binding to FKBP-12, and subsequently inhibiting mTOR activation, halting the cell cycle at the G1 phase. Also reduces angiogenesis by inhibiting VEGF and HIF-1 expression. Temsirolimus is the prodrug of sirolimus, the active metabolite. Everolimus is a sirolimus derivative	Peripheral edema, hypertension, angina pectoris, atrial fibrillation, HF, deep vein thrombosis, hypotension, pulmonary embolism, renal artery thrombosis, syncope, tachycardia
	Temsirolimus	<1% (Minor)	*Renal cell cancer*		

Abbreviations: AHA, American Heart Association; AV, atrioventricular; DNA, deoxyribonucleic acid; ECG, electrocardiogram; ESC, European Society of Cardiology; GIST, gastrointestinal stromal tumor; PNET, primitive neuroectodermal tumor.

Data from Refs.[22,23,35–41]

increased risk of developing HF after 3 decades.[42] This risk is higher in patients with left-sided chest radiation and concomitant chemotherapy.[43] This increase is likely related to the higher incidence of radiation-induced coronary artery disease in the left anterior descending and distal diagonal arteries, which normally irrigate the LV.[44] It has recently been shown that the cumulative cardiac radiation dose is proportionally correlated with the rate of major acute coronary events; the ensuing increased mortality risk is intensified by additional coexistent cardiovascular risk factors.[45]

Radiotherapy-induced cardiomyopathy is commonly accompanied by interstitial myocardial fibrosis with various degrees of severity.[46] These pathologic changes may also account for the higher incidence of cardiac autonomic dysfunction, impaired exercise performance, and mortality in cancer survivors who underwent chest radiation.[47] Furthermore, these patients also have an increased incidence of diastolic LV dysfunction[48] and subtle LV contractile impairment as detected by echocardiographic strain imaging.[49] In addition, cardiac irradiation can lead to complex stenotic and regurgitant valvular heart disease, which may progress to dilated cardiomyopathy and HFrEF.[50] Constrictive pericarditis, restrictive cardiomyopathy, and conduction abnormalities have also been associated with chest radiotherapy.[47]

Heart Failure Related to Cancer

There rare occasions in which HF can be a direct consequence of benign or malignant tumors. For example, AL amyloidosis coexistent with multiple myeloma or plasma cell dyscrasias may lead to infiltrative restrictive cardiomyopathy through the myocardial deposition of free light chains.[51] Carcinoid heart disease, thought to be caused by vasoactive substances released by pulmonary or hepatic neuroendocrine (carcinoid) tumors, results in preferentially right-sided valvular fibrosis, stenosis, and/or regurgitation, leading to right-sided congestive HF syndrome.[52] Some primary and secondary cardiac tumors, such as myxomas and angiosarcomas, can also lead to an HF syndrome through external compression or intracavitary inflow/outflow obstructions; however, this is extraordinarily rare.[53]

MANAGEMENT OF HEART FAILURE IN PATIENTS WITH CANCER AND CANCER SURVIVORS

Despite the increasing preponderance of cardio-oncology patients worldwide and the inherent obligation to optimize their care,[23,25] there are no unified and universally accepted evidence-based practice guidelines on the management of HF in this population. An increasing number of cardiology and oncology expert consensuses from Europe and North America have recently been published in this regard, each addressing different facets of the cardiovascular health care of these patients.[1,23,34,54–60] Table 4 lists and systematizes these recommendations, providing a condensed but comprehensive synopsis on the evaluation and management of acute and chronic HF in patients with cancer and cancer survivors. In addition, important aspects pertaining to this specific complex patient population are discussed later.

Cardioprotection for Patients with Cancer at Risk of Heart Failure

Most of the experimental and clinical research efforts in the area of cardio-oncology have been put into preventing cancer therapeutics–related cardiac dysfunction (CTCD), particularly in the setting of concomitant anthracycline and/or trastuzumab use. Although Table 4 summarizes the current guideline-directed evaluation and management (GDEM) recommendations for patients with stage A HF, several other cardioprotective strategies are building momentum.

Heart failure pharmacotherapy
For example, within the β-blocker family, carvedilol manifests a consistent cardioprotective role in the literature, preventing left ventricular strain imaging abnormalities,[61] preserving both systolic and diastolic LV functions,[62] and decreasing the incidence of symptomatic HF in patients with cancer.[63,64] This cardioprotective effect cannot be extrapolated to the entire drug family, but it seems to be limited to those agents with inherent antioxidant activity. In experimental research, carvedilol prevents the oxidative stress, mitochondrial dysfunction, and histopathologic myocardial toxic lesions caused by doxorubicin.[65] Nebivolol also seems to preserve LV systolic dysfunction and its associated increase in N-terminus pro-brain natriuretic peptide (NT-proBNP) level during anthracycline therapy.[66] In contrast, atenolol, which lacks antioxidant properties, does not seem to have cardioprotective effects.[65] In a similar way, metoprolol has either failed to show a beneficial effect,[67] or has yielded inadequate results to extract reliable conclusions.[68]

The cardioprotective role of angiotensin-converting enzyme inhibitors (ACEIs), enalapril in particular, has also been encouraging, albeit inconsistent. When serum troponin level increase is used as a marker of risk, early enalapril therapy seems to prevent the development of AIC,[69] and the combination of enalapril and carvedilol was recently shown to prevent the decrease of LVEF,

Table 4
Current guidelines for the management of heart failure in patients with cancer and cancer survivors

Guideline-Derived Evaluation		Guideline-Derived Management	
Stage A Chronic HF			
General	Baseline assessment of HF risk factors (hypertension, lipid disorders, obesity, diabetes mellitus, tobacco use, and known cardiotoxic agents) to identify patients at risk of CTCD. [1,23,34]	Cardio-oncology referral	Patients at high risk of CTCD (either high-risk patients due to their inherent cardiovascular risk factor burden, or planned high-risk chemotherapy, such as high-dose anthracyclines) should be referred to a cardio-oncology specialist for prevention, surveillance, and early management of cardiomyopathy. [23,34,56]
ECG	ECG is recommended in all patients before and during cancer treatment to detect signs of cardiac toxicity, including resting tachycardia, ST-T wave changes, conduction disturbances, QT interval prolongation or arrhythmias. [23,54,56]	General	HF risk factors should be controlled or avoided, before, during and after cancer therapies, tailored on the basis of goals of care (eg, curative vs palliative), in accordance with contemporary guidelines. [1,56]
Imaging	Evaluation of systolic and diastolic LV function, before initiation and after completion of known cardiotoxic cancer therapies, irrespective of baseline cardiovascular risk. [23,54,56] Serial evaluation of LVEF should be ideally performed by the same observer, using the same modality, with the same equipment, to reduce variability. [23,55,56] Echocardiography, and in particularly 3D echocardiography, is the method of choice for baseline and serial assessment of systolic ventricular function. [23,55,56,58] If 2D Echocardiography is used for baseline and serial assessments of LV function, the LVEF should be estimated using the Biplane Simpson's method. [55] Serial GLSI should be considered for early detection of subclinical CTCD; a reduction of >15% from baseline would be considered abnormal. [23,54–56,59]	Physical Activity	Daily physical activity should be encouraged in all patients before, during and after chemotherapy. [56] Dexrazoxane should be used in women with metastatic breast cancer who have received a cumulative dose of 300 mg/m^2 of Doxorubicin, and who will continue to receive it to maintain tumor control. [54]
		Cardioprotective pharmacotherapy	Cardioprotective agents (ie, ACEI, ARB, and b-blockers) may be initiated if subclinical LV dysfunction biomarkers are elevated. [23,54,56] Cardioprotective agents (ie, ACEI, ARB, and b-blockers) may be used in patients deemed to be at high risk of CTCD. [56]

Patients receiving anthracyclines and/or ERBB2 inhibitors should have serial monitoring of LV function every 3 months for at least 18 months after the initiation of treatment. Alternatively, surveillance in low risk patients should be considered every 4 cycles of anti-ERBB2 treatment or after 200 mg/m^2 of doxorubicin (or equivalent anthracycline cumulative dose); more frequent surveillance may be considered for patients with abnormal baseline echocardiography and those with higher baseline clinical risk (eg, prior anthracycline use, previous myocardial infarction (MI), treated HF).[23,54,57]

Cardiac function surveillance should be infrequent in asymptomatic patients with metastatic disease.[54]

If systolic dysfunction is found on baseline imaging prior to anthracycline use, options of non-anthracycline chemotherapy and/or cardioprotection agents should be discussed.[23]

Assessment of cardiac function is recommended at 1, 4, and 10 y after anthracycline therapy in patients who were treated at <15 y of age, or even at age >15 y but with cumulative dose of doxorubicin of >240 (or >300) mg/m^2 (or equivalent anthracycline dose), or those who developed symptomatic HF during chemotherapy.[23,34,54]

Cancer survivors exposed to high cumulative anthracycline doses and/or chest radiotherapy should be offered lifelong cardiac surveillance.[23,59]

For patients receiving VEGF inhibitors, assessment of LVEF is reasonable at baseline, after 2–4 wk, and every 6 mo, until stability of LVEF values is achieved.[23]

Biomarkers   Baseline and periodic measurement of cardiac biomarkers (Troponins and BNP/NT-proBNP) should be considered for early detection of subclinical CTCD.[23,54,56]

(continued on next page)

Table 4
(continued)

Guideline-Derived Evaluation		Guideline-Derived Management
Stage B Chronic HF		
Imaging	CTCD is defined as a decrease in the LVEF of >10%, to a point below the lower limit of normal (50%–53%), in two consecutive studies.[23,54,55] A decrease in the LVEF of >10%, to a point above the lower limit of normal (50%–53%) should undergo reevaluation in 2–4 wk.[23,54,55]	Chemotherapy discontinuation	If LV dysfunction is confirmed, chemotherapy should be held (with exception of ERBB2 inhibitors); standard HF therapy, frequent clinical and echocardiographic assessments should be implemented, and other causes of LV dysfunction should be excluded.[54,56] If the risk of progressive CTCD during cardiotoxic chemotherapy exceeds the risk of cancer recurrence without the agent, the agent should be discontinued.[56] If LVEF declines to <40%, chemotherapy should be stopped (including ERBB2 inhibitors); alternatives cancer therapies should be discussed, standard HF therapy should be implemented, and other causes of LV dysfunction should be excluded.[54,56]
		Cardio-oncology referral	Cancer patients and cancer survivors with LV dysfunction should be referred to a Cardio-Oncology specialist for early management and recovery of cardiomyopathy.[23,34,56]

General	Cancer patients who develop LV dysfunction should be aggressively treated with standard HF GDMT, just as any other HF patient, especially if the neoplasia allows a long-term survival.[54]
Therapeutic pharmacotherapy	β-blockers (bisoprolol, carvedilol, or metoprolol succinate) should be used in all patients with reduced LVEF, unless contraindicated.[1,23,54]
	ACEI (or ARB if ACEI intolerant) should be used in all patients with reduced LVEF, unless contraindicated.[1,23,55]
	Statins should be used in all patients with history of ACS and reduced LVEF.[1]
	Nondihydropyridine calcium channel blockers with negative inotropic effects should not be used in patients with low LVEF.[1]
Device therapy	An ICD may be implanted in patients on appropriate HF medical therapy with LVEF <30%, who are at least 40 d post-MI, and have reasonable expectation of survival with a good functional status for more than 1 y.[1]

(continued on next page)

Table 4
(continued)

	Guideline-Derived Evaluation	Guideline-Derived Management
Stage C Chronic HF		
	Cardio-oncology referral	Cancer patients and cancer survivors with HF should be referred to a Cardio-Oncology specialist for implementation of GDEM.[23,34,56]
	Chemotherapy discontinuation	Drugs known to adversely affect the clinical status of patients with current or prior symptoms of HFrEF should be avoided or withdrawn whenever possible (see Table 3).[1]
		If the risk of worsening HF during cardiotoxic chemotherapy exceeds the risk of cancer recurrence without the agent, the agent should be discontinued.[56]
		If symptomatic HFrEF develops during cardiotoxic cancer therapy, chemotherapy should be stopped, alternatives cancer therapies should be discussed, standard HF therapy should be implemented, and other causes of LV dysfunction should be excluded.[23,54,56]
	HF pharmacotherapy discontinuation	HF therapy should be continued indefinitely unless normal systolic LV function remains stable after cessation of HF therapy and no further cardiotoxic cancer therapy is planned.[23]
		In the particular case of Anti-ERBB2-induced cardiac dysfunction, cessation of HF treatment after normalization of LVEF may be considered.[23]
	Lifestyle interventions	HF patients should receive specific education to facilitate HF self-care.[1]
		Dietary sodium restriction is reasonable in HF patients.[1]

	Cardiac rehabilitation, exercise training, or regular physical activity is recommended in clinically stable HF patients.[1]
Therapeutic pharmacotherapy	Continuous positive airway pressure (C-PAP) is recommended in HF patients with sleep apnea.[1] Diuretics are recommended when there is evidence of fluid retention, unless contraindicated.[1] β-blockers (bisoprolol, carvedilol, or metoprolol succinate) should be used in all patients with HFrEF, unless contraindicated.[1,23,54] ACEI, or ARB if ACEI intolerant, should be used in all patients with HFrEF, unless contraindicated.[1,23,53] In patients with HFrEF NYHA class II-III who tolerate an ACEI or ARB, replacement by an angiotensin receptor–neprilysin inhibitor (ARNI), such as valsartan-sacubitril, is recommended, unless contraindicated (angioedema). ARNIs should not be administered concomitantly with ACEI, or within 36 h of the last dose of an ACEI.[60] Mineralocorticoid receptor antagonists are recommended in patients with NYHA II–IV HFrEF with an LVEF ≤ 35% (or LVEF <40% following an acute MI), unless contraindicated (Creatinine > 2.5 mg% or Potassium > 5 mEq/L).[1] The combination of hydralazine and isosorbide dinitrate is recommended for African American patients with NYHA III–IV HFrEF receiving optimal therapy, unless contraindicated.[1] Digoxin can be beneficial in patients with HFrEF, unless contraindicated[1] Ivabradine can be beneficial for patients with NYHA II-III HFrEF (LVEF ≤35%) on GDMT, including a beta blocker at maximum tolerated dose, and who are in sinus rhythm with a resting heart rate of ≥70 bpm.[60] Chronic anticoagulant therapy is reasonable for HF patients with chronic atrial fibrillation, and it is especially recommended if they have an additional risk factor for cardioembolic stroke (history of hypertension, diabetes mellitus, previous stroke or transient ischemic attack, or ≥75 y of age), unless contraindicated.[1]

(continued on next page)

Table 4
(continued)

	Guideline-Derived Evaluation		Guideline-Derived Management
		Device therapies	Omega-3 polyunsaturated fatty acid supplementation is reasonable for patients with NYHA II–IV HFrEF or HFpEF, unless contraindicated.[1]
			ICD therapy is recommended in patients with NYHA II–III HFrEF with LVEF ≤35% (and > 40 d post-MI) on chronic GDMT, who have reasonable expectation of meaningful survival for more than 1 y.[1]
			CRT is recommended in patients with NYHA II–IV HFrEF with LVEF ≤35%, with either LBBB and QRS duration of 120–149 ms, or with a QRS duration of ≥150 ms, on GDMT, who have reasonable expectation of meaningful survival for more than 1 y[1]
		Surgical therapies	Coronary artery revascularization via CABG or PCI is indicated for all patients with HF on GDMT with angina and suitable coronary anatomy, especially for a left main stenosis (>50%) or left main equivalent disease.[1]
			CABG, in addition to HF GDMT, is reasonable for patients with HF with severe LV dysfunction (LVEF <35%) and significant coronary artery disease[1]
			Surgical aortic valve replacement is reasonable for patients with critical aortic stenosis and a predicted surgical mortality <10%; otherwise, transcatheter aortic valve replacement after careful candidate consideration is reasonable[1]
			Transcatheter mitral valve repair or mitral valve surgery for functional mitral insufficiency is of uncertain benefit, but it could be considered on carefully selected patients on GDMT[1]
			LV aneurysmectomy may be considered in carefully selected patients with HFrEF for specific indications, including intractable HF and ventricular arrhythmias[1]

Stage D Chronic HF		
	Lifestyle interventions	Fluid restriction (1.5–2 L/d) is reasonable in patients with advanced HF with hyponatremia[1]
	Inotropic IV pharmacotherapy	Patients with cardiogenic shock should receive temporary IV inotropic support to maintain systemic perfusion and preserve end-organ performance, until definitive therapy (eg, coronary revascularization, MCS, heart transplant) or resolution of the acute precipitating problem[1]
		Long-term, continuous IV inotropic support may be considered as palliative therapy in patients with advanced HF who are not eligible for either MCS or cardiac transplant[1]
	Mechanical circulatory support	Either durable or nondurable MCS is reasonable in carefully selected patients with advanced HF, in whom definitive management (eg, cardiac transplant) or cardiac recovery is anticipated or planned[1]
		Durable MCS is reasonable as destination therapy in carefully selected patients with advanced HF ineligible for cardiac transplant[1]
	Heart transplant	Evaluation for cardiac transplant is indicated for carefully selected patients with stage D HF despite GDMT, device, and surgical management[1]
	Palliative care	Palliative and supportive care is effective for patients with symptomatic advanced HF to improve quality of life[1]

(continued on next page)

Table 4
(continued)

	Guideline-Derived Evaluation		Guideline-Derived Management
Acute HF			
General	Common precipitating factors for acute HF should be promptly identified (ACS, cardiotoxic chemotherapy, and so forth)[1]	General	Common precipitating factors for acute HF should be treated optimally as appropriate to the overall condition and prognosis of the patient[1]
		Chemotherapy discontinuation	If symptomatic HFrEF develops during cardiotoxic cancer therapy, chemotherapy should be stopped, alternative cancer therapies should be discussed, standard HF therapy should be implemented, and other causes of LV dysfunction should be excluded[23,54,56]
		Therapeutic pharmacotherapy	Chronic HF GDMT should be continued in hospitalized patients with AHF, in the absence of hemodynamic instability or contraindications[1]
			Hospitalized patients with AHF with significant fluid overload should be promptly treated with IV loop diuretics as either intermittent boluses or continuous infusion, at a dose that equals or exceeds their chronic oral daily dose[1]
			Low-dose dopamine infusion may be considered in hospitalized patients with AHF to improve diuresis and better preserve renal function and renal blood flow[1]

	In the absence of hypotension, IV nitroglycerin, nitroprusside, or nesiritide may be considered an adjuvant to diuretic therapy in patients admitted with acutely decompensated HF[1]
	Hospitalized patients with AHF should receive venous thromboembolism prophylaxis with an anticoagulant medication if the risk/benefit ratio is favorable[1]
	In hospitalized patients with AHF with volume overload who have persistent severe hyponatremia despite water restriction and maximization of GDMT, vasopressin antagonists may be considered in the short term to improve serum sodium[1]
Device therapy	Ultrafiltration may be considered for patients with HF with obvious volume overload to alleviate congestive symptoms and fluid weight, in particular in those with refractory congestion not responding to medical therapy[1]

Abbreviations: 2D, two dimensional; 3D, three dimensional; ACS, acute coronary syndrome; AHF, acute HF; BNP, brain natriuretic peptide; CABG, coronary artery bypass graft; CRT, cardiac resynchronization therapy; CTCD, cancer therapeutics–related cardiac dysfunction; ECG, electrocardiogram; GDEM, guideline-directed evaluation and management; GDMT, guideline-directed medical therapy; GLSI, global longitudinal myocardial strain imaging; HFpEF, HF with preserved ejection fraction; HFrEF, HF with reduced ejection fraction; ICD, implantable cardiac defibrillator; IV, intravenous; LBBB, left bundle branch block; LV, left ventricular; LVEF, left ventricular ejection fraction; MCS, mechanical circulatory support; NT-proBNP, N-terminus pro-brain natriuretic peptide; NYHA, New York Heart Association; PCI, percutaneous coronary intervention.

Data from Refs.[1,23,34,54–60]

and the incidence of death or HF in patients with malignant hemopathies undergoing anthracycline-based chemotherapy.[70] However, enalapril therapy on a pediatric population with history of apparently recovered AIC was not associated with improvements in exercise performance or LVEF.[71] Its effect on another adult lymphoma study population was also inconclusive.[68]

Angiotensin receptor blockers (ARBs) have had a similar mixed performance. Candesartan was shown to provide protection against early decline of global LV function in patients treated with adjuvant anthracycline-containing regimens, with or without trastuzumab and radiation.[67] However, in a larger multicenter study, prophylactic candesartan use in an early ERBB2-positive breast cancer population undergoing treatment with anthracycline-containing chemotherapy followed by trastuzumab did not affect changes in LVEF or cardiac biomarkers of injury and wall stress (NT-proBNP and high sensitivity troponin T (hs-TnT)).[72] In contrast, valsartan prevented LV end-diastolic diameter, corrected QT interval (QTc), and brain natriuretic peptide (BNP) level increases in a small patient cohort receiving CHOP, with no significant changes in blood pressure or heart rate.[73] Telmisartan was shown to reduce circulating reactive oxygen species and interleukin-6 levels, and to preserve myocardial strain-rate peak after high-dose anthracycline chemotherapy.[74] In addition, from within the renin-angiotensin-aldosterone system physiologic pathway, spironolactone is so far the only mineralocorticoid receptor antagonist clinically studied as a cardioprotectant in patients with cancer; it was found to prevent systolic and diastolic impairment, but the clinical effect was minimal.[75]

Statins (hydroxymethylglutaryl–coenzyme A reductase inhibitors) are yet to show cardioprotective benefit in prospective clinical trials. In a retrospective study, statin use was associated with a lower risk for incident HF in female patients with breast cancer treated with anthracyclines.[76] However, in another contemporary prospective trial atorvastatin failed to show preservation of LVEF and LV diameter in a similar population.[77]

Natural supplements

Clinical cardioprotective data involving natural supplements are scarce, but growing. Coenzyme Q10 administration in children receiving anthracyclines was associated with a lesser degree of LV dysfunction and remodeling.[78] N-acetylcysteine, either alone or in combination with vitamin E and vitamin C, prevented the development of LV dysfunction in patients undergoing doxorubicin therapy and high-dose chemotherapy or radiotherapy, respectively.[79,80] Many other agents have been shown to ameliorate cardiac toxicity in animal models receiving cancer therapies, such as metformin, melatonin, sesame oil, and nicorandil; however, these therapies have not been yet translated into the clinical setting, because of lack of evidence or effectiveness (Table 5 provides a complete list of preclinical cardioprotective agents).[81]

Dexrazoxane

Dexrazoxane is a metal chelating agent associated with statistically significant risk reductions for most cardiotoxic outcomes related to doxorubicin use,[82] without compromising its therapeutic efficacy, both in pediatric and adult populations.[83–86] In the United States, dexrazoxane is the only cardioprotective agent approved to reduce the incidence or severity of AIC.[87] Although it is only approved for used in women with metastatic breast cancer who have received a cumulative dose of 300 mg/m^2 and who will continue to receive doxorubicin to maintain tumor control,[87,88] it has also been recommended by expert-derived guidelines for use in other malignancies.[89] It needs to be administered within 30 minutes before doxorubicin infusion, in a 10:1 (dexrazoxane/doxorubicin) intravenous dosing ratio.[83,85] Despite its consistent cardioprotective effects in multiple clinical trials, survival improvement with its use is yet to be shown.[82]

Dexrazoxane use in pediatric patients with Hodgkin disease has been associated with a probable increased risk of acute myeloid leukemia, myelodysplastic syndrome, and second malignant neoplasms.[90] However, many subsequent studies have not been able to reproduce these initial results, finding no statistically significant association between dexrazoxane use and secondary malignancies.[82,91–93] In addition, because of early, and not yet reproduced, concerns of impairing tumor response rate to chemotherapy, dexrazoxane is not currently recommended for routine use with the initiation of doxorubicin therapy, for either primary or metastatic disease.[89,94,95] However, contemporary data from pediatric populations have shown that use of dexrazoxane with the initiation of doxorubicin therapy was cardioprotective, did not compromise antitumor efficacy, did not increase the frequencies of toxicities, and was not associated with a significant increase in second malignancies.[96]

Other preventive strategies

With the exception of dexrazoxane, these multiple clinical and preclinical investigative agents, although promising, are not yet universally accepted as efficacious for the prevention of CTCD.[91,97] Consequently, most expert consensuses currently limit their recommendations to the use of HF pharmacotherapy (in particular, carvedilol and enalapril)

Table 5
Cardioprotective agents for chemotherapy-induced cardiomyopathy

Agent Type	Preclinical Studies	Clinical Studies	Approved for Clinical Use (FDA)
Chelating agent	Dexrazoxane	Dexrazoxane	Dexrazoxane
β-Blockers	Carvedilol Nebivolol	Carvedilol Nebivolol	
ACEI	Enalapril	Enalapril	
ARB	Valsartan	Valsartan Candesartan Telmisartan	
MRA		Spironolactone	
Statins	Atorvastatin	Atorvastatin	
Natural antioxidants	Coenzyme Q10 Vitamin E Vitamin C Dihydromyricetin Oleuropein Hydroxytyrosol Sesame oil Sesamin Salidroside Melatonin Glutathione Quercetin Isorhamnetin Carabidiol Resveratrol	Coenzyme Q10 Vitamin E Vitamin C	
Others	N-acetylcysteine Mdivi-1 Metformin Prenylamine Amifostine Prostacyclin (prostaglandin I2) Meloxicam Diazoxide Ferric carboxymaltose PC-SOD Ghrelin L-Carnitine Molsidomine Didox α-Linolenic acid Nicorandil	N-acetylcysteine	

Abbreviations: ACEI, angiotensin-converting enzyme inhibitor; ARB, angiotensin receptor blocker; FDA, US Food and Drug Administration; MRA, mineralocorticoid receptor antagonist; PC-SOD, lecithinized human recombinant superoxide dismutase.
Data from Refs.[61–89]

in high-risk patients or in the setting of increased serum troponin or BNP levels during cardiotoxic chemotherapy (see Table 4).[23,54,56] Nevertheless, the number of upcoming clinical trials focused on prevention strategies for CTCD is increasing rapidly; Table 6 lists some of the currently active preventive research endeavors, both diagnostic and therapeutic.

Early Diagnosis and Recovery of Cardiac Dysfunction in Patients with Cancer

It has been shown that close monitoring of cardiac function during cardiotoxic chemotherapy permits early detection of LV dysfunction, and subsequent early initiation of HF therapy, which can in turn lead to LV recovery.[31,69,98,99] As would be expected,

Table 6
Active chemotherapy-induced cardiomyopathy prevention clinical trials

	Preventive Strategy	Registration Number	Registration Agency
Surveillance LV imaging	CMR	NCT01022086	ClinicalTrials.gov
		NCT02666378	
		NCT01719562	
		NCT02306538	
	Strain echocardiography	NCT02423356	
		NCT02080390	
		ACTRN12614000341628	anzctr.org.au
Pharmacology	Carvedilol	NCT01724450	ClinicalTrials.gov
	ACEI + β-blockers	NCT02236806	
		NCT01016886	
	Eplerenone	NCT01708798	
	Simvastatin	NCT02096588	
	Metformin	NCT02472353	
Aerobic physical activity	Exercise program	NCT02796365	
		NCT02471053	
		NCT02006979	

Abbreviation: CMR, cardiac magnetic resonance.

the percentage of responders progressively decreases as initiation of HF therapy is delayed.[98] The likelihood of LV recovery decreases when there is overt myocardial damage, as shown by increased serum troponin level,[99,100] and when initiation of HF therapy is delayed beyond 6 months from the end of chemotherapy.[98] Younger age, smaller left atrium volume under echocardiography, and lower BNP levels seem to be additional predictors of recoverability.[101] Unsurprisingly, responders have a lower rate of cumulative cardiac events than partial responders and nonresponders.[98]

Management of Symptomatic Cardiac Dysfunction in Patients with Cancer

AIC is the archetype of CTCD, and the most extensively studied.[24] It has historically carried a very poor prognosis,[24,32] although less so in the modern era.[33] As with any other type of cardiomyopathy leading to an HFrEF syndrome, early addition of ACEI/ARB and β-blockers in patients with AIC has led to improved symptoms, and even recovery of cardiac systolic function.[33] Likewise, patients with AIC derive a significant echocardiographic and symptomatic benefit from cardiac resynchronization therapy (CRT), similar to that seen in other forms of nonischemic cardiomyopathy.[102] Consequently, AIC and any other type of CTCD should be approached in accordance with the current general HF management guidelines, until new evidence dictates otherwise (see Table 4).[23,54,56]

Despite efforts to improve symptoms and recover LV function, AIC often progresses to advanced HFrEF, accounting for ~2.6% of all patients with nonischemic cardiomyopathy who undergo cardiac transplant.[103] These patients seem to be twice as likely to require biventricular mechanical circulatory support as bridge to transplant, compared with patients with idiopathic nonischemic cardiomyopathy, and they have a higher incidence of infections and malignancies after cardiac transplant.[103] However, these complications seem not to alter expected short-term and long-term posttransplant survival.[103,104] More frequently than cardiac transplant, patients with end-stage AIC undergo mechanical circulatory device support as destination therapy.[105] These patients, mostly female, are more prone to bleeding and right ventricular failure requiring mechanical circulatory support; nevertheless, survival does not seem to be affected by these compliations.[105]

Regrettably, no medical or surgical intervention has yet shown survival improvement in patients with HFpEF[1]; this may be, at least in part, related to long-term survival in this population mostly being driven by noncardiovascular causes.[16] New therapies for HFpEF are currently in development, such as the InterAtrial Shunt Device, which is already showing promising initial results.[106]

Acute HF is characterized by a decompensated, highly symptomatic state that usually requires hospitalization for decongestion and improvement of end-organ perfusion.[1] Standard HF therapies should be implemented in patients with cancer and survivors with acute HF, as summarized in Table 4. Discontinuation of cardiotoxic chemotherapy leading to this condition is paramount.[54]

MANAGEMENT OF OTHER HEART FAILURE SYNDROMES

Disorders of the right ventricle (RV), pericardium, heart valves, and great vessels can also elicit HF syndromes; however, their management can be distinct from management of conditions caused by LV dysfunction.[107–110]

Significant cardiac irradiation may lead to both stenotic and regurgitant complex valvular heart disease, which can in turn cause a dilated cardiomyopathy and an HF syndrome.[23,46] Although many of the general HF management strategies apply to these conditions, specific medical and surgical recommendations for the management of valvular heart disease have recently been released by the AHA and ACC.[107]

Constrictive pericarditis, likewise associated with cardiac irradiation in patients with cancer, presents with a congestive syndrome in the setting of a nondilated heart and thickened, and often calcified, pericardium.[46,111] Decongestion with diuretics can provide temporary symptom relief, but pericardiectomy is usually the only definitive treatment.[108,111]

Pulmonary hypertension (PH) can lead to tricuspid and pulmonary regurgitation, and progressive RV dilatation and failure, manifesting as a syndrome of dyspnea on exertion and peripheral edema.[109] Outside of the common PH secondary to LV dysfunction (group II), PH groups I and V of the World Health Organization (WHO) classification can be associated with cancer and cancer therapies. In particular, dasatinib has recently been linked with a high incidence of precapillary PH that improves with discontinuation of the agent.[112] Extensive oncologic surgeries, such as pneumonectomies, can also lead to mild compensatory PH, carrying suboptimal clinical outcomes.[113] The evaluation and management of PH has become increasingly complex in recent years; specific management guidelines have been developed for this purpose, involving use of diuretics, calcium channel blockers, anticoagulants, and novel pulmonary artery vasodilators, among others.[109]

In addition, hypertrophic cardiomyopathy (HCM) is a familial condition that characterizes an abnormal and/or disproportional myocardium growth, sometimes causing obstruction of the LV outflow tract and impeding blood from exiting the heart.[114] It affects ~1 in every 500 people, and could be concurrent with patients with cancer

and survivors.[110] Dyspnea on exertion, angina, palpitations, and syncope are the most common presenting symptoms; sudden cardiac death (SCD) is the principal cardiovascular mortality associated with this condition.[110] Nonobstructive HCM is usually asymptomatic, and seems to have a more benign clinical course.[114] As with other complex conditions, specific guidelines have been developed for its management[110]; these involve medications (β-blockers, nondihydropyridine calcium channel blockers, disopyramide), procedural options such as septal ablation or septal myomectomy, and implantable cardiac defibrillators for primary prevention of SCD.[110]

HEART FAILURE PHARMACOTHERAPY AND CANCER OUTCOMES

It has recently come to light that patients with HF are at increased risk of incident cancers[115–117]; the reasons behind these findings have not been yet elucidated. Although some data suggest that HF pharmacotherapy is not responsible for these findings,[97] and can even contribute to favorable cancer outcomes, other data suggest the contrary.

For example, digoxin has been associated with increased risk of breast cancer, attributed to its estrogenic effects.[118,119] However, spironolactone was not associated with an increased risk of breast cancer, despite its more potent estrogenic effects.[120] In 2010, a small meta-analysis linked the use of ARBs with an increased risk of incident cancer.[121] However, 3 other subsequent studies could not replicate these findings.[97,122,123] Conclusively, the US Food and Drug Administration (FDA) conducted the largest meta-analysis to date, including 156,000 patients from 31 trials, with an average follow-up of 39 months, finding no association between ARBs and incident cancer or cancer-related death.[124] Similarly, exposure to ACEIs has been associated with increased breast cancer relapse[125]; however, other investigators found no association between ACEI use and cancer or cancer death.[126]

On the positive side, β-blockers seem to reduce the rate of relapse-free survival in breast cancer,[125,127] and educe the mortality associated with prostate cancer.[128,129] Aspirin has likewise been associated with decreased risk of breast cancer recurrence and cancer death.[130] Hydrophilic statins, such as rosuvastatin, pravastatin, and fluvastatin, have similarly been linked with decreased incidence of progression-free survival in patients with inflammatory breast cancer.[131]

THE ART OF CARDIO-ONCOLOGY PRACTICE

Cardio-oncology is a young specialty intended to amalgamate both the scientific and the artistic aspects of 2 distinct medical fields. Although evidence-based guidelines to assist health care providers are already in development, as summarized earlier, practice-based patient care guidelines are elusive. Because this component is of vital importance, a few practical recommendations for the management of HF in patients with cancer and cancer survivors are provided later.

Applying the Basic Principles of Patient Care

The general physician behaviors shown to promote patient satisfaction and improve health outcomes should be especially applied in the care of these complex patients.[132,133] Some of these principles are: (1) focus on the patient; (2) establish an interpersonal and intellectual connection; (3) assess the patient's response to illness and suffering; (4) communicate congruence, acceptance, and understanding; (5) use physical touch, when appropriate; (6) use subtle humor, when appropriate; (7) show explicit empathy.[132]

Estimating of the Likelihood of Heart Failure Based on Concomitant Cancer Types

When patients are referred to a cardio-oncology specialist for the evaluation and management of HF, the consultation request is often triggered by unspecific symptoms such as dyspnea, palpitations, and peripheral edema. In addition to general HF epidemiology, the type of cancer that is affecting or has affected the patient can serve as an initial clue to estimate the likelihood of CTCD. Sarcomas, hematopoietic and lymphoid malignancies (including subsequent bone marrow transplant), and breast cancer, are frequently treated with anthracyclines and alkylating agents, and probably carry the highest HF risk. Renal cell cancers are often treated with VEGF inhibitors, gastrointestinal cancers with antimetabolites, and melanoma with cardiotoxic immunomodulators; these agents have also been associated with CTCD.[41]

Establishing a Comprehensive Differential Diagnosis

Just as correlation does not always imply causation, cardiomyopathy diagnosed after cardiotoxic chemotherapy does not always imply chemotherapy-induced cardiomyopathy. However, a vigilant mindset toward cardiotoxicity often overshadows the comprehensive differential diagnosis clinicians ought to do, leading to premature and unfounded conclusions. Common HF causes, such as myocardial ischemia and infarction, hypertension, valvular heart disease, arrhythmias, thyroid disorders, sleep apnea, and alcoholism always need to be considered.[6] Sometimes, HF can be indirectly caused by risk factors induced by cancer therapies, such as hypertension related to VEGF inhibitors, or coronary vasospasm related to antimetabolites.[41]

Personal Interpretation of Primary Clinical Data

Like few other examples in contemporary medicine, cardio-oncology specialists deal with clinical data that often determine the continuation or discontinuation of life-prolonging treatment; misinterpretation may indirectly lead to worsening survival. Therefore, a personal examination of the primary clinical data, in particular imaging and electrocardiographic data (ie, QTc), is highly recommended. Alleged abnormalities in echocardiographic imaging or strain can often be explained by poor data quality or common measurement errors.

Heart Failure Pharmacotherapy Concurrent with Chemotherapy

The use of cardioprotective and therapeutic HF agents is becoming customary, even though there are few data supporting their safety, tolerability, and efficacy. In contrast with the general HF population, patients with cancer undergoing chemotherapy often have several noncardiac adverse effects that may threaten the tolerability of HF agents, such as hypotension, nausea and vomiting, dehydration, diarrhea, and asthenia.[41] In one study, cardioprotective medications had to be discontinued in one-third of patients with cancer undergoing chemotherapy.[63] Therefore, until more robust data are generated, common sense should guide the cardio-oncology practice in this regard. Sodium restriction, diuretics, and medications that reduce blood pressure should be used with caution during times when gastrointestinal side effects limit oral intake or absorption. In a similar way, antihypertensive agents prescribed to counteract the effects of VEGF inhibitors may need to be held when the drug is likewise held, and anticoagulants may need to be stopped in the context of severe thrombocytopenia and bleeding diathesis.

Clinical Discernment and Discontinuation of Chemotherapy

There is little evidence-based guidance regarding the permanent discontinuation of cardiotoxic chemotherapy, especially when no equally effective agents are available. It is recommended that, if the risk of HF during cardiotoxic chemotherapy exceeds the risk of cancer recurrence without the chemotherapy agent, this should be discontinued.[56] Similarly, expert consensus also agrees that chemotherapy should probably be stopped when symptomatic HFrEF develops during cardiotoxic cancer therapy, after exclusion of other causes of LV dysfunction.[23,54,56] However, there are no data to suggest that this strategy is always the most beneficial for patients in the long term. It seems reasonable to believe, in general terms, that residual mild LV dysfunction in a cancer survivor would be associated with better prognosis than metastatic cancer in a patient with a normal or recovered LV function. Although the degree of LV dysfunction does correlate with severity of HF and mortality,[11,12] as does hypertension,[6] it is difficult to predict what the final extent of cardiovascular toxicity would be, and its health outcomes, if the chemotherapy agent were to be continued after the incipient cardiovascular damage. Therefore, a fluid communication between the oncology and the cardio-oncology specialist must be paramount, also involving the patient in the decision-making process, with the goal of a consensual, patient-satisfactory decision.

Keeping the Big Picture Always in Mind

The relief of suffering, both present and future, is considered the primary goal of medicine.[134] The diagnostic and therapeutic armamentarium should be tailored to patients, and not isolated diseases; this requires an in-depth knowledge of the patient, the disease, and the situation.[135] The management of HF in patients with cancer and cancer survivors has to abide by these foundational principles, in which the maximization of function takes priority over prolongation of life.

SUMMARY

The number of cancer survivors continues to increase annually, bringing forth a concomitant increase in CTCD. This article surveys the epidemiologic impact of this condition, and its most significant mediators. In addition, it collects and systematizes the available health care recommendations in this regard, providing a condensed but comprehensive synopsis on the evaluation and management of acute and chronic HF in patients with cancer and cancer survivors. The ultimate goal is to improve the overall morbidity and mortality of these patients through a durable collaboration between oncology and cardiology health care providers.

REFERENCES

1. Yancy CW, Jessup M, Bozkurt B, et al. 2013 ACCF/AHA guideline for the management of heart failure: a report of the American College of Cardiology Foundation/American Heart Association Task Force on Practice Guidelines. Circulation 2013;128(16): e240–327.
2. Stevenson LW, Pagani FD, Young JB, et al. INTERMACS profiles of advanced heart failure: the current picture. J Heart Lung Transplant 2009;28(6): 535–41.
3. Stehlik J, Edwards LB, Kucheryavaya AY, et al. The registry of the International Society for Heart and Lung Transplantation: 29th official adult heart transplant report–2012. The J Heart Lung Transplant 2012;31(10):1052–64.
4. Djousse L, Driver JA, Gaziano JM. Relation between modifiable lifestyle factors and lifetime risk of heart failure. JAMA 2009;302(4):394–400.
5. Curtis LH, Whellan DJ, Hammill BG, et al. Incidence and prevalence of heart failure in elderly persons, 1994-2003. Arch Intern Med 2008; 168(4):418–24.
6. Mozaffarian D, Benjamin EJ, Go AS, et al. Heart disease and stroke statistics-2016 update: a report from the American Heart Association. Circulation 2016;133(4):e38–360.
7. Heidenreich PA, Albert NM, Allen LA, et al. Forecasting the impact of heart failure in the United States: a policy statement from the American Heart Association. Circ Heart Fail 2013;6(3):606–19.
8. Gerber Y, Weston SA, Redfield MM, et al. A contemporary appraisal of the heart failure epidemic in Olmsted County, Minnesota, 2000 to 2010. JAMA Intern Med 2015;175(6):996–1004.
9. Roger VL, Weston SA, Redfield MM, et al. Trends in heart failure incidence and survival in a community-based population. JAMA 2004;292(3):344–50.
10. Merlo M, Pivetta A, Pinamonti B, et al. Long-term prognostic impact of therapeutic strategies in patients with idiopathic dilated cardiomyopathy: changing mortality over the last 30 years. Eur J Heart Fail 2014;16(3):317–24.
11. Lam CS, Lyass A, Kraigher-Krainer E, et al. Cardiac dysfunction and noncardiac dysfunction as precursors of heart failure with reduced and preserved ejection fraction in the community. Circulation 2011;124(1):24–30.
12. Yeboah J, Rodriguez CJ, Stacey B, et al. Prognosis of individuals with asymptomatic left ventricular systolic dysfunction in the Multi-ethnic Study of Atherosclerosis (MESA). Circulation 2012;126(23):2713–9.
13. Zile MR, Brutsaert DL. New concepts in diastolic dysfunction and diastolic heart failure: Part I: diagnosis, prognosis, and measurements of diastolic function. Circulation 2002;105(11):1387–93.

14. Lindenfeld J, Fiske KS, Stevens BR, et al. Age, but not sex, influences the measurement of ejection fraction in elderly patients hospitalized for heart failure. J Card Fail 2003;9(2):100–6.

15. Bursi F, Weston SA, Redfield MM, et al. Systolic and diastolic heart failure in the community. JAMA 2006;296(18):2209–16.

16. Senni M, Redfield MM. Heart failure with preserved systolic function. A different natural history? J Am Coll Cardiol 2001;38(5):1277–82.

17. Yancy CW, Lopatin M, Stevenson LW, et al. Clinical presentation, management, and in-hospital outcomes of patients admitted with acute decompensated heart failure with preserved systolic function: a report from the Acute Decompensated Heart Failure National Registry (ADHERE) database. J Am Coll Cardiol 2006;47(1):76–84.

18. Siegel RL, Miller KD, Jemal A. Cancer statistics, 2016. CA Cancer J Clin 2016;66(1):7–30.

19. Giovannucci E, Harlan DM, Archer MC, et al. Diabetes and cancer: a consensus report. CA Cancer J Clin 2010;60(4):207–21.

20. Koene RJ, Prizment AE, Blaes A, et al. Shared risk factors in cardiovascular disease and cancer. Circulation 2016;133(11):1104–14.

21. Askoxylakis V, Thieke C, Pleger ST, et al. Long-term survival of cancer patients compared to heart failure and stroke: a systematic review. BMC Cancer 2010;10:105.

22. Page RL 2nd, O'Bryant CL, Cheng D, et al. Drugs that may cause or exacerbate heart failure: a scientific statement from the American Heart Association. Circulation 2016;134(6):e32–69.

23. Zamorano JL, Lancellotti P, Rodriguez Munoz D, et al. 2016 ESC position paper on cancer treatments and cardiovascular toxicity developed under the auspices of the ESC Committee for Practice Guidelines: the Task Force for Cancer Treatments and Cardiovascular Toxicity of the European Society of Cardiology (ESC). Eur Heart J 2016;37(36):2768–801.

24. Von Hoff DD, Layard MW, Basa P, et al. Risk factors for doxorubicin-induced congestive heart failure. Ann Intern Med 1979;91(5):710–7.

25. Miller KD, Siegel RL, Lin CC, et al. Cancer treatment and survivorship statistics, 2016. CA Cancer J Clin 2016;66(4):271–89.

26. Ferlay J, Steliarova-Foucher E, Lortet-Tieulent J, et al. Cancer incidence and mortality patterns in Europe: estimates for 40 countries in 2012. Eur J Cancer 2013;49(6):1374–403.

27. Carver JR, Shapiro CL, Ng A, et al. American Society of Clinical Oncology clinical evidence review on the ongoing care of adult cancer survivors: cardiac and pulmonary late effects. J Clin Oncol 2007; 25(25):3991–4008.

28. Tashakkor AY, Moghaddamjou A, Chen L, et al. Predicting the risk of cardiovascular comorbidities in adult cancer survivors. Curr Oncol 2013;20(5): e360–70.

29. Oeffinger KC, Mertens AC, Sklar CA, et al. Chronic health conditions in adult survivors of childhood cancer. N Engl J Med 2006;355(15):1572–82.

30. Limat S, Daguindau E, Cahn JY, et al. Incidence and risk-factors of CHOP/R-CHOP-related cardiotoxicity in patients with aggressive non-Hodgkin's lymphoma. J Clin Pharm Ther 2014;39(2):168–74.

31. Cardinale D, Colombo A, Bacchiani G, et al. Early detection of anthracycline cardiotoxicity and improvement with heart failure therapy. Circulation 2015;131(22):1981–8.

32. Felker GM, Thompson RE, Hare JM, et al. Underlying causes and long-term survival in patients with initially unexplained cardiomyopathy. N Engl J Med 2000;342(15):1077–84.

33. Tallaj JA, Franco V, Rayburn BK, et al. Response of doxorubicin-induced cardiomyopathy to the current management strategy of heart failure. The J Heart Lung Transplant 2005;24(12):2196–201.

34. Denlinger CS, LJ, Are M, et al. NCCN guidelines version 2.2015. Survivorship: Anthracycline-Induced Cardiac Toxicity (SCARDIO-2). 2015.

35. Pai VB, Nahata MC. Cardiotoxicity of chemotherapeutic agents: incidence, treatment and prevention. Drug Saf 2000;22(4):263–302.

36. Cerny J, Hassan A, Smith C, et al. Coronary vasospasm with myocardial stunning in a patient with colon cancer receiving adjuvant chemotherapy with FOLFOX regimen. Clin Colorectal Cancer 2009;8(1):55–8.

37. Kruit WH, Punt KJ, Goey SH, et al. Cardiotoxicity as a dose-limiting factor in a schedule of high dose bolus therapy with interleukin-2 and alpha-interferon. An unexpectedly frequent complication. Cancer 1994;74(10):2850–6.

38. Misawa S, Sato Y, Katayama K, et al. Safety and efficacy of thalidomide in patients with POEMS syndrome: a multicentre, randomised, double-blind, placebo-controlled trial. Lancet Neurol 2016; 15(11):1129–37.

39. Feijen EA, Leisenring WM, Stratton KL, et al. Equivalence ratio for daunorubicin to doxorubicin in relation to late heart failure in survivors of childhood cancer. J Clin Oncol 2015;33(32):3774–80.

40. Ullenhag GJ, Rossmann E, Liljefors M. A phase I dose-escalation study of lenalidomide in combination with gemcitabine in patients with advanced pancreatic cancer. PLoS One 2015;10(4):e0121197.

41. Wolters Kluwer Clinical Drug Information, Inc. (Lexi-Drugs). Wolters Kluwer Drug Information, Inc. Available at: http://www.wolterskluwercdi.com/drug-reference/online/. Accessed September 1, 2016.

42. Aleman BM, van den Belt-Dusebout AW, De Bruin ML, et al. Late cardiotoxicity after treatment for Hodgkin lymphoma. Blood 2007;109(5):1878–86.

43. Hooning MJ, Botma A, Aleman BM, et al. Long-term risk of cardiovascular disease in 10-year survivors of breast cancer. J Natl Cancer Inst 2007; 99(5):365–75.

44. Nilsson G, Holmberg L, Garmo H, et al. Distribution of coronary artery stenosis after radiation for breast cancer. J Clin Oncol 2012;30(4):380–6.

45. Darby SC, Ewertz M, McGale P, et al. Risk of ischemic heart disease in women after radiotherapy for breast cancer. N Engl J Med 2013; 368(11):987–98.

46. Jaworski C, Mariani JA, Wheeler G, et al. Cardiac complications of thoracic irradiation. J Am Coll Cardiol 2013;61(23):2319–28.

47. Groarke JD, Tanguturi VK, Hainer J, et al. Abnormal exercise response in long-term survivors of Hodgkin lymphoma treated with thoracic irradiation: evidence of cardiac autonomic dysfunction and impact on outcomes. J Am Coll Cardiol 2015; 65(6):573–83.

48. Heidenreich PA, Hancock SL, Vagelos RH, et al. Diastolic dysfunction after mediastinal irradiation. Am Heart J 2005;150(5):977–82.

49. Armstrong GT, Joshi VM, Ness KK, et al. Comprehensive echocardiographic detection of treatment-related cardiac dysfunction in adult survivors of childhood cancer: results from the St. Jude Lifetime Cohort Study. J Am Coll Cardiol 2015;65(23): 2511–22.

50. Heidenreich PA, Hancock SL, Lee BK, et al. Asymptomatic cardiac disease following mediastinal irradiation. J Am Coll Cardiol 2003;42(4): 743–9.

51. Falk RH, Alexander KM, Liao R, et al. AL (light-chain) cardiac amyloidosis: a review of diagnosis and therapy. J Am Coll Cardiol 2016;68(12):1323–41.

52. Luis SA, Pellikka PA. Carcinoid heart disease: diagnosis and management. Best Pract Res Clin Endocrinol Metab 2016;30(1):149–58.

53. Burke A, Tavora F. The 2015 WHO classification of tumors of the heart and pericardium. J Thorac Oncol 2016;11(4):441–52.

54. Curigliano G, Cardinale D, Suter T, et al. Cardiovascular toxicity induced by chemotherapy, targeted agents and radiotherapy: ESMO clinical practice guidelines. Ann Oncol 2012;23(Suppl 7):vii155–66.

55. Plana JC, Galderisi M, Barac A, et al. Expert consensus for multimodality imaging evaluation of adult patients during and after cancer therapy: a report from the American Society of Echocardiography and the European Association of Cardiovascular Imaging. J Am Soc Echocardiogr 2014;27(9): 911–39.

56. Virani SA, Dent S, Brezden-Masley C, et al. Canadian Cardiovascular Society guidelines for evaluation and management of cardiovascular complications of cancer therapy. Can J Cardiol 2016;32(7):831–41.

57. Mackey JR, Clemons M, Cote MA, et al. Cardiac management during adjuvant trastuzumab therapy: recommendations of the Canadian Trastuzumab Working Group. Curr Oncol 2008;15(1):24–35.

58. Lancellotti P, Nkomo VT, Badano LP, et al. Expert consensus for multi-modality imaging evaluation of cardiovascular complications of radiotherapy in adults: a report from the European Association of Cardiovascular Imaging and the American Society of Echocardiography. Eur Heart J Cardiovasc Imaging 2013;14(8):721–40.

59. Armenian SH, Hudson MM, Mulder RL, et al. Recommendations for cardiomyopathy surveillance for survivors of childhood cancer: a report from the International Late Effects of Childhood Cancer Guideline Harmonization Group. Lancet Oncol 2015;16(3):e123–36.

60. Yancy CW, Jessup M, Bozkurt B, et al. 2016 ACC/AHA/HFSA focused update on new pharmacological therapy for heart failure: an update of the 2013 ACCF/AHA guideline for the management of heart failure: a report of the American College of Cardiology/American Heart Association Task Force on Clinical Practice Guidelines and the Heart Failure Society of America. Circulation 2016;68(13):1476–88.

61. Elitok A, Oz F, Cizgici AY, et al. Effect of carvedilol on silent anthracycline-induced cardiotoxicity assessed by strain imaging: a prospective randomized controlled study with six-month follow-up. Cardiol J 2014;21(5):509–15.

62. Kalay N, Basar E, Ozdogru I, et al. Protective effects of carvedilol against anthracycline-induced cardiomyopathy. J Am Coll Cardiol 2006;48(11): 2258–62.

63. Negishi K, Negishi T, Haluska BA, et al. Use of speckle strain to assess left ventricular responses to cardiotoxic chemotherapy and cardioprotection. Eur Heart J Cardiovasc Imaging 2014;15(3):324–31.

64. Seicean S, Seicean A, Alan N, et al. Cardioprotective effect of beta-adrenoceptor blockade in patients with breast cancer undergoing chemotherapy: follow-up study of heart failure. Circ Heart Fail 2013;6(3):420–6.

65. Oliveira PJ, Bjork JA, Santos MS, et al. Carvedilol-mediated antioxidant protection against doxorubicin-induced cardiac mitochondrial toxicity. Toxicol Appl Pharmacol 2004;200(2):159–68.

66. Kaya MG, Ozkan M, Gunebakmaz O, et al. Protective effects of nebivolol against anthracycline-induced cardiomyopathy: a randomized control study. Int J Cardiol 2013;167(5):2306–10.

67. Gulati G, Heck SL, Ree AH, et al. Prevention of cardiac dysfunction during adjuvant breast cancer therapy (PRADA): a 2 x 2 factorial, randomized, placebo-controlled, double-blind clinical trial of candesartan and metoprolol. Eur Heart J 2016; 37(21):1671–80.

68. Georgakopoulos P, Roussou P, Matsakas E, et al. Cardioprotective effect of metoprolol and enalapril in doxorubicin-treated lymphoma patients: a prospective, parallel-group, randomized, controlled study with 36-month follow-up. Am J Hematol 2010;85(11):894–6.

69. Cardinale D, Colombo A, Sandri MT, et al. Prevention of high-dose chemotherapy-induced cardiotoxicity in high-risk patients by angiotensin-converting enzyme inhibition. Circulation 2006;114(23): 2474–81.

70. Bosch X, Rovira M, Sitges M, et al. Enalapril and carvedilol for preventing chemotherapy-induced left ventricular systolic dysfunction in patients with malignant hemopathies: the OVERCOME trial (preventiOn of left Ventricular dysfunction with Enalapril and caRvedilol in patients submitted to intensive ChemOtherapy for the treatment of Malignant hEmopathies). J Am Coll Cardiol 2013;61(23): 2355–62.

71. Silber JH, Cnaan A, Clark BJ, et al. Enalapril to prevent cardiac function decline in long-term survivors of pediatric cancer exposed to anthracyclines. J Clin Oncol 2004;22(5):820–8.

72. Boekhout AH, Gietema JA, Milojkovic Kerklaan B, et al. Angiotensin II-receptor inhibition with candesartan to prevent trastuzumab-related cardiotoxic effects in patients with early breast cancer: a randomized clinical trial. JAMA Oncol 2016;2(8): 1030–7.

73. Nakamae H, Tsumura K, Terada Y, et al. Notable effects of angiotensin II receptor blocker, valsartan, on acute cardiotoxic changes after standard chemotherapy with cyclophosphamide, doxorubicin, vincristine, and prednisolone. Cancer 2005; 104(11):2492–8.

74. Cadeddu C, Piras A, Mantovani G, et al. Protective effects of the angiotensin II receptor blocker telmisartan on epirubicin-induced inflammation, oxidative stress, and early ventricular impairment. Am Heart J 2010;160(3):487.e1-7.

75. Akpek M, Ozdogru I, Sahin O, et al. Protective effects of spironolactone against anthracycline-induced cardiomyopathy. Eur J Heart Fail 2015; 17(1):81–9.

76. Seicean S, Seicean A, Plana JC, et al. Effect of statin therapy on the risk for incident heart failure in patients with breast cancer receiving anthracycline chemotherapy: an observational clinical cohort study. J Am Coll Cardiol 2012;60(23): 2384–90.

77. Acar Z, Kale A, Turgut M, et al. Efficiency of atorvastatin in the protection of anthracycline-induced cardiomyopathy. J Am Coll Cardiol 2011;58(9): 988–9.

78. Iarussi D, Auricchio U, Agretto A, et al. Protective effect of coenzyme Q10 on anthracyclines cardiotoxicity: control study in children with acute lymphoblastic leukemia and non-Hodgkin lymphoma. Mol Aspects Med 1994;15(Suppl): s207–12.

79. Wagdi P, Rouvinez G, Fluri M, et al. Cardioprotection in chemo- and radiotherapy for malignant diseases–an echocardiographic pilot study. Praxis (Bern 1994) 1995;84(43):1220–3 [in German].

80. Myers C, Bonow R, Palmeri S, et al. A randomized controlled trial assessing the prevention of doxorubicin cardiomyopathy by N-acetylcysteine. Semin Oncol 1983;10(1 Suppl 1):53–5.

81. Zhang J, Cui X, Yan Y, et al. Research progress of cardioprotective agents for prevention of anthracycline cardiotoxicity. Am J Transl Res 2016;8(7): 2862–75.

82. Shaikh F, Dupuis LL, Alexander S, et al. Cardioprotection and second malignant neoplasms associated with dexrazoxane in children receiving anthracycline chemotherapy: a systematic review and meta-analysis. J Natl Cancer Inst 2016;108(4).

83. Venturini M, Michelotti A, Del Mastro L, et al. Multicenter randomized controlled clinical trial to evaluate cardioprotection of dexrazoxane versus no cardioprotection in women receiving epirubicin chemotherapy for advanced breast cancer. J Clin Oncol 1996;14(12):3112–20.

84. Marty M, Espie M, Llombart A, et al. Multicenter randomized phase III study of the cardioprotective effect of dexrazoxane (Cardioxane) in ·advanced/ metastatic breast cancer patients treated with anthracycline-based chemotherapy. Ann Oncol 2006;17(4):614–22.

85. Choi HS, Park ES, Kang HJ, et al. Dexrazoxane for preventing anthracycline cardiotoxicity in children with solid tumors. J Korean Med Sci 2010;25(9): 1336–42.

86. Lipshultz SE, Rifai N, Dalton VM, et al. The effect of dexrazoxane on myocardial injury in doxorubicin-treated children with acute lymphoblastic leukemia. N Engl J Med 2004;351(2):145–53.

87. FDA statement on dexrazoxane. 2011. Available at: http://www.fda.gov/drugs/drugsafety/ucm263 729.htm. Accessed September 1, 2016.

88. Swain SM, Whaley FS, Gerber MC, et al. Delayed administration of dexrazoxane provides cardioprotection for patients with advanced breast cancer treated with doxorubicin-containing therapy. J Clin Oncol 1997;15(4):1333–40.

89. Hensley ML, Hagerty KL, Kewalramani T, et al. American Society of Clinical Oncology 2008 clinical practice guideline update: use of chemotherapy and radiation therapy protectants. J Clin Oncol 2009;27(1):127–45.

90. Tebbi CK, London WB, Friedman D, et al. Dexrazoxane-associated risk for acute myeloid leukemia/ myelodysplastic syndrome and other secondary

malignancies in pediatric Hodgkin's disease. J Clin Oncol 2007;25(5):493–500.

91. van Dalen EC, Caron HN, Dickinson HO, et al. Cardioprotective interventions for cancer patients receiving anthracyclines. Cochrane Database Syst Rev 2011;(6):CD003917.

92. Barry EV, Vrooman LM, Dahlberg SE, et al. Absence of secondary malignant neoplasms in children with high-risk acute lymphoblastic leukemia treated with dexrazoxane. J Clin Oncol 2008; 26(7):1106–11.

93. Seif AE, Walker DM, Li Y, et al. Dexrazoxane exposure and risk of secondary acute myeloid leukemia in pediatric oncology patients. Pediatr Blood Cancer 2015;62(4):704–9.

94. FDA drug safety: Zinecard. 2012. Available at: http://www.accessdata.fda.gov/drugsatfda_docs/label/2012/020212s013lbl.pdf. Accessed September 1, 2016.

95. Swain SM, Whaley FS, Gerber MC, et al. Cardioprotection with dexrazoxane for doxorubicin-containing therapy in advanced breast cancer. J Clin Oncol 1997;15(4):1318–32.

96. Asselin BL, Devidas M, Chen L, et al. Cardioprotection and safety of dexrazoxane in patients treated for newly diagnosed T-cell acute lymphoblastic leukemia or advanced-stage lymphoblastic non-Hodgkin lymphoma: a report of the Children's Oncology Group Randomized Trial Pediatric Oncology Group 9404. J Clin Oncol 2016;34(8): 854–62.

97. Bangalore S, Kumar S, Kjeldsen SE, et al. Antihypertensive drugs and risk of cancer: network meta-analyses and trial sequential analyses of 324,168 participants from randomised trials. Lancet Oncol 2011;12(1):65–82.

98. Cardinale D, Colombo A, Lamantia G, et al. Anthracycline-induced cardiomyopathy: clinical relevance and response to pharmacologic therapy. J Am Coll Cardiol 2010;55(3):213–20.

99. Cardinale D, Colombo A, Torrisi R, et al. Trastuzumab-induced cardiotoxicity: clinical and prognostic implications of troponin I evaluation. J Clin Oncol 2010;28(25):3910–6.

100. Cardinale D, Sandri MT, Martinoni A, et al. Left ventricular dysfunction predicted by early troponin I release after high-dose chemotherapy. J Am Coll Cardiol 2000;36(2):517–22.

101. Oliveira GH, Mukerji S, Hernandez AV, et al. Incidence, predictors, and impact on survival of left ventricular systolic dysfunction and recovery in advanced cancer patients. Am J Cardiol 2014; 113(11):1893–8.

102. Rickard J, Kumbhani DJ, Baranowski B, et al. Usefulness of cardiac resynchronization therapy in patients with Adriamycin-induced cardiomyopathy. Am J Cardiol 2010;105(4):522–6.

103. Oliveira GH, Hardaway BW, Kucheryavaya AY, et al. Characteristics and survival of patients with chemotherapy-induced cardiomyopathy undergoing heart transplantation. The J Heart Lung Transplant 2012;31(8):805–10.

104. Lenneman AJ, Wang L, Wigger M, et al. Heart transplant survival outcomes for Adriamycin-dilated cardiomyopathy. Am J Cardiol 2013; 111(4):609–12.

105. Oliveira GH, Dupont M, Naftel D, et al. Increased need for right ventricular support in patients with chemotherapy-induced cardiomyopathy undergoing mechanical circulatory support: outcomes from the INTERMACS Registry (Interagency Registry for Mechanically Assisted Circulatory Support). J Am Coll Cardiol 2014; 63(3):240–8.

106. Hasenfuss G, Hayward C, Burkhoff D, et al. A transcatheter intracardiac shunt device for heart failure with preserved ejection fraction (REDUCE LAP-HF): a multicentre, open-label, single-arm, phase 1 trial. Lancet 2016;387(10025):1298–304.

107. Nishimura RA, Otto CM, Bonow RO, et al. 2014 AHA/ACC guideline for the management of patients with valvular heart disease: a report of the American College of Cardiology/American Heart Association Task Force on Practice Guidelines. J Am Coll Cardiol 2014;63(22):e57–185.

108. Adler Y, Charron P, Imazio M, et al. 2015 ESC Guidelines for the diagnosis and management of pericardial diseases: the Task Force for the Diagnosis and Management of Pericardial Diseases of the European Society of Cardiology (ESC) Endorsed by: The European Association for Cardio-Thoracic Surgery (EACTS). Eur Heart J 2015;36(42):2921–64.

109. McLaughlin VV, Archer SL, Badesch DB, et al. ACCF/AHA 2009 expert consensus document on pulmonary hypertension a report of the American College of Cardiology Foundation Task Force on Expert Consensus Documents and the American Heart Association developed in collaboration with the American College of Chest Physicians; American Thoracic Society, Inc.; and the Pulmonary Hypertension Association. J Am Coll Cardiol 2009; 53(17):1573–619.

110. Gersh BJ, Maron BJ, Bonow RO, et al. 2011 ACCF/AHA guideline for the diagnosis and treatment of hypertrophic cardiomyopathy: a report of the American College of Cardiology Foundation/American Heart Association Task Force on Practice Guidelines. Developed in collaboration with the American Association for Thoracic Surgery, American Society of Echocardiography, American Society of Nuclear Cardiology, Heart Failure Society of America, Heart Rhythm Society, Society for Cardiovascular Angiography and Interventions, and

Society of Thoracic Surgeons. J Am Coll Cardiol 2011;58(25):e212–60.

111. Barbetakis N, Xenikakis T, Paliouras D, et al. Pericardiectomy for radiation-induced constrictive pericarditis. Hellenic J Cardiol 2010;51(3):214–8.

112. Montani D, Bergot E, Gunther S, et al. Pulmonary arterial hypertension in patients treated by dasatinib. Circulation 2012;125(17):2128–37.

113. Potaris K, Athanasiou A, Konstantinou M, et al. Pulmonary hypertension after pneumonectomy for lung cancer. Asian Cardiovasc Thorac Ann 2014; 22(9):1072–9.

114. Maron MS, Rowin EJ, Olivotto I, et al. Contemporary natural history and management of nonobstructive hypertrophic cardiomyopathy. J Am Coll Cardiol 2016;67(12):1399–409.

115. Banke A, Schou M, Videbaek L, et al. Incidence of cancer in patients with chronic heart failure: a long-term follow-up study. Eur J Heart Fail 2016;18(3): 260–6.

116. Hasin T, Gerber Y, McNallan SM, et al. Patients with heart failure have an increased risk of incident cancer. J Am Coll Cardiol 2013;62(10):881–6.

117. Hasin T, Gerber Y, Weston SA, et al. Heart failure after myocardial infarction is associated with increased risk of cancer. J Am Coll Cardiol 2016; 68(3):265–71.

118. Ahern TP, Lash TL, Sorensen HT, et al. Digoxin treatment is associated with an increased incidence of breast cancer: a population-based case-control study. Breast Cancer Res 2008; 10(6):R102.

119. Biggar RJ, Wohlfahrt J, Oudin A, et al. Digoxin use and the risk of breast cancer in women. J Clin Oncol 2011;29(16):2165–70.

120. Mackenzie IS, Macdonald TM, Thompson A, et al. Spironolactone and risk of incident breast cancer in women older than 55 years: retrospective, matched cohort study. BMJ 2012;345:e4447.

121. Sipahi I, Debanne SM, Rowland DY, et al. Angiotensin-receptor blockade and risk of cancer: meta-analysis of randomised controlled trials. Lancet Oncol 2010;11(7):627–36.

122. Collaboration ARBT. Effects of telmisartan, irbesartan, valsartan, candesartan, and losartan on cancers in 15 trials enrolling 138,769 individuals. J Hypertens 2011;29(4):623–35.

123. Pasternak B, Svanstrom H, Callreus T, et al. Use of angiotensin receptor blockers and the risk of cancer. Circulation 2011;123(16):1729–36.

124. FDA drug safety communication: no increase in risk of cancer with certain blood pressure drugs – Angiotensive Receptor Blockers (ARBs). 2011. Available at: http://www.fda.gov/Drugs/DrugSafety/ucm257516.htm. Accessed September 1, 2016.

125. Ganz PA, Habel LA, Weltzien EK, et al. Examining the influence of beta blockers and ACE inhibitors on the risk for breast cancer recurrence: results from the LACE cohort. Breast Cancer Res Treat 2011;129(2):549–56.

126. Sipahi I, Chou J, Mishra P, et al. Meta-analysis of randomized controlled trials on effect of angiotensin-converting enzyme inhibitors on cancer risk. Am J Cardiol 2011;108(2):294–301.

127. Melhem-Bertrandt A, Chavez-Macgregor M, Lei X, et al. Beta-blocker use is associated with improved relapse-free survival in patients with triple-negative breast cancer. J Clin Oncol 2011;29(19):2645–52.

128. Grytli HH, Fagerland MW, Fossa SD, et al. Use of beta-blockers is associated with prostate cancer-specific survival in prostate cancer patients on androgen deprivation therapy. Prostate 2013; 73(3):250–60.

129. Grytli HH, Fagerland MW, Fossa SD, et al. Association between use of beta-blockers and prostate cancer-specific survival: a cohort study of 3561 prostate cancer patients with high-risk or metastatic disease. Eur Urol 2014;65(3):635–41.

130. Holmes MD, Chen WY, Li L, et al. Aspirin intake and survival after breast cancer. J Clin Oncol 2010; 28(9):1467–72.

131. Brewer TM, Masuda H, Liu DD, et al. Statin use in primary inflammatory breast cancer: a cohort study. Br J Cancer 2013;109(2):318–24.

132. Egnew TR. The art of medicine: seven skills that promote mastery. Fam Pract Manag 2014;21(4): 25–30.

133. Stewart M, Brown JB, Boon H, et al. Evidence on patient-doctor communication. Cancer Prev Control 1999;3(1):25–30.

134. Cassel EJ. The nature of suffering and the goals of medicine. N Engl J Med 1982;306(11):639–45.

135. Cassell EJ. The relief of suffering. Arch Intern Med 1983;143(3):522–3.

Proteasome Inhibitors as a Potential Cause of Heart Failure

Georgios Koulaouzidis, MD[a], Alexander R. Lyon, MD, PhD[a,b],*

KEYWORDS

- Proteasome inhibitors • Heart failure • Myocardium • Multiple myeloma

KEY POINTS

- Proteasome inhibitors have become an important drug class in the treatment of multiple myeloma, and currently 3 have received regulatory approval.
- In addition to its role in myeloma cells, the proteasome plays a critical role in the myocardium, particularly in the context of cardiac stress.
- The growing awareness of the cardiovascular toxicity of proteasome inhibitors is emerging following the phase 3 trials and the transition into real-world practice.

INTRODUCTION

Proteasomes are protease complexes that are responsible for degrading endogenous proteins and protein recycling within cellular metabolism. Proteins to be destroyed are recognized by proteasomes because of the presence of ubiquitin moieties as posttranslational modifications.[1] The ubiquitin proteasome pathway represents the major intracellular pathway for intracellular protein degradation, with more than 80% of cellular proteins degraded through this pathway as part of natural turnover in cellular metabolism.[2,3] This pathway is active in the cardiomyocytes of ventricular myocardium under basal conditions; it is upregulated in various disease states, including myocardial stress, left ventricular hypertrophy, and heart failure (HF). It has become increasingly clear that defects within this pathway are associated with several noncardiac diseases, including several cancers.[4,5]

Proteasome inhibitors (PIs) have been developed to block the action of proteasomes. PIs have been studied in the treatment of cancer, and they are approved for use in both the United States and Europe for the treatment of multiple myeloma and mantle cell lymphoma.[6–8] Bortezomib (Velcade) is a first-in-class PI, acting as a reversible inhibitor, and has been approved for the treatment of multiple myeloma and also relapsed and refractory mantle cell lymphoma.[9] Carfilzomib (Kyprolis) is a modified epoxyketone PI that selectively targets the proteasome enzymes within the cell. It is more potent than bortezomib and irreversibly binds to the active sites of the 20S proteasome as well as the core component within the 26S proteasome.[10,11] Ixazomib (Ninlaro) is the first oral PI and has recently received a license for relapsed and refractory multiple myeloma.[12] It is a reversible PI that preferentially binds to the beta 5 subunit of the 20S

A.R. Lyon is supported by the NIHR Cardiovascular Biomedical Research Unit at the Royal Brompton Hospital and British Heart Foundation (FS/11/67/28954).

Disclosures: A.R. Lyon has been a specialist advisor to Onyx Pharmaceuticals and AMGEN.

[a] NIHR Cardiovascular Biomedical Research Unit, Royal Brompton Hospital, London SW3 6NP, UK; [b] Imperial College London, London, UK

* Corresponding author. Department of Cardiology, Royal Brompton Hospital, London SW3 6NP, UK.

E-mail address: a.lyon@imperial.ac.uk

proteasome and inhibits its chymotrypsinlike activity.

The aim of this article is to review the cardiovascular toxicity in patients receiving PIs.

PHASE III RANDOMIZED CONTROLLED TRIALS
Bortezomib

There have been 2 major phase 3 trials of bortezomib in multiple myeloma including 677 patients receiving bortezomib, usually in combination with dexamethasone and immune modulators, for example, lenalidomide. Bortezomib treatment was also included in the ENDEAVOR trial as the comparator arm to carfilzomib (see later discussion). There has also been a meta-analysis of 25 trials and 4330 patients treated with bortezomib, which provides the most accurate estimate of cardiotoxicity rates in patients with multiple myeloma.

APEX Trial (2005)

The APEX trial was a phase 3 randomized trial that compared bortezomib with high-dose dexamethasone in patients with multiple myeloma who had a relapse after one to 3 other therapies.[13] A total of 669 patients with relapsed multiple myeloma were randomly assigned to receive bortezomib (n = 333) or high-dose dexamethasone (n = 336).

Efficacy

The median time to disease progression was 6.22 months in the bortezomib group and 3.49 months in the dexamethasone group (hazard ratio for the bortezomib group, 0.55; $P<.001$). At 1 year of follow-up, patients who received bortezomib had a higher rate of overall survival (80%) than those who received dexamethasone (66%, $P = .003$).

Cardiotoxicity

The incidence of cardiac events during treatment with bortezomib and dexamethasone was 15% and 13%, respectively. Five percent of patients in the bortezomib arm developed congestive cardiac failure compared with 4% in the dexamethasone arm. These data show a high rate of cardiac events including HF in this patient population but did not suggest bortezomib was increasing the rate significantly. Dyspnea is a commonly reported adverse event (AE) in PI trials; perhaps insufficient data prevent adjudication committees to define as cardiac, for example, HF or pulmonary (including pulmonary embolus and pulmonary hypertension). Dyspnea without cause specified was reported in 20% of patients receiving bortezomib and 17% in the control arm.

VISTA Trial (2008)

This trial was a phase III trial for comparison bortezomib plus melphalan-prednisone (bortezomib group) with melphalan-prednisone alone (control group) in patients with newly diagnosed myeloma who were ineligible for high-dose therapy.[14] This study was an open-label study in which 344 patients were randomly assigned in the bortezomib group and 338 in the control group.

Efficacy

The rates of partial response or better were 71% in the bortezomib group as compared with 35% in the control group ($P<.001$), and the complete-response rates were 30% and 4%, respectively ($P<.001$). After a median follow-up of 16.3 months, 45 patients (13%) in the bortezomib group and 76 patients (22%) in the control group had died (hazard ratio in the bortezomib group, 0.61, $P = .008$).

Cardiotoxicity

The rate of all serious AEs in the bortezomib group was higher than that in the control group (46% vs 36%). HF-related symptoms were more common in the bortezomib group: dyspnea was observed in 15% in the bortezomib group versus 13% in the melphalan group, whereas peripheral edema was twice as common in the bortezomib arm (20% vs 10%). It is not clear if the edema was bilateral (eg, cardiac or renal) or unilateral, raising the possibility of deep vein thrombosis. Together with data from the APEX trial, there is a suggestion that bortezomib may increase the risk of cardiac events and these trials may have been underpowered to detect a significant effect. The absolute increase, if real, is relatively modest; what is more relevant is the identification of a high background rate of cardiac events suggesting patients with multiple myeloma are a high-risk population for cardiovascular disease per se.

Meta-analysis

Xiao and colleagues[15] in a meta-analysis investigated the incidence and risk of cardiotoxicity in patients treated with bortezomib. They included in their analysis 4330 patients who received bortezomib from 11 phase III and 14 phase II trials, for the purpose of analysis. The incidence of all-grade cardiotoxicity was ranged from 0% to 17.9% with the highest incidence observed in elderly patients with mantle cell lymphoma. Using a random-effects model, the summary incidence of all-grade cardiotoxicity in all patients was 3.8% (95% confidence interval [CI]: 2.6%–5.6%). The incidence of high-grade cardiotoxicity ranged from 0% to 7.7% across the trials evaluated, with the highest incidence seen in the trial of elderly patients with mantle cell lymphoma, whereas no events of cardiotoxicity were observed in 3 trials. Among patients with bortezomib-associated high-grade cardiotoxicity, this meta-analysis showed that the mortality of cardiotoxicity was 3.0%. High-grade cardiovascular toxicity, including HF and sudden cardiac death, was seen in 2.3% patients receiving bortezomib. The rate was higher in the multiple myeloma trials (4.3%), perhaps reflecting the higher incidence of preexisting cardiovascular comorbidities.

Carfilzomib

Carfilzomib is a more potent and irreversible PI. The first two phase 3 trials have demonstrated increased efficacy of carfilzomib as a second-line PI in patients with progressive multiple myeloma despite first-line bortezomib against different comparator arms. The latest phase 3 trial recently published compared carfilzomib head-to-head with bortezomib as first-line PI strategy, with superior efficacy of the more potent carfilzomib. Aligned to the increased efficacy, the higher potency is also reflected in a higher risk of cardiovascular toxicity in patients receiving carfilzomib treatment compared with bortezomib.

ASPIRE Trial (2015)

The ASPIRE trial was a randomized, open-label, multicenter, phase 3 study that evaluated the safety and efficacy of carfilzomib with lenalidomide and weekly dexamethasone (carfilzomib group) compared with lenalidomide and weekly dexamethasone alone (control group).[16] In this trial, 792 patients with relapsed multiple myeloma were randomly assigned, in a 1:1 ratio.

Efficacy
The median progression-free survival (PFS) was 26.3 months (95% CI, 23.3–30.5) in the carfilzomib group as compared with 17.6 months (95% CI, 15.0–20.6) in the control group (P = .0001). The Kaplan-Meier 24-month overall survival rates were 73.3% (95% CI, 68.6–77.5) in the carfilzomib group and 65.0% (95% CI, 59.9–69.5) in the control group.

Cardiovascular toxicity
Cardiac AEs were common in this trial and increased in carfilzomib (26.6%) compared with the control arm (15.6%). Severe cardiac AEs (>grade 3) were twice as frequent in the carfilzomib arm (11.4% vs 5.7%). HF related to treatment was reported in 25 patients in the carfilzomib group (6.4%) versus 16 patients in the control arm

(4.1%). Severe HF was also higher in the carfilzomib arm (3.8% vs 1.8% in the control group).

Vascular toxicity, including ischemic heart disease events, mainly reflecting troponin-positive acute coronary syndromes, was also higher in the carfilzomib group (5.9% in the carfilzomib group and 4.6% in control arm). Hypertension was another cardiovascular complication increased by carfilzomib (14.3% vs 6.9% in the control group). Dyspnea without a specific cause was very common; with the assumption that some were cardiac in origin, the overall rate of cardiac AEs plus new dyspnea was reported in 46.0% of patients in the carfilzomib arm compared with 30.5% in the control group.

FOCUS Trial (2016)

The FOCUS trial is a phase 3 trial of carfilzomib versus low-dose corticosteroids and optional cyclophosphamide in patients with relapsed and refractory multiple myeloma.[17] Three hundred fifteen patients were recruited and randomized to carfilzomib (n = 157) versus control (n = 158), with 95% of the control arm receiving cyclophosphamide. All patients had previously received bortezomib treatment, and approximately 76% of patients recruited had received prior anthracycline chemotherapy.

Efficacy
Median overall survival was similar between study arms (10.2 months carfilzomib vs 10.0 months in controls). PFS was also similar, but the overall response rate with significantly higher in the carfilzomib arm (19.1% vs 11.4%).

Cardiovascular toxicity
Hypertension was the most common cardiovascular AE and increased in the carfilzomib arm (15% vs 6% in controls). This finding may reflect a higher rate of renal failure in the carfilzomib arm (24% vs 9% in controls). HF was reported in 7 patients in the carfilzomib arm (4.5%) and only one patient in the control arm (0.6%), with severe HF in 3 patients treated with carfilzomib.

ENDEAVOR Trial (2016)

The ENDEAVOR trial is the largest phase 3 trial of PIs and tested carfilzomib head-to-head with bortezomib in advanced multiple myeloma.[18] In the ENDEAVOR trial 929 patients with relapsed or refractory multiple myeloma and a median of 2 prior lines of therapy were randomized to either carfilzomib with dexamethasone (n = 464) or bortezomib-dexamethasone (n = 465). Prior PI therapy was allowed providing a partial response had been reported and no prior PI-related serious AEs were reported. Patients with HF and reduced left ventricular ejection fraction (LVEF) (<40%) or recent myocardial infarction (MI) were excluded.

Efficacy

At a median follow-up of 12 months, PFS was significantly longer in the carfilzomib arm (median 18.7 months vs 9.4 months in the bortezomib arm, P<.0001). The superiority of carfilzomib was seen in both bortezomib-exposed and bortezomib-naïve patients, although PFS was longer in bortezomib-naïve patients in both arms.

Cardiovascular toxicity and general safety

Mortality due to AEs was relatively high and numerically higher in the carfilzomib arm (4.3% vs 3.1%). Treatment discontinuation due to AEs was common in patients who had received 1 prior line of treatment (17.2% vs 18.5%, respectively) and even higher in those patients enrolled who had received 2 or more prior lines of treatment (22.5% vs 23.1%).

Severe cardiac AEs (grade >3 HF, hypertension) and grade 3 dyspnea occurred in 76 patients in the carfilzomib arm (16.3%) compared with 25 patients in the bortezomib arm (5.4%). Serious HF (grade 3+) occurred more frequently in carfilzomib-treated patients (10 [2.2%] versus 3 patients [0.6%]). Deep vein thrombosis and pulmonary emboli were also more common in the carfilzomib arm compared with bortezomib (10.2% vs 6.2%).

In an echocardiographic substudy, serial echocardiograms were performed at baseline (pretreatment) and 12 weekly intervals from 151 patients (75 from the carfilzomib group and 76 from the bortezomib group). This substudy only identified one patient (in the bortezomib group) with significant LVEF reduction within the first 24 weeks of study treatment; yet the rate of cardiovascular AEs was similar to the overall study, suggesting this strategy failed to detect the carfilzomib-induced left ventricular dysfunction before clinical presentation. Further information regarding the data quality and scientific details of the echocardiographic substudy has been presented in abstract form, and more details in the main substudy publication are awaited. Three additional patients (2 from the carfilzomib group and one from the bortezomib group) had a significant reduction in LVEF at any time during the study. All patients but one (in the carfilzomib group) had resolution to normal LVEF on follow-up.

RECENT PHASE II STUDIES
CYCLONE Trial

CYKLONE was a multicenter, single-arm, open-label, phase Ib/II study assessing the efficacy and safety of carfilzomib in newly diagnosed MM.[19] Patients received carfilzomib by intravenous infusion over 30 minutes on days 1, 2, 8, 9, 15, and 16 of a 28-day cycle. All patients received cyclophosphamide 300 mg/m^2 orally on days 1, 8, and 15; thalidomide 100 mg orally on days 1 to 28; and dexamethasone 40 mg orally on days 1, 8, 15, and 22. Patients received CYKLONE treatment for 4 cycles or more, followed by a stem cell transplant. Sixty-four patients were evaluated for response. Sixteen percent of patients receiving carfilzomib had a cardiovascular AE, with severe cardiac AEs in 6% patients. Dyspnea (20%) was also common in the patients with multiple myeloma receiving carfilzomib.

Integrated Safety Profile of Single-agent Carfilzomib: Experience from 526 Patients Enrolled in 4 Phase II Clinical Studies

Siegel and colleagues[20] analyzed safety data for carfilzomib from 526 patients with advanced multiple myeloma who took part in one of 4 phase II studies (PX-171-003-A0, PX-171-003-A1, PX-171-004, and PX-171-005) before FOCUS and ENDEAVOR.

Overall, 73.6% of patients had a past medical history of cardiovascular events and 70.0% had baseline cardiac risk factors. Cardiac AEs were reported in 22.1% of patients receiving carfilzomib, and severe grade 3 or greater cardiac AEs were observed in 9.5% patients treated with carfilzomib. Cardiac failure events were reported in 32 patients (7.2%). The overall mortality rate, including due to disease progression, was the same (7%) in patients who had baseline cardiac risk factors as it was for patients without these risk factors. Hypertension (mainly grade 1–2) was reported in 14.3% of patients, more than half of whom had a history of hypertension. Dyspnea was also a commonly reported treatment-emergent AE in patients receiving carfilzomib (42%), raising the question of a specific cause, with undiagnosed pulmonary edema or pulmonary emboli as potential explanations.

In response to a cardiac-related AE, 6 patients (1.1%) had a carfilzomib dose reduction. Cardiac events leading to treatment discontinuation were noted in 23 patients (4.4%) and included congestive HF (CHF) (1.5%), cardiac arrest (1.0%), and myocardial ischemia (0.6%). The main cluster of cardiovascular toxicity events are early after treatment, with cardiac AEs occurring within 1 day of dosing in 62 patients (11.8%). The rate of cardiac AEs did not increase later in the cycles.

REAL-WORLD STUDIES

Atrash and colleagues[21] reported the cardiotoxicity data associated with carfilzomib in 130 patients with relapsed and/or refractory multiple myeloma, either on a phase 2 compassionate carfilzomib protocol ($n = 118$) or as single-patient treatment with an investigational new drug ($n = 12$). Twenty-six patients out of the total 130 patients (20%) developed cardiac AEs. Eleven patients were hospitalized for CHF and a further 4 patients were admitted for CHF with hypotension, the total new HF incidence of 11.5%. Pulmonary edema led to the hospitalization of 2 patients and included one case of severe hypertensive crisis. Serious cardiac arrhythmia was also reported. Three patients presented with significant arrhythmias complicated by hypotension, and a fourth patient required hospitalization arrhythmia without hypotension. Among the 4 patients who were hospitalized for arrhythmia, 2 had cardiac arrest due to arrhythmias.

Echocardiograms were performed at baseline and as symptom-driven follow-ups ($n = 93$ [72%]). The median LVEF as assessed by echocardiogram reduced from 55% to 33% during carfilzomib treatment. Sixty-nine of 130 patients (53%) also had baseline B-type natriuretic peptide (BNP) measurements and measurements during the first cycle of carfilzomib. Among these patients, a median increase of 407 pg/mL BNP from baseline was observed ($P<.001$). Elevation of BNP did not seem to correlate with clinical symptoms or hospitalization but may be a useful marker for detecting subclinical carfilzomib cardiotoxicity.

Danhof and colleagues[22] in a single-center retrospective study of 22 patients with relapsed/refractory multiple myeloma examined the efficacy and safety of carfilzomib combination therapy in a nontrial clinical practice setting. All patients received carfilzomib with a starting dose of 20 mg/m^2 on days 1, 2, 8, 9, 15, and 16 during the first 28-day cycle and a target dose of 27 mg/m^2 per scheduled treatment day thereafter. All patients also received concomitant low-dose dexamethasone at a maximum of 160 mg per cycle, and 5 patients received lenalidomide with a target dose of 25 mg on days 1 through 21.

The second most common group of nonhematologic severe AEs was cardiac. Five patients developed symptomatic HF. They presented with shortness of breath, weight gain, edema, and pleural effusions and had increased N-terminal-pro-BNP (NT-proBNP) levels (median: 28,447, range: 23,018–31,620 pg/mL) and reduced LVEF (median: 30, range 18%–45%). All patients required oxygen and intravenous diuretic therapy. In some patients, inotropic support was given and 2 patients required intensive care treatment. The period to full recovery was usually short after suspension of myeloma treatment. One patient who had experienced an MI 25 years previously had persistent left ventricular impairment with reduced LVEF of 30%.

Finally, Grandin and colleagues[23] described the clinical presentation and management of 6 patients with relapsed and/or refractory multiple myeloma who experienced significant cardiac toxicity associated with carfilzomib treatment. According with the investigators, elevated BNP levels seemed to correlate with the development of cardiac dysfunction and BNP levels declined with recovery of cardiac function.

ORAL PROTEASOME INHIBITOR

The safety and efficacy of ixazomib were demonstrated in the TOURMALINE-MM1 study, an international, phase 3, double-blind clinical trial.[24] More than 720 patients with relapsed and/or refractory multiple myeloma were randomized to ixazomib plus lenalidomide and dexamethasone or to placebo plus lenalidomide and dexamethasone.

The median time to response was 1.1 months in the ixazomib group and 1.9 months in the placebo group, and the corresponding median duration of response was 20.5 months and 15.0 months. At a median follow-up of approximately 23 months, the median overall survival has not been reached in either study group, and follow-up is ongoing. The rates of serious AEs were similar in the two study groups (47% in the ixazomib group and 49% in the placebo group), as were the rates of death during the study period (4% and 6%, respectively). The rate of HF-related symptoms was similar in both groups, with a trend to higher rates in the ixazomib arm (25% vs 18%).

SUMMARY

PIs are associated with an elevated risk of cardiovascular toxicity, probably as a direct result of reduced proteasome activity in the cardiac myocytes, given the important role of the proteasome in protein degradation in both normal metabolism and in particular in the ventricular myocardium following myocardial stress.

Bortezomib is the first therapeutic PI to be licensed for treatment; carfilzomib is a more potent, irreversible PI, which seems to be more effective in treating refractory Multiple myeloma but also portends a greater cardiovascular risk. Ixazomib is a new oral PI and may also have an increased cardiovascular risk.

Bortezomib has been reported to be cardiotoxic, but with more than 10 years of wide-scale use this incidence is apparently very low. Carfilzomib-associated cardiac toxicity was reported as any of the following: new-onset or worsening CHF, arrhythmia (mostly of low grade), MI, pulmonary hypertension, deep vein thrombosis and pulmonary emboli, sudden cardiac death, and an asymptomatic decrease in LVEF. Elevation in the cardiac biomarkers (BNP, NT-proBNP) from baseline was reported in most patients treated with carfilzomib but with no apparent correlation to symptoms.

A head-to-head comparison of cardiovascular toxicity with carfilzomib and bortezomib is available through the ENDEAVOR trial.[18] In that trial in the setting of relapsed/refractory disease, any cardiac event of any grade was reported in 12% of patients in the carfilzomib arm compared with 4% in the bortezomib arm. Regarding the cardiotoxicity of ixazomib, the clinical experience is very limited and further trials required for safety data, but concerns regarding cardiotoxicity are present given the class-associated risk and results from the TOURMALINE-MM1 trial.[24]

Most cardiac AEs occurred relatively early in the course of treatment (2–3 months from treatment initiation) and mostly in patients with cardiovascular comorbidities or prior exposure to other cardiotoxic agents, raising the possibility of a synergistic effect with background cardiac risk factors, which are common in this patient group.[25]

Treatment strategies should involve risk stratification at baseline diagnosis before starting PI treatment and medical optimization of preexisting cardiovascular comorbidities, including hypertension, ischemic heart disease, and preexisting left ventricular dysfunction. Minimizing fluid loads associated with treatments, avoiding concomitant cardiotoxic and nephrotoxic drugs, and use of diuretics to optimize fluid balance are pragmatic approaches that can be delivered in current clinical practice. Cardio-oncology services have been developed to advance expertise in managing cardiovascular toxicity and complications in patients receiving cancer therapies. Cardio-oncology services are supporting hemato-oncology specialists to help manage PI-associated cardiotoxicity, with an important emphasis on communication and education between cardiologists and hemato-oncologists. The role of echocardiography and cardiac biomarkers, including natriuretic peptides, in patients treated with PIs for cardiotoxicity surveillance and optimal treatment of cardiotoxicity to support ongoing PI treatment in patients with responsive disease remain to be determined and are important goals of future work.

REFERENCES

1. Adams J. The development of proteasome inhibitors as anticancer drugs. Cancer Cell 2004;5(5):417–21.
2. Voorhees PM, Dees EC, O'Neil B, et al. The proteasome as a target for cancer therapy. Clin Cancer Res 2003;9(17):6316–25.
3. Adams J. Proteasome inhibitors as new anticancer drugs. Curr Opin Oncol 2002;14(6):628–34.
4. DeMartino GN. Proteasome inhibition: mechanism of action. J Natl Compr Canc Netw 2004;2(Suppl 4): S5–9.
5. Johnson DE. The ubiquitin-proteasome system: opportunities for therapeutic intervention in solid tumors. Endocr Relat Cancer 2015;22(1):T1–17.
6. Faiman B, Richards T. Innovative agents in multiple myeloma. J Adv Pract Oncol 2014;5(3):193–202.
7. Kubiczkova L, Pour L, Sedlarikova L, et al. Proteasome inhibitors - molecular basis and current perspectives in multiple myeloma. J Cell Mol Med 2014;18(6):947–61.
8. Hideshima T, Richardson P, Chauhan D, et al. The proteasome inhibitor PS-341 inhibits growth, induces apoptosis, and overcomes drug resistance in human multiple myeloma cells. Cancer Res 2001;61(7):3071–6.
9. Richardson PG, Hideshima T, Anderson KC. Bortezomib (PS-341): a novel, first-in-class proteasome inhibitor for the treatment of multiple myeloma and other cancers. Cancer Control 2003;10(5):361–9.
10. McBride A, Klaus JO, Stockerl-Goldstein K. Carfilzomib: a second-generation proteasome inhibitor for the treatment of multiple myeloma. Am J Health Syst Pharm 2015;72(5):353–60.
11. Jakubowiak AJ. Evolution of carfilzomib dose and schedule in patients with multiple myeloma: a historical overview. Cancer Treat Rev 2014;40(6): 781–90.
12. Raedler LA. Ninlaro (ixazomib): first oral proteasome inhibitor approved for the treatment of patients with relapsed or refractory multiple myeloma. Am Health Drug Benefits 2016;9(Spec Feature):102–5.
13. Richardson PG, Sonneveld P, Schuster MW, et al, Assessment of Proteasome Inhibition for Extending Remissions (APEX) Investigators. Bortezomib or high-dose dexamethasone for relapsed multiple myeloma. N Engl J Med 2005;352(24):2487–98.
14. San Miguel JF, Schlag R, Khuageva NK, et al, VISTA Trial Investigators. Bortezomib plus melphalan and prednisone for initial treatment of multiple myeloma. N Engl J Med 2008;359(9):906–17.
15. Xiao Y, Yin J, Wei J, et al. Incidence and risk of cardiotoxicity associated with bortezomib in the treatment of cancer: a systematic review and meta-analysis. PLoS One 2014;9(1):e87671.
16. Stewart AK, Rajkumar SV, Dimopoulos MA, et al, ASPIRE Investigators. Carfilzomib, lenalidomide,

and dexamethasone for relapsed multiple myeloma. N Engl J Med 2015;372(2):142–52.

17. Hájek R, Bryce R, Ro S, et al. Design and rationale of FOCUS (PX-171-011): a randomized, open-label, phase 3 studies of carfilzomib versus best supportive care regimen in patients with relapsed and refractory multiple myeloma (R/R MM). BMC Cancer 2012;12:415.

18. Dimopoulos MA, Moreau P, Palumbo A, et al, ENDEAVOR Investigators. Carfilzomib and dexamethasone versus bortezomib and dexamethasone for patients with relapsed or refractory multiple myeloma (ENDEAVOR): a randomised, phase 3, open-label, multicentre study. Lancet Oncol 2016; 17(1):27–38.

19. Mikhael JR, Reeder CB, Libby EN, et al. Phase Ib/II trial of CYKLONE (cyclophosphamide, carfilzomib, thalidomide and dexamethasone) for newly diagnosed myeloma. Br J Haematol 2015;169(2): 219–27.

20. Siegel D, Martin T, Nooka A, et al. Integrated safety profile of single-agent carfilzomib: experience from 526 patients enrolled in 4 phase II clinical studies. Haematologica 2013;98(11):1753–61.

21. Atrash S, Tullos A, Panozzo S, et al. Cardiac complications in relapsed and refractory multiple myeloma patients treated with carfilzomib. Blood Cancer J 2015;5:e272.

22. Danhof S, Schreder M, Rasche L, et al. 'Real-life' experience of preapproval carfilzomib-based therapy in myeloma - analysis of cardiac toxicity and predisposing factors. Eur J Haematol 2016;97(1): 25–32.

23. Grandin EW, Ky B, Cornell RF, et al. Patterns of cardiac toxicity associated with irreversible proteasome inhibition in the treatment of multiple myeloma. J Card Fail 2015;21(2):138–44.

24. Moreau P, Masszi T, Grzasko N, et al, TOURMALINE-MM1 Study Group. Oral ixazomib, lenalidomide, and dexamethasone for multiple myeloma. N Engl J Med 2016;374(17):1621–34.

25. Mikhael J. Management of carfilzomib-associated cardiac adverse events. Clin Lymphoma Myeloma Leuk 2016;16(5):241–5.

Cardio-oncology Related to Heart Failure

Epidermal Growth Factor Receptor Target-Based Therapy

Benjamin Kenigsberg, MD, Varun Jain, MD, Ana Barac, MD, PhD*

KEYWORDS

- Targeted cancer therapeutics • EGFR signaling • HER2 pathways • Heart failure
- Cardiovascular toxicity • Cancer • Cardiac therapies

KEY POINTS

- Cancer therapy targeting the epidermal growth factor receptor (EGFR)/erythroblastic leukemia viral oncogene B (ErbB)/human EGFR (HER) receptor family of tyrosine kinases has been successfully used in treatment of several malignancies.
- The ErbB pathways also play a role in the maintenance of cardiac homeostasis, and their inhibition can lead to left ventricular systolic dysfunction and overt heart failure.
- This article summarizes the current knowledge about EGFR/ErbB/HER receptor-targeted cancer therapeutics with focus on their cardiotoxicity profiles, molecular mechanisms, and implications in clinical cardio-oncology.
- The article discusses challenges in predicting, monitoring, and treating cardiac dysfunction and heart failure associated with ErbB-targeted cancer therapeutics and highlights opportunities for researchers and clinical investigators in this field.

INTRODUCTION

Cancer therapy targeting the cellular pathways of the epidermal growth factor receptor (EGFR)/erythroblastic leukemia viral oncogene B (ErbB) family of tyrosine kinases has been successfully used in treatment of subtypes of breast[1] and lung[2] cancer and is increasingly explored in a variety of malignancies, including gliomas,[3] ovarian,[4] pancreatic,[5] colorectal,[6] prostate,[7] and head and neck cancer.[8] However, these same ErbB pathways also play a role in the maintenance of cardiac homeostasis; their inhibition can have important cardiovascular adverse effects, most prominently leading to left ventricular (LV) systolic dysfunction and overt heart failure (HF).

The EGFR/ErbB/human EGFR (HER) receptor family comprises 4 membrane-bound protein tyrosine kinases that are often recognized under different names reflecting their paths of discovery and distinct receptor functions. ErbB1, named after the erythroblastic leukemia viral oncogene to which these receptors are homologous, is most commonly known as the EGFR and less often as HER1. ErbB2 or EGFR2 is best known as HER2 or HER2/neu (after proto-oncogene Neu), whereas dual names may often be found for ErbB3/HER3 and ErbB4/HER4. In addition to their key roles in physiologic development and homeostasis, members of the EGFR/ErbB/HER family have been identified as important regulators of the

MedStar Washington Hospital Center, MedStar Heart and Vascular Institute, Washington, DC, USA
* Corresponding author. MedStar Washington Hospital Center, MedStar Heart and Vascular Institute, 110 Irving Street, Northwest, Suite 1F1218, Washington, DC.
E-mail address: ana.barac@medstar.net

Heart Failure Clin 13 (2017) 297–309
http://dx.doi.org/10.1016/j.hfc.2016.12.002
1551-7136/17/© 2016 Elsevier Inc. All rights reserved.

development and progression of several cancers[9] and have become attractive targets for anticancer drug development.

This review summarizes the current knowledge about EGFR/ErbB/HER receptor-targeted cancer therapeutics with focus on their cardiotoxicity profiles, molecular mechanisms, and implications in clinical cardio-oncology. The authors discuss challenges in predicting, monitoring, and treating cardiac dysfunction and HF associated with ErbB-targeted cancer therapeutics and highlight opportunities for researchers and clinical investigators in this field.

ERYTHROBLASTIC LEUKEMIA VIRAL ONCOGENE B RECEPTORS AND THEIR MECHANISM OF ACTION

The 4 ErbB1 to 4 family members are encoded by the corresponding *ErbB1* to 4 genes and share a common transmembrane receptor tyrosine kinase structure including an extracellular region, a single transmembrane-spanning region, and a cytoplasmic tyrosine kinase domain (Fig. 1). For simplicity, in this review, the authors use the most frequently cited names for each of the receptors as follows: ErbB1/EGFR for ErbB1/EGFR/HER1, ErbB2/HER2 for ErbB2/EGFR2/HER2, and ErbB3 and ErbB4 for ErbB3/EGFR3/HER3 and ErbB4/EGFR4/HER4, respectively.

Each ErbB receptor has specific ligand binding characteristics causing receptor homo-dimerization or hetero-dimerization and the activation of intrinsic tyrosine kinase domains, resulting in phosphorylation of specific tyrosine kinases within the cytoplasmic domain. The epidermal growth factor (EGF) family of ligands can be divided into 3 groups (see Fig. 1). None of the ligands bind directly to ErbB2, but ErbB2 is the preferred dimerization partner for all other ErbB receptors. ErbB3 has impaired kinase

activity and only acquires signaling potential when it is dimerized with another ErbB receptor, such as ErbB2.[10] After ErbB receptor dimerization, tyrosine kinase phosphorylation leads to activation of the intracellular signaling cascade mechanism. There are 3 main pathways that can be stimulated on activation of ErbBs, the mitogen-activated protein kinase (MAPK)–rat sarcoma virus oncogene (Ras)–extracellular signal-regulated kinase (ERK) pathway, the phosphatidylinositol 3-kinase (PI3K)–protein kinase B (Akt), and the Janus kinase–signal transducer and activator of transcription protein (STAT) pathway, all responsible for the regulation of the cellular metabolism, growth, and survival.[11–14]

ERYTHROBLASTIC LEUKEMIA VIRAL ONCOGENE B RECEPTORS AND CANCER

The ErbB pathway can lead to cancer by various mechanisms, including overproduction of the binding ligands, overexpression of the ErbB receptors, or mutation causing constitutive activation of the receptors. Many tumors also produce the EGF-related growth factors themselves or induce the surrounding stromal cells to produce it.[15] Receptor amplification is associated with higher tumor grade, increased proliferation potential, and increased mortality due to the cancer.[10] The ErbB2 pathway is most frequently associated with carcinogenesis, as it is overexpressed in 20% to 30% of breast cancers because of gene amplification[16] and can also be pathogenic in ovarian, gastric, and bladder cancer.[17] In some breast cancer cells, the overexpressed ErbB2 receptor undergoes proteolytic cleavage of the extracellular domain leading to a constitutively activated truncated membrane-bound fragment, called p95, which is the active form of the receptor.[18] Mutations in the kinase domains of the ErbB2 have also been identified in non–small-cell lung cancers

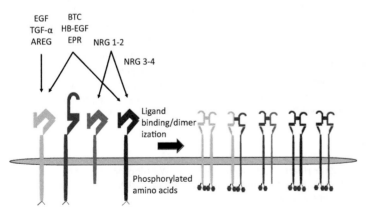

EGF　BTC
TGF-α　HB-EGF
AREG　EPR　NRG 1-2
NRG 3-4

Ligand binding/dimerization

Phosphorylated amino acids

ErbB1　ErbB2　ErbB3　ErbB4

Fig. 1. ErbB receptors and their specific binding ligands. Ligand binding induces the dimerization, phosphorylation, and activation of the ErbB receptors. AREG, amphiregulin; BTC, Betacellulin; EGF, epidermal growth factor; EPR, Epiregulin; HB-EGF, heparin-binding EGF-like growth factor; NRG, neuregulin; TGF-α, transforming growth factor α.

(NSCLCs).[19] ErbB3/ErbB2 heterodimers are usually associated with ErbB2 overexpressed cancer cells.

ERYTHROBLASTIC LEUKEMIA VIRAL ONCOGENE B RECEPTORS AS TARGETS FOR CANCER CHEMOTHERAPY

Cancer therapeutics target ErbB pathways mostly using one of 2 strategies: administration of humanized monoclonal antibodies against the extracellular receptor domains or utilization of small molecule tyrosine-kinase inhibitors (TKIs) that may target both receptor and nonreceptor tyrosine kinases. Additionally, newer antibody-drug conjugates combine conventional chemotherapeutic agents bound to targeted monoclonal antibodies as delivery vehicles. Most pharmacologic research has focused on the targeting of the EGFR and HER2 receptors.

The monoclonal antibodies trastuzumab, pertuzumab, cetuximab, and panitumumab are large molecules that bind to the extracellular domain of ErbB receptors, thus, blocking ligand binding and/or receptor dimerization. Antibody binding inhibits activation of the downstream signaling pathways, induces receptor internalization, and decreases the expression of the receptors on the cell surface. The monoclonal antibodies also bind to the Fc receptor of immunoglobulins and activate neutrophils, macrophages, and natural killers cells leading to complement-induced cytotoxicity or antibody-dependent cell-mediated cytotoxicity.[20]

The small-molecule TKIs function as adenosine triphosphate (ATP) analogues and inhibit downstream intracellular signaling by competing with the ATP binding sites on the catalytic domain of the receptor tyrosine kinase.[21] An important effect of interruption of the ErBB receptor downstream signaling is the reversal of the Bcl-2–antagonist of cell death (BAD) inhibition, which leads to a decrease in antiapoptotic B-cell lymphoma-extra large (Bcl-xL) expression, release of cytochrome C (Cyt C) from the mitochondria, and ultimately activation of caspases with cell death[10] (Fig. 2).

The newer antibody drug conjugate ado-trastuzumab emtansine (T-DM1) is the monoclonal antibody trastuzumab linked to several molecules

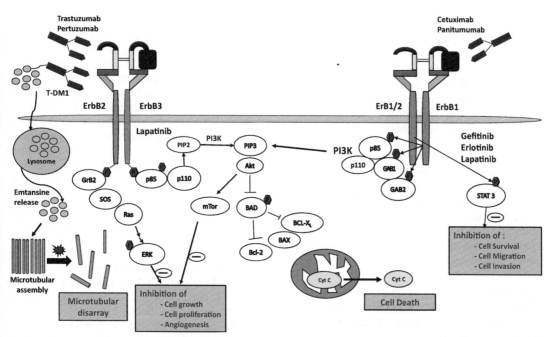

Fig. 2. ErbB-targeted cancer therapeutics and their mechanisms of actions in cancer cell. Monoclonal antibodies (trastuzumab, pertuzumab, cetuximab, panitumumab, and ado-trastuzumab emtansine [T-DM1]) bind extracellularly and receptor TKIs (gefitinib, lapatinib, erlotinib) bind to the intracellular kinase domain. Drug binding leads to the inhibition of downstream cell signaling pathways and cell death. Emtansine, a cytotoxic agent, causes breakdown of the microtubular assembly leading to inhibition of cell division and cell death. Akt, protein kinase B; BAX, Bcl-2–like protein 4 encoded by BAX gene; Bcl-2, B-cell lymphoma family of regulator protein; Bcl-X_L, B-cell lymphoma-extra large; ErbB2, named after the erythroblastic leukemia viral oncogene B/*EGFR-2*/HER2/ *Neu* (proto-oncogene Neu); ErbB3, named after the erythroblastic leukemia viral oncogene/*EGFR 3*/HER-3; mToR, mechanistic target of rapamycin; PIP2, phosphatidylinositol 4,5 biphosphate; PIP3, phosphatidylinositol 3,4,5 triphosphate.

of the highly cytotoxic agent emtansine. T-DM1 is activated through trastuzumab binding to HER2, following which the ligand-bound receptor complex gets internalized and delivered to the lysosome. Emtansine then undergoes lysosomal proteolytic degradation and is released to the cytoplasm where it binds to the vinca site at microtubules resulting in the inhibition of polymerization, cell cycle arrest, and ultimately apoptotic cell death[22] (see Fig. 2).

TKIs are generally less specific than monoclonal antibodies, which is potentially advantageous as TKIs have the ability to inhibit several tyrosine kinases with similar homology, although with some increased risk of toxicity. Of note, TKIs may show more potent antitumor effects when used in combination with a selective antibody,[23] suggesting that TKIs may further modulate intracellular signaling that is not fully blocked by the extracellularly bound monoclonal antibody.[10]

CARDIOTOXICITY OF ERYTHROBLASTIC LEUKEMIA VIRAL ONCOGENE B/EPIDERMAL GROWTH FACTOR RECEPTOR–TARGETED THERAPIES

Cardiovascular effects of targeted therapeutics, including ErbB-targeted agents, are divided in 2 broad categories based on the molecular mechanism underlying the effects. On-target toxicity occurs when the tyrosine kinase target (such as ErbB receptor) regulating cancer cell survival and/or proliferation also serves an important role in normal cardiovascular cell survival or homeostasis leading to the expected outcome of cardiovascular toxicity. Off-target toxicity, on the other hand, describes events when ErbB or other cancer target-directed agent also affects other key cellular molecules not intended as the primary target of the drug.[10] Although important, this concept has become harder to apply with the evolution of multi-targeted agents, therapeutics that are designed to affect numerous kinases with different levels of activity.[24]

CARDIOTOXICITY RELATED TO TARGETING OF ERYTHROBLASTIC LEUKEMIA VIRAL ONCOGENE B 1/EPIDERMAL GROWTH FACTOR RECEPTOR

Cetuximab is an immunoglobulin G 1 (IgG1) monoclonal antibody with high affinity for ErbB1/EGFR. It is approved for use in locally advanced head and neck cancers and metastatic EFGR-positive colorectal carcinomas.[25] Cetuximab has been associated with rare events of sudden cardiac death and myocardial infarctions in clinical trials resulting in the Food and Drug Administration (FDA)

package insert boxed warning regarding cardiopulmonary arrest,[25] recommending particular caution in patients with a history of coronary artery disease, arrhythmias, and/or HF. Another, Ig2 monoclonal antibody against ErbB1/EGFR is panitumumab that is approved for treatment of EGFR-expressing metastatic colorectal carcinomas.[26] Clinical trial data suggest relative safety of panitumumab with minimal cardiotoxic effects.

Gefitinib and erlotinib are small molecule TKIs targeting ErbB1/EGFR that are currently in use against EGFR-expressing NSCLCs, gliomas, and other cancers. Gefitinib and erlotinib have no significant cardiovascular toxicity noted in clinical trials.

CARDIOTOXICITY RELATED TO TARGETING OF ERYTHROBLASTIC LEUKEMIA VIRAL ONCOGENE B 2/HUMAN EPIDERMAL GROWTH FACTOR RECEPTOR 2
Trastuzumab

Trastuzumab is a humanized monoclonal antibody that selectively binds to the extracellular subdomain IV of ErbB2/HER2 and inhibits its signaling through several mechanisms. It is approved for use in HER2-overexpressing breast, metastatic gastric, or gastroesophageal junction adenocarcinoma and has an FDA serious adverse effect warning for cardiomyopathy.[27] Although molecular details of trastuzumab-related cardiac injury remain subject of investigations, increased knowledge about tumor and cardiomyocyte cell biology continues to offer-potential insights. The trastuzumab target, ErbB2, does not have a known high-affinity ligand; however, in cancer cells its kinase activity can be activated by receptor overexpression or by hetero-association with other members of the ErbB family. In cardiomyocytes, ErbB2-preferred coreceptor ErbB4 serves as a ligand of neuregulin 1 (NRG-1) and NRG1-ErbB4/ErbB2 pathway plays an important role in cardiac homeostasis and cellular responses to stress and injury.[28] Blockade of NRG-1/ErbB4/ErbB2 signaling cascade by trastuzumab may alter protective myocardial cellular responses to pressure overload and/or anthracycline injury and lead to activation of apoptotic pathways.[29] This concept is supported by the clinical practice observations whereby concurrent therapy with trastuzumab and anthracyclines increases the risk of cardiotoxicity more than either agent alone.[30]

Pertuzumab

Pertuzumab is recombinant humanized monoclonal antibody directed against the extracellular dimerization domain (subdomain II) of ErbB2/HER2 receptor and acts by preventing the association of ErbB2 with other ErbB family members.

Inhibition of HER2 dimerization is complementary to the actions of trastuzumab and pertuzumab augments cancer therapeutic efficacy when given in combination with trastuzumab.[31,32] Pertuzumab is approved for treatment of HER2 overexpressing breast cancer in combination with trastuzumab and docetaxel.[33] In meta-analysis of pertuzumab trials cardiac dysfunction was reported in 4.5% to 14.5% patients; however, no apparent additive risk of cardiotoxicity was noted with the addition of pertuzumab to trastuzumab therapy, and cardiac dysfunction was predominantly attributed to the concurrent trastuzumab.[34]

Lapatinib

Lapatinib is a small molecule TKI approved for treatment of HER2-positive breast cancer.[35,36] It is an orally administered dual inhibitor of ErbB2/HER2 and ErbB1/EGFR that acts by binding to the intracellular kinase component of the receptor. Lapatinib has shown minimal cardiac toxicity in clinical trials and subsequent FDA monitoring.[34,37] In phase III clinical trials both with and without trastuzumab pretreatment, lapatinib therapy was associated with 2.5% incidence of asymptomatic decrease in LV ejection fraction (LVEF) and no symptomatic HF.[38,39] At present, lapatinib use in patients with HER2-positive breast cancer is limited to second line treatments but no cardiotoxicity surveillance is mandated by the FDA[40] (Table 1).

Ado-Trastuzumab Emtansine

T-DM1 is an antibody drug conjugate approved in 2013 for HER2-positive metastatic breast cancer.[41] T-DM1 combines the monoclonal antibody trastuzumab and the cytotoxic activity of the microtubule inhibitor emtansine (DM1) and was found to prolong progression-free and overall survival in patients with advanced HER2-positive breast cancer.[42] Clinical trials that introduced T-DM1 to clinical practice followed similar cardiac safety design as trastuzumab trials and did not demonstrate excess toxicity. Based on this evidence T-DM1 cardiotoxicity profile is considered similar to the one of trastuzumab, and recommendations for cardiac monitoring and exclusion of patients with reduced LVEF are similar[41] (see Table 1).

TRANSLATION INTO CLINICAL PRACTICE

ErbB receptor, in particular ErbB2/HER2-target, based therapy has revolutionized cancer care and epitomizes the remarkable effectiveness of molecularly targeted oncologic treatment. The seminal study of trastuzumab-combination therapy in HER2-positive metastatic breast cancer found a remarkable 20% relative risk reduction of mortality at 30 months of follow-up.[1] Unexpectedly, however, cardiac dysfunction developed in 27% of participants on trastuzumab and doxorubicin, 13% on trastuzumab and paclitaxel, and only 1% on paclitaxel monotherapy.[1] A subsequent meta-analysis similarly found that the incidence of trastuzumab-associated cardiotoxicity was highest with concurrent anthracycline use.[43] These findings were a surprise as no cardiotoxicity signal was seen in preclinical trastuzumab studies. In light of the dramatic improvement in progression-free survival and overall survival of patients with metastatic HER2-positive breast cancer, trastuzumab was approved for clinical use in this population with important caution regarding its cardiac risk. More importantly, these observations critically influenced the design of ensuing adjuvant trials in early HER2-positive breast cancer that introduced the following elements: (1) change in drug administration to ensure no concomitant dosing of trastuzumab with anthracyclines, (2) exclusion of patients with abnormal cardiac function before receipt of trastuzumab, and (3) implementation of LVEF with strict holding and stopping criteria based on the changes in LVEF and/or HF symptoms.

As a result, incidence of cardiac dysfunction with trastuzumab administration in adjuvant HER2-positive breast cancer trials was significantly decreased, with symptomatic HF and asymptomatic decreased LV function developing in 2% to 4% and 7% to 14%, respectively.[44,45] The varied incidence of trastuzumab-related cardiac dysfunction can be attributed to alterations in eligibility criteria, chemotherapy regimen, definitions of cardiotoxicity, and the subsequent initiation of routine cardiac monitoring. A contemporary meta-analysis of 12,000 patients with early breast cancer noted relative risks of 5.1 and 1.8 for the development of LV dysfunction and HF, respectively, with continuing improvement in breast cancer–free survival and overall survival with trastuzumab therapy, highlighting the continued overall benefit of HER2-targeted therapy.[46]

NEUREGULIN AS HEART FAILURE THERAPY AND EXAMPLE OF NEW PARADIGMS IN CARDIO-ONCOLOGY

The discovery of ErbB2/HER2 therapy–related LV dysfunction and research into molecular pathways of ErbB signaling have revealed a new role of NRG in heart homeostasis. NRG is a peptide and growth factor that binds and activates ErbB4/ErbB4 and ErbB4/ErbB2 homodimers and heterodimers leading to activation of downstream kinases

Table 1
Current erythroblastic leukemia viral oncogene B/epidermal growth factor receptor –targeted therapies in clinical use and toxicity profiles

Class	Agent	Target	Malignancy	Cardiotoxicity Profile	Other Toxicity
Monoclonal antibody	Trastuzumab	ErbB2/HER2	HER2-positive breast cancer	Known cardiac toxicity particularly in patients with abnormal LV function: recommended on treatment LV function monitoring	Infusion reactions, neutropenia
	Pertuzumab	ErbB2/HER2	ErbB2-positive breast cancer, ovarian, prostate cancer, NSCLC	When given with trastuzumab no evidence of worsening of trastuzumab cardiotoxicity profile: recommended on treatment LV function monitoring	Skin rash, diarrhea
	Panitumumab	ErbB1/EGFR	CRC	Rare, no routine cardiac monitoring	Skin rash
	Cetuximab	ErbB1/EGFR	CRC, squamous cell carcinoma of head/neck	Rare, no routine cardiac monitoring	Skin rash, infusion reactions, interstitial lung disease, electrolyte imbalances, cardiopulmonary arrest
Small molecule TKIs	Lapatinib	ErbB2/HER2 and ErbB1/EGFR	erbB2-positive breast cancer, ovarian cancer, gliomas, NSCLC	Rare, no routine cardiac monitoring	Skin rash, diarrhea
	Gefitinib	ErbB1/EGFR	NSCLC, gliomas	Rare, no routine cardiac monitoring	Skin rash, nausea, diarrhea, interstitial lung disease
	Erlotinib	ErbB1/EGFR	NSCLC, pancreatic cancer, gliomas	Rare, no routine cardiac monitoring	Skin rash, nausea, diarrhea, interstitial lung disease
Antibody drug conjugate	T-DM1	ErbB2/HER2	HER2-positive late-stage breast cancer	Cardiotoxicity considered similar to trastuzumab, no excess toxicity seen in clinical trials; recommended on treatment LV function	Hemorrhage, hepatotoxicity, teratogenicity, infusion reaction, pancytopenia, interstitial lung disease

(Fig. 3). During embryogenesis, NRG pathway regulates growth, proliferation, and differentiation of neonatal cardiomyocytes, whereas in the adult heart, NRG signaling has been implicated in maintaining the myocardial architecture and preventing pathologic remodeling.[47,48] It was the discovery of NRG as a stress-activated mediator of cardiac repair that led to the investigations of the recombinant NRG-1beta as a possible treatment of systolic HF,[49] thus, providing an exciting example of unique opportunities in cardio-oncology research to advance identification of new cardiovascular disease targets. NRG is also being investigated as a biomarker in patients receiving anthracyclines and HER2-targeted therapies as a higher baseline NRG level has been proposed to identify patients at higher risk for significant cardiotoxicity.[50,51]

MONITORING AND EARLY IDENTIFICATION OF ERYTHROBLASTIC LEUKEMIA VIRAL ONCOGENE B 2/HUMAN EPIDERMAL GROWTH FACTOR RECEPTOR 2 THERAPY–RELATED CARDIOTOXICITY

Cardiac monitoring prior and during cancer treatment predominantly focuses on cardiac imaging modalities, such as nuclear multiple gated acquisition scans, cardiac MRI, and echocardiography, to assess changes in LV function. Currently, a preexisting cardiomyopathy generally precludes HER2-targeted therapy, as the American Society of Clinical Oncology's clinical practice guidelines list decreased LVEF or clinical HF as the single most important contraindication to trastuzumab therapy.[52] Once begun on HER2-targeted therapy,

contemporary studies prioritize cardiac screening and frequently mandate serial imaging of LV function.[53] Adopting the trastuzumab clinical trial design, routine LVEF assessment is recommended by clinical practice guidelines and the FDA at baseline and every 3 months during the first year of trastuzumab therapy.[54,55] Patients with decreases in LVEF less than the specified cutoffs are recommended not to continue trastuzumab therapy until LV function returns to normal. Similarly adopting the trial design, trastuzumab is typically held for 4 weeks if LVEF decreases 16 or more percentage points from baseline or 10% to 15% points from baseline to less than the lower limit of normal; trastuzumab is permanently discontinued if the LVEF remains less than these levels or if patients had symptomatic HF while receiving therapy.[56] Two other currently approved HER2-targeted therapies, pertuzumab and T-DMI, have similar recommendations for cardiac monitoring and therapy holding or discontinuation.

Novel imaging parameters and biomarkers have been investigated to identify early markers of myocardial injury before outright LVEF changes. Global longitudinal strain (GLS) assessment, or myocardial strain, using speckle tracking echocardiography has become the most promising predictor of future LVEF decline. A meta-analysis of relatively small studies of patients treated with anthracyclines and frequently trastuzumab therapy noted an absolute decrease in GLS (expressed as percentage of myocardial shortening in longitudinal direction during systole) between 10% and 15% predicts subsequent cardiotoxicity, including both asymptomatic LV dysfunction and symptomatic

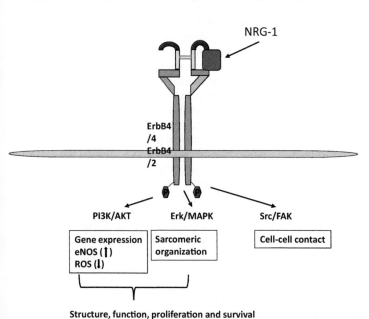

Fig. 3. Role of NRG-1/ErbB signaling in the adult cardiovascular system. The interaction of NRG with ErbB4/4 homodimers and ErbB2/4 heterodimers in a cardiomyocyte. ErbB2/4 and ErbB4/4, ErbB receptor heterodimers; FAK, focal adhesion kinase; Src, SRC gene-encoded nonreceptor tyrosine kinase. (*Adapted from* Galindo CL, Ryzhov S, Sawyer DB. Neuregulin as a heart failure therapy and mediator of reverse remodeling. Curr Heart Fail Rep 2014;11(1):41; with permission.)

HF.[57] Based on these small studies, the American Society of Echocardiography (ASE) and the European Association of Cardiovascular Imaging jointly recommended using speckle-tracking echocardiography–derived strain imaging for the evaluation of subclinical LV systolic dysfunction in patients at risk for cancer treatment–related cardiomyopathy.[58] This recommendation was based on the expert consensus, as clinical use of GLS in patients undergoing potentially cardiotoxic cancer treatments continues to be an area of active investigation. The ongoing Strain sUrveillance during Chemotherapy for improving Cardiovascular OUtcomes (SUCCOR) trial, for example, assesses the utility of serial GLS measurements during breast cancer treatment to trigger initiation of HF pharmacotherapy and is expected to inform the use of GLS in clinical decision-making in patients with breast cancer undergoing HER2-targeted therapy.[59]

Several studies have indicated that early increases in biomarkers, such as cardiac troponin, during doxorubicin and trastuzumab therapy may predict subsequent cardiotoxicity[60]; the consideration of biomarkers is recommended in patients at potentially higher risk or unclear clinical presentation. However, evidence to support the routine use of cardiac biomarker assessment during HER2 therapy is still missing; this area requires further investigation through outcome-driven, randomized multicenter clinical trials.

TREATMENT OF ERYTHROBLASTIC LEUKEMIA VIRAL ONCOGENE B 2/HUMAN EPIDERMAL GROWTH FACTOR RECEPTOR 2 THERAPY–RELATED CARDIOTOXICITY

Fortunately, most patients with HER2 therapy–related cardiotoxicity have recovery of myocardial function with appropriate monitoring, early cardiotoxicity identification, and treatment.[61,62] In addition to temporarily discontinuing HER2-targeted therapy, standard HF therapies, including beta-blockers (BBs) and renin-angiotensin-aldosterone system antagonists, are the main treatments for HER2-related cardiac toxicity.[63] Reports indicate that up to 50% of patients with on-treatment LVEF decreases have sufficient subsequent myocardial recovery to be restarted on trastuzumab.[64] LVEF recovery has also been observed after prolonged trastuzumab therapy, in which 28% of patients developed cardiac toxicity and 94% of these patients had improved LVEF or HF symptoms with discontinuation of trastuzumab and with appropriate medical therapy.[65] Despite overall encouraging reports, a smaller proportion of patients will have sustained reductions in LVEF despite appropriate monitoring and cardiac treatment[66]; long cardiac outcomes in these patients remain important investigational focus.

PREVENTION OF HUMAN EPIDERMAL GROWTH FACTOR RECEPTOR 2 THERAPY–RELATED CARDIOTOXICITY

Persistent LV dysfunction and the potential morbidity from delays and alterations in cancer treatment regimens make prophylactic therapy to prevent myocardial dysfunction desirable. Three recently published trials, along with several ongoing trials, initiated BB or angiotensin-converting enzyme inhibitor (ACEi) or angiotensin receptor blocker (ARB) concurrently with chemotherapy in an attempt to address this clinical question. The Prevention of Cardiac Dysfunction During Adjuvant Breast Cancer Therapy (PRADA) trial randomized 130 patients starting adjuvant anthracycline therapy with or without trastuzumab to candesartan (ARB), metoprolol succinate (BB), or placebo and found that candesartan, but not metoprolol, provided a small but statistically significant protection against early decline in LVEF.[67] The similarly designed the Multidisciplinary Approach to Novel Therapies in Cardiology Oncology Research (MANTICORE) trial randomized patients starting trastuzumab therapy to concomitant perindopril (ACEi), bisoprolol (BB), or placebo.[68] Contradicting the PRADA trial results, MANTICORE demonstrated that bisoprolol was more effective than perindopril in preventing reduction in LVEF.[69] These trials differed in their target population; in the PRADA trial, all patients received anthracycline-based treatment with epirubicin followed by adjuvant trastuzumab in HER2-positive patients (only a fraction of study population), whereas MANTICORE included only HER2-positive patients receiving trastuzumab and favored a nonanthracycline-based regimen. In addition to opening a question whether different neurohormonal antagonists, namely, BB and ACEi/ARBs, may specifically benefit injury resulting from anthracyclines versus HER2-targeted agents, the outcomes of these trials focused on attenuation of small changes in LVEF, thus, making the impact of their findings on clinical practice unclear.[70]

Most recently, a third trial assessed 206 patients getting adjuvant anthracycline-containing chemotherapy followed by trastuzumab and found no LVEF difference between candesartan or placebo as measured by echocardiography or multiple gate acquisition radionuclide imaging.[71] Initiation of cardiac therapy at the time of trastuzumab start, after completion of anthracycline, was suggested as one possible explanation of negative results, in addition to reliance on clinical LVEF reports lacking the precision of single laboratory cardiac magnetic resonance assessment used in PRADA and MANTICORE.[70]

Until further data are available, aggressive control of cardiac risk factors and avoidance of concomitant cardiotoxic therapies remain standard preventative therapy (Fig. 4). This approach is further supported by the retrospective analyses of trastuzumab trials and epidemiology studies indicating that advanced age, prior anthracycline treatment, presence of hypertension, and mildly reduced LVEF (in trastuzumab trials) or other cardiovascular risk factors (in epidemiology studies) remain statistically significant risk factors for subsequent development of trastuzumab-induced cardiac events.[61,72]

SURVIVORSHIP

The remarkable effectiveness of novel cancer treatment regimens has increased the number of cancer survivors and incidentally also led to an increased need for longitudinal onco-cardiology care focused on managing cardiovascular complications of therapy.[73,74] Fortunately, the risk of incident HF seems to decline after completion of EGFR-targeted treatment.[75] Notably though, clinicians should remain mindful about other cardiovascular complications of chemotherapy and radiation treatment, including coronary atherosclerosis, valvular heart disease,[76] and systemic hypertension during therapy. Over long-term follow-up, breast cancer survivors remain at elevated risk of death from cardiovascular disease, especially when treated with radiotherapy at a younger age.[77]

FUTURE RESEARCH

Although there has already been tremendous effort over the past 2 decades, clearly there are more areas for clinical inquiry and discovery to help further refine clinical care both preceding and during EGFR-targeted therapy. Should patients with baseline LV dysfunction continue to be excluded from EGFR-targeted therapy and, thus, restricted from potentially curative or life-sustaining treatment options? The ongoing Pilot Study Assessing the Cardiac SAFEty of HER2 Targeted Therapy in Patients With HER2 Positive Breast Cancer and Reduced Left Ventricular Function (SAFE-HEaRt)[78] trial will address this question by enrolling patients with a

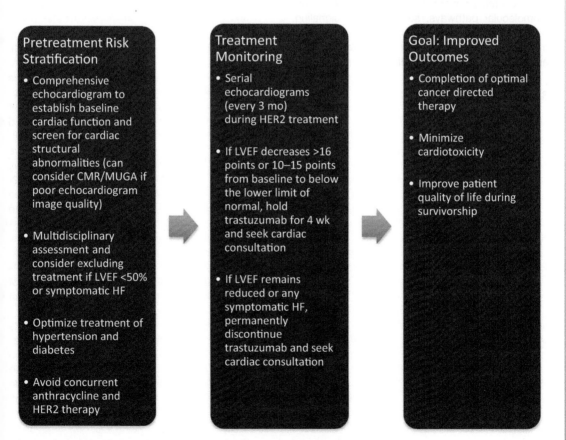

Fig. 4. Current clinical management recommendations for HER2/trastuzumab therapy.

baseline LVEF between 40% and 50% on echocardiogram before HER2-targeted therapies and monitoring cardiac function during cancer therapy along with concomitant BB and ACEi treatment.[78] Further investigation is also needed regarding cardiac surveillance, as current guidelines may not be appropriate for all patients and may lead to potentially unnecessary cardiac testing and alterations in oncologic care.[79] Additional imaging parameters, such as GLS, may better inform clinical treatment during cancer therapy and are undergoing further evaluation.[59] Another major area of further investigation is the need for systemic anthracycline-based chemotherapy, given the expanding role of molecularly targeted therapy. Ten-year follow-up of the BCIRG trial demonstrated statistically similar survival rates with AC-TH (doxorubicin and cyclophosphamide followed by docetaxel and 1 year of trastuzumab) versus TCH (docetaxel and carboplatin with 1 year of trastuzumab); however, the AC-TH group had 5 times more cases of HF than TCH (2.0% vs 0.4%).[80] This study indicates that nonanthracycline-based therapy could further reduce adverse cardiac events without compromising oncology outcomes in patients with HER2-positive breast cancer. Lastly, novel insights into biomolecular pathways, such as NRG signaling, offer an exciting example of how targeted oncologic therapies may advance our understanding and approach to cardiovascular disease treatment.[81]

REFERENCES

1. Slamon DJ, Leyland-Jones B, Shak S, et al. Use of chemotherapy plus a monoclonal antibody against HER2 for metastatic breast cancer that overexpresses HER2. N Engl J Med 2001;344:783–92.

2. Lee CK, Brown C, Gralla RJ, et al. Impact of EGFR inhibitor in non-small cell lung cancer on progression-free and overall survival: a meta-analysis. J Natl Cancer Inst 2013;105(9):595–605.

3. Stupp R, Hegi ME, van den Bent MJ, et al, European Organisation for Research and Treatment of Cancer Brain Tumor and Radiotherapy Groups; National Cancer Institute of Canada Clinical Trials Group. Changing paradigms–an update on the multidisciplinary management of malignant glioma. Oncologist 2006;11(2):165–80.

4. Yap TA, Carden CP, Kaye SB. Beyond chemotherapy: targeted therapies in ovarian cancer. Nat Rev Cancer 2009;9(3):167–81.

5. Starling N, Neoptolemos J, Cunningham D. Role of erlotinib in the management of pancreatic cancer. Ther Clin Risk Manag 2006;2(4):435–45.

6. Chung KY, Shia J, Kemeny NE, et al. Cetuximab shows activity in colorectal cancer patients with tumors that do not express the epidermal growth factor receptor by immunohistochemistry. J Clin Oncol 2005;23(9):1803–10.

7. Agus DB, Sweeney CJ, Morris MJ, et al. Efficacy and safety of single-agent pertuzumab (rhuMAb 2C4), a human epidermal growth factor receptor dimerization inhibitor, in castration-resistant prostate cancer after progression from taxane-based therapy. J Clin Oncol 2007;25(6):675–81.

8. Bonner JA, Harari PM, Giralt J, et al. Radiotherapy plus cetuximab for squamous-cell carcinoma of the head and neck. N Engl J Med 2006;354(6):567–78.

9. Arteaga CL, Engelman JA. ERBB receptors: from oncogene discovery to basic science to mechanism-based cancer therapeutics. Cancer Cell 2014;25(3):282–303.

10. Holbro T, Hynes NE. ErbB receptors: directing key signaling networks throughout life. Annu Rev Pharmacol Toxicol 2004;44:195–217.

11. Yarden Y, Sliwkowski MX. Untangling the ErbB signalling network. Nat Rev Mol Cell Biol 2001;2(2):127–37.

12. Burden S, Yarden Y. Neuregulins and their receptors: a versatile signaling module in organogenesis and oncogenesis. Neuron 1997;18(6):847–55.

13. Earp HS 3rd, Calvo BF, Sartor CI. The EGF receptor family–multiple roles in proliferation, differentiation, and neoplasia with an emphasis on HER4. Trans Am Clin Climatol Assoc 2003;114:315–33 [discussion: 333–4].

14. Schlessinger J. Common and distinct elements in cellular signaling via EGF and FGF receptors. Science 2004;306(5701):1506–7.

15. Salomon DS, Brandt R, Ciardiello F, et al. Epidermal growth factor-related peptides and their receptors in human malignancies. Crit Rev Oncol Hematol 1995;19(3):183–232.

16. Borg A, Baldetorp B, Fernö M, et al. ERBB2 amplification in breast cancer with a high rate of proliferation. Oncogene 1991;6(1):137–43.

17. Hynes NE, Stern DF. The biology of erbB-2/neu/HER-2 and its role in cancer. Biochim Biophys Acta 1994;1198(2–3):165–84.

18. Christianson TA, Doherty JK, Lin YJ, et al. NH2-terminally truncated HER-2/neu protein: relationship with shedding of the extracellular domain and with prognostic factors in breast cancer. Cancer Res 1998;58(22):5123–9.

19. Stephens P, Hunter C, Bignell G, et al. Lung cancer: intragenic ERBB2 kinase mutations in tumours. Nature 2004;431(7008):525–6.

20. Iannello A, Ahmad A. Role of antibody-dependent cell-mediated cytotoxicity in the efficacy of therapeutic anti-cancer monoclonal antibodies. Cancer Metastasis Rev 2005;24(4):487–99.

21. Imai K, Takaoka A. Comparing antibody and small-molecule therapies for cancer. Nat Rev Cancer 2006;6(9):714–27.

22. Recondo G, de la Vega M, Galanternik F, et al. Novel approaches to target HER2-positive breast cancer: trastuzumab emtansine. Cancer Manag Res 2016; 8:57–65.

23. Xia W, Gerard CM, Liu L, et al. Combining lapatinib (GW572016), a small molecule inhibitor of ErbB1 and ErbB2 tyrosine kinases, with therapeutic anti-ErbB2 antibodies enhances apoptosis of ErbB2-overexpressing breast cancer cells. Oncogene 2005;24(41):6213–21.

24. Maitland ML, Ratain MJ. Terminal ballistics of kinase inhibitors: there are no magic bullets. Ann Intern Med 2006;145(9):702–3.

25. Cetuximab [package insert]. Branchburg, NJ: ImClone LLC; 2015. Available at: http://www.accessdata.fda.gov/drugsatfda_docs/label/2015/125084s262lbl.pdf. Accessed September 10, 2016.

26. Panitimumab [package insert]. Thousand Oaks, CA: Amgen Inc; 2009. Available at: http://www.accessdata.fda.gov/drugsatfda_docs/label/2009/125147s080lbl.pdf. Accessed September 10, 2016.

27. Trastuzumab [package insert]. South San Francisco, CA: Genentech, Inc; 2010. Available at: http://www.accessdata.fda.gov/drugsatfda_docs/label/2010/103792s5256lbl.pdf. Accessed September 10, 2016.

28. Odiete O, Hill MF, Sawyer DB. Neuregulin in cardiovascular development and disease. Circ Res 2012; 111(10):1376–85.

29. Crone SA, Zhao YY, Fan L, et al. ErbB2 is essential in the prevention of dilated cardiomyopathy. Nat Med 2002;8(5):459–65.

30. Gianni L, Salvatorelli E, Minotti G. Anthracycline cardiotoxicity in breast cancer patients: synergism with trastuzumab and taxanes. Cardiovasc Toxicol 2007; 7(2):67–71.

31. Baselga J, Cortés J, Kim SB, et al, CLEOPATRA Study Group. Pertuzumab plus trastuzumab plus docetaxel for metastatic breast cancer. N Engl J Med 2012;366(2):109–19.

32. Swain SM, Baselga J, Kim SB, et al, CLEOPATRA Study Group. Pertuzumab, trastuzumab, and docetaxel in HER2-positive metastatic breast cancer. N Engl J Med 2015;372(8):724–34.

33. Pertuzumab [package insert]. South San Francisco, CA: Genentech, Inc; 2013. Available at: http://www.accessdata.fda.gov/drugsatfda_docs/label/2013/125409s051lbl.pdf. Accessed September 10, 2016.

34. Sendur MA, Aksoy S, Altundag K. Cardiotoxicity of novel HER2-targeted therapies. Curr Med Res Opin 2013;29(8):1015–24.

35. Lapatinib [package insert]. Research Triangle Park, NC: GlaxoSmithKline; 2012. Available at: http://www.accessdata.fda.gov/drugsatfda_docs/label/2012/022059s013lbl.pdf. Accessed September 10, 2016.

36. Cameron DA, Stein S. Drug insight: intracellular inhibitors of HER2–clinical development of lapatinib in breast cancer. Nat Clin Pract Oncol 2008;5(9):512–20.

37. Wittayanukorn S, Qian J, Johnson BS, et al. Cardiotoxicity in targeted therapy for breast cancer: a study of the FDA adverse event reporting system (FAERS). J Oncol Pharm Pract 2015. [Epub ahead of print].

38. Burris HA 3rd, Hurwitz HI, Dees EC, et al. Phase I safety, pharmacokinetics, and clinical activity study of lapatinib (GW572016), a reversible dual inhibitor of epidermal growth factor receptor tyrosine kinases, in heavily pretreated patients with metastatic carcinomas. J Clin Oncol 2005;23(23):5305–13.

39. Geyer CE, Forster J, Lindquist D, et al. Lapatinib plus capecitabine for HER2-positive advanced breast cancer. N Engl J Med 2006;355(26):2733–43.

40. de Azambuja E, Bedard PL, Suter T, et al. Cardiac toxicity with anti-HER-2 therapies: what have we learned so far? Target Oncol 2009;4(2):77–88.

41. Ado-trastuzumab emtansine [package insert]. South San Francisco, CA: Genentech, Inc; 2013. Available at: http://www.accessdata.fda.gov/drugsatfda_docs/label/2013/125427lbl.pdf. Accessed September 10, 2016.

42. Verma S, Miles D, Gianni L, et al. Trastuzumab emtansine for HER2-positive advanced breast cancer. N Engl J Med 2012;367(19):1783–91.

43. Seidman A, Hudis C, Pierri MK, et al. Cardiac dysfunction in the trastuzumab clinical trials experience. J Clin Oncol 2002;20(5):1215–21.

44. Piccart-Gebhart MJ, Procter M, Leyland-Jones B, et al. Trastuzumab after adjuvant chemotherapy in HER2-positive breast cancer. N Engl J Med 2005; 353(16):1659–72.

45. Tan-Chiu E, Yothers G, Romond E, et al. Assessment of cardiac dysfunction in a randomized trial comparing doxorubicin and cyclophosphamide followed by paclitaxel, with or without trastuzumab as adjuvant therapy in node-positive, human epidermal growth factor receptor 2-overexpressing breast cancer: NSABP B-31. J Clin Oncol 2005; 23(31):7811–9.

46. Moja L, Tagliabue L, Balduzzi S, et al. Trastuzumab containing regimens for early breast cancer. Cochrane Database Syst Rev 2012;(4):CD006243.

47. Galindo CL, Ryzhov S, Sawyer DB. Neuregulin as a heart failure therapy and mediator of reverse remodeling. Curr Heart Fail Rep 2014;11(1):40–9.

48. Cote GM, Sawyer DB, Chabner BA. ERBB2 inhibition and heart failure. N Engl J Med 2012;367(22): 2150–3.

49. Galindo CL, Kasasbeh E, Murphy A, et al. Anti-remodeling and anti-fibrotic effects of the neuregulin-1β glial growth factor 2 in a large animal model of heart failure. J Am Heart Assoc 2014;3(5):e000773.

50. Geisberg CA, Abdallah WM, da Silva M, et al. Circulating neuregulin during the transition from stage A to stage B/C heart failure in a breast cancer cohort. J Card Fail 2013;19(1):10–5.

51. Eschenhagen T, Force T, Ewer MS, et al. Cardiovascular side effects of cancer therapies: a position statement from the Heart Failure Association of the European Society of Cardiology. Eur J Heart Fail 2011;13(1):1–10.

52. Giordano SH, Temin S, Kirshner JJ, et al, American Society of Clinical Oncology. Systemic therapy for patients with advanced human epidermal growth factor receptor 2-positive breast cancer: American Society of Clinical Oncology clinical practice guideline. J Clin Oncol 2014;32(19):2078–99.

53. Slamon DJ, Eiermann W, Robert N, et al. Adjuvant trastuzumab in HER2-positive breast cancer. N Engl J Med 2011;365:1273–83.

54. Mackey JR, Clemons M, Côté MA, et al. Cardiac management during adjuvant trastuzumab therapy: recommendations of the Canadian Trastuzumab Working Group. Curr Oncol 2008;15(1):24–35.

55. US Food and Drug Administration. HERCEPTIN® (trastuzumab) intravenous infusion. Available at: http://www.accessdata.fda.gov/drugsatfda_docs/label/2010/103792s5250lbl.pdf. Accessed August 25, 2016.

56. Romond EH, Perez EA, Bryant J, et al. Trastuzumab plus adjuvant chemotherapy for operable HER2-positive breast cancer. N Engl J Med 2005; 353(16):1673–84.

57. Thavendiranathan P, Poulin F, Lim KD, et al. Use of myocardial strain imaging by echocardiography for the early detection of cardiotoxicity in patients during and after cancer chemotherapy: a systematic review. J Am Coll Cardiol 2014;63(25 Pt A):2751–68.

58. Plana JC, Galderisi M, Barac A, et al. Expert consensus for multimodality imaging evaluation of adult patients during and after cancer therapy: a report from the American Society of Echocardiography and the European Association of Cardiovascular Imaging. J Am Soc Echocardiogr 2014;27(9):911–39.

59. Australian and New Zealand Clinical Trials Registry [internet]: Sydney (NSW): NHMRC Clinical Trials Centre, University of Sydney (Australia); 2014 – Identifier ACTRN12614000341628. Randomised controlled trial (RCT) of chemotherapy patients at risk of cardiotoxicity undergoing cardioprotection guided by measurement of LV strain compared with cardioprotection guided by measurement of left ventricular (LV) ejection fraction for avoidance of cardiotoxicity. Available at: https://www.anzctr.org.au/Trial/Registration/TrialReview.aspx?id=366020. Accessed September 11, 2016.

60. Ky B, Putt M, Sawaya H, et al. Early increases in multiple biomarkers predict subsequent cardiotoxicity in patients with breast cancer treated with doxorubicin, taxanes, and trastuzumab. J Am Coll Cardiol 2014; 63(8):809–16.

61. Romond EH, Jeong JH, Rastogi P, et al. Seven-year follow-up assessment of cardiac function in NSABP B-31, a randomized trial comparing doxorubicin and cyclophosphamide followed by paclitaxel (ACP) with ACP plus trastuzumab as adjuvant therapy for patients with node-positive, human epidermal growth factor receptor 2-positive breast cancer. J Clin Oncol 2012;30(31):3792–9.

62. Russell SD, Blackwell KL, Lawrence J, et al. Independent adjudication of symptomatic heart failure with the use of doxorubicin and cyclophosphamide followed by trastuzumab adjuvant therapy: a combined review of cardiac data from the National Surgical Adjuvant Breast and Bowel Project B-31 and the North Central Cancer Treatment Group N9831 clinical trials. J Clin Oncol 2010;28(21):3416–21.

63. Martín M, Esteva FJ, Alba E, et al. Minimizing cardiotoxicity while optimizing treatment efficacy with trastuzumab: review and expert recommendations. Oncologist 2009;14(1):1–11.

64. Perez EA, Suman VJ, Davidson NE, et al. Cardiac safety analysis of doxorubicin and cyclophosphamide followed by paclitaxel with or without trastuzumab in the North Central Cancer Treatment Group N9831 adjuvant breast cancer trial. J Clin Oncol 2008;26(8):1231–8.

65. Guarneri V, Lenihan DJ, Valero V, et al. Long-term cardiac tolerability of trastuzumab in metastatic breast cancer: the M.D. Anderson Cancer Center experience. J Clin Oncol 2006;24(25):4107–15.

66. Telli ML, Hunt SA, Carlson RW, et al. Trastuzumab-related cardiotoxicity: calling into question the concept of reversibility. J Clin Oncol 2007;25(23): 3525–33.

67. Gulati G, Heck SL, Ree AH, et al. Prevention of cardiac dysfunction during adjuvant breast cancer therapy (PRADA): a 2 × 2 factorial, randomized, placebo-controlled, double-blind clinical trial of candesartan and metoprolol. Eur Heart J 2016;37(21): 1671–80.

68. Pituskin E, Haykowsky M, Mackey JR, et al. Rationale and design of the Multidisciplinary Approach to Novel Therapies in Cardiology Oncology Research Trial (MANTICORE 101–Breast): a randomized, placebo-controlled trial to determine if conventional heart failure pharmacotherapy can prevent trastuzumab-mediated left ventricular remodeling among patients with HER2+ early breast cancer using cardiac MRI. BMC Cancer 2011;11:318.

69. Pituskin E. Prophylactic beta blockade preserves left ventricular ejection fraction in HER2-overexpressing breast cancer patients receiving trastuzumab: Primary results of the MANTICORE randomized controlled trial. Proceedings of the 36th Annual CTRC-AACR San Antonio Breast Cancer Symposium. San Antonio (TX): 2015.

70. Barac A, Swain SM. Cardiac protection in HER2-targeted treatment: how should we measure new strategies? JAMA Oncol 2016;2(8):1037–9.

71. Boekhout AH, Gietema JA, Milojkovic Kerklaan B, et al. Angiotensin II-receptor inhibition with candesartan to prevent trastuzumab-related cardiotoxic effects in patients with early breast cancer: a randomized clinical trial. JAMA Oncol 2016;2(8): 1030–7.

72. Ezaz G, Long JB, Gross CP, et al. Risk prediction model for heart failure and cardiomyopathy after adjuvant trastuzumab therapy for breast cancer. J Am Heart Assoc 2014;3(1):e000472.

73. Barac A, Murtagh G, Carver JR, et al. Cardiovascular health of patients with cancer and cancer survivors: a roadmap to the next level. J Am Coll Cardiol 2015;65(25):2739–46.

74. Yeh ET, Chang HM. Oncocardiology-past, present, and future: a review. JAMA Cardiol 2016. http://dx. doi.org/10.1001/jamacardio.2016.2132.

75. Goldhar HA, Yan AT, Ko DT, et al. The temporal risk of heart failure associated with adjuvant trastuzumab in breast cancer patients: a population study. J Natl Cancer Inst 2015;108(1) [pii: djv301].

76. Bouillon K, Haddy N, Delaloge S, et al. Long-term cardiovascular mortality after radiotherapy for breast cancer. J Am Coll Cardiol 2011;57(4):445–52.

77. Hooning MJ, Aleman BM, van Rosmalen AJ, et al. Cause-specific mortality in long-term survivors of breast cancer: a 25-year follow-up study. Int J Radiat Oncol Biol Phys 2006;64(4):1081–91.

78. Washington Hospital Center. Cardiac safety study in patients with HER2 + breast cancer (SAFE-HEaRt). In: ClinicalTrials.gov [Internet]. Bethesda (MD): National Library of Medicine (US); 2000. Available at: https:// clinicaltrials.gov/ct2/show/NCT01904903. Accessed August 28, 2016.

79. Dang CT, Yu AF, Jones LW, et al. Cardiac surveillance guidelines for trastuzumab-containing therapy in early-stage breast cancer: getting to the heart of the matter. J Clin Oncol 2016;34(10):1030–3.

80. Slamon DJ, Eiermann W, Robert NJ, et al. Ten year follow-up of BCIRG-006 comparing doxorubicin plus cyclophosphamide followed by docetaxel (AC→T) with doxorubicin plus cyclophosphamide followed by docetaxel and trastuzumab (AC→TH) with docetaxel, carboplatin and trastuzumab (TCH) in HER2+ early breast cancer. Oral presentation at: San Antonio Breast Cancer Symposium 2015.

81. Vermeulen Z, Segers VF, De Keulenaer GW. ErbB2 signaling at the crossing between heart failure and cancer. Basic Res Cardiol 2016;111(6):60.

Cardio-oncology Related to Heart Failure

Pediatric Considerations for Cardiac Dysfunction

Kirsten Rose-Felker, MD[a,b,*],
William L. Border, MBChB, MPH[a,b], Borah J. Hong, MD[c],
Eric J. Chow, MD, MPH[d]

KEYWORDS

• Childhood cancer survivors • Anthracyclines • Cardiac dysfunction • Cardiotoxicity

KEY POINTS

• Although tremendous advances in pediatric cancer treatment have improved survival, they remain at increased risk of early morbidity and mortality.
• Increased surveillance and improvement in cardiovascular imaging modalities have led to earlier detection of cardiac dysfunction, but the outcomes remain poor once this has developed.
• A great deal of work remains to be done to refine screening and identify high-risk patients more precisely.
• It is necessary to develop more evidence-based strategies for effective primary and secondary cardioprotection and treatment.

INTRODUCTION

The overall 5-year survival rates for childhood cancers now exceed 80%.[1] This translates to nearly 400,000 childhood cancer survivors in the United States as of January 2011, a number that continues to increase.[2] Although this marks tremendous success in cancer treatment, it also represents a large population of survivors who will require special attention and treatment owing to the adverse health and quality of life outcomes that survivors face.[3] A number of studies have shown that childhood cancer survivors are at increased risk of chronic health conditions and poorer general health.[4] The greatest cause of morbidity and mortality after cancer recurrence and secondary malignancies is cardiovascular disease, owing to a number of factors, including the limited regenerative capacity of myocardial cells.[5] The risk of early cardiac death in cancer survivors has been reported at more than 8 times greater than expected.[6] Both chemotherapy and radiation therapy can be cardiotoxic.[7,8] Nearly 60% of childhood cancer survivors are at risk for the development of cardiovascular disease based solely on exposure to these modalities.[9] Among adult

The authors have nothing to disclose.
[a] Department of Pediatrics, Sibley Heart Center Cardiology, 201 Dowman Drive, Atlanta, GA 30322, USA;
[b] Division of Pediatric Cardiology, Department of Pediatrics, Emory University School of Medicine, 1405 Clifton Road Northeast, Atlanta, GA 30322, USA; [c] Division of Pediatric Cardiology, Department of Pediatrics, Seattle Children's Hospital, University of Washington School of Medicine, University of Washington, 4800 Sand Point Way Northeast, Seattle, WA 98105, USA; [d] Clinical Research Division, Fred Hutchinson Cancer Research Center, University of Washington, PO Box 19024, Seattle, WA 98109, USA
* Corresponding author. Division of Pediatric Cardiology, Emory University School of Medicine, 1405 Clifton Road Northeast, Atlanta, GA 30322.
E-mail address: rosefelkerk@kidsheart.com

survivors of childhood cancer who are age 40 years or greater, the prevalences of cardiomyopathy, coronary artery disease, and arrhythmias have been reported to be each approximately 10%, whereas more than one-third of survivors have been found to have valvular disease.[10]

TREATMENT RISK FACTORS
Radiation

Radiation therapy damages all structures of the heart, including the myocardium, pericardium, valves, coronary vessels, and conduction system.[11] Patients at greatest risk are those exposed to high total doses of radiation (35–40 Gy), higher fractionated dose, younger age at exposure, and concomitant use of cardiotoxic chemotherapy.[8] However, doses as low as 5 Gy have been associated with increased cardiovascular mortality.[12] Radiation fields that place patients most at risk are not only mediastinal and thoracic, but those in which the heart is in the field including spinal, left or whole upper abdominal, and total body irradiation.

Acute effects include endothelial damage, lipid and inflammatory cell infiltration, and lysosomal activation.[13,14] The common pathway for these has been demonstrated in animal studies to be microcirculatory damage.[15] Potential mechanisms of such damage include oxidative stress[16] and generation of proinflammatory cytokines interleukin-6, C-reactive protein, tumor necrosis factor-α, and interferon-γ, all of which have been shown to be significantly increased in atomic bomb survivors exposed to 1 Gy or more of radiation after adjustment for other risk factors.[17] Interstitial fibrosis is the hallmark of late damage from irradiation, marked by the replacement of healthy myocardium with scar tissue. Studies from patients treated for postirradiation pericarditis show an increase in overall collagen with a disproportionate increase in type I collagen, which may contribute to the diastolic dysfunction seen in these patients.[18] Studies also have documented rhythm disturbances after radiation therapy, including advanced heart block.[19]

Anthracyclines

Anthracyclines are a class of antitumor antibiotics that interfere with DNA replication and transcription, especially in rapidly dividing cells. They also have a number of cardiotoxic effects, many of which are thought to be separate from their antitumor effects. Anthracyclines approved by the US Food and Drug Administration include doxorubicin, daunorubicin, epirubicin and idarubicin. Their actions include (1) inhibition of both DNA replication and RNA transcription, (2) free radical generation, leading to DNA damage or lipid peroxidation, (3) DNA alkylation, (4) DNA cross-linking, (5) interference with DNA unwinding of DNA strand separation and helicase activity, (6) direct membrane damage owing to lipid oxidation, and (7) inhibition of topoisomerase II.[20] It is unclear which of these mechanisms is the most harmful to myocytes, but the final common pathway is thought to be myocyte death.[21] This has been demonstrated in biopsies obtained immediately after anthracycline exposure showing mitochondrial swelling and chromatin contraction, key features of apoptosis.[22] The limited capacity of myocytes to regenerate leads to hypertrophy of surviving myocytes to maintain cardiac output.[23] This hypertrophy in conjunction with reduced wall thickness and interstitial fibrosis leads to eventual pathologic ventricular remodeling.[24]

Anthracycline toxicity is divided into 3 categories: (1) acute, which occurs within 1 week of anthracycline exposure, (2) early onset chronic progressive, which occurs between 1 week and 1 year, and (3) late onset chronic progressive, which occurs after the first year.[25] Acute toxicity is rare and marked by a reversible decrease in myocardial function or new arrhythmias. The most common rhythm alteration is sinus tachycardia, thought to represent autonomic dysfunction, but nonspecific ST segment and T wave changes, decreased QRS amplitude, and prolonged QTc interval can also be seen.[26] The long-term risk for cardiac dysfunction is greatest in those who continue to have dysfunction after treatment is completed.[25] Early onset chronic progressive toxicity is more common than acute toxicity. In a study of patients diagnosed with acute lymphoblastic leukemia treated with anthracyclines, 11 of 115 had heart failure within 1 year of therapy completion, all of whom had improvement with medical management. However, 5 of these 11 patients developed later recurrent congestive heart failure, 2 of whom went on to undergo cardiac transplantation.[24] Early and late onset cardiac dysfunction is generally asymptomatic initially, with evidence of systolic or diastolic dysfunction by echocardiogram, but can become progressive if untreated. Studies have shown that anthracycline-related heart failure carries a poor prognosis with a 2-year mortality of 50% in those with untreated symptomatic left ventricular (LV) dysfunction.[27] Both early and late onset chronic progressive toxicity is characterized by progressive myocyte loss with LV wall thinning and progressive LV dilation as well as the onset of coronary artery disease and rhythm disturbances.[10,28] Lipshultz and colleagues[28] found that significant changes emerged in all cardiac measures studied when patients were followed 6 or more years after diagnosis, including significant decreases in contractility, wall thickness, LV mass, and fractional shortening (FS), but increases in LV end-diastolic dimension and afterload.

There is a dose-dependent association between cardiomyopathy and anthracycline dose with doses of 250 mg/m^2 or more presenting the greatest risk.[8,10,24,27,29] However, there is also evidence to suggest that even lower doses can cause similar cardiomyopathy, suggesting there is no safe dose of anthracyclines.[30] Lipshultz and colleagues[28] reported that some patients who received doses as low as 45 mg/m^2 eventually experienced cardiac abnormalities, including significantly reduced LV mass and dimension when followed for longer than 5 years after completing therapy.

Different anthracyclines may have different cardiotoxicity profiles. Many published cardiotoxicity equivalence ratios are based on anthracycline agents' hematologic toxicities, from which cardiotoxicity is extrapolated.[31] A recent such study directly assessing the incidence of heart failure in more than 15,000 childhood cancer survivors by treatment exposure found the cardiotoxicity equivalence ratio of daunorubicin to be only 0.4 to 0.5 times that of doxorubicin after correcting for radiation exposure and total dose delivered.[32] Adult studies have found decreased clinical and subclinical cardiotoxicity with epirubicin compared with doxorubicin as well.[33]

There has also been concern that high peak serum concentrations of anthracyclines are more cardiotoxic, leading some to examine continuous infusion strategies.[34,35] However, a randomized trial by Lipshultz[36] compared bolus doses of doxorubicin (given over 1 hour) with continuous infusion (given over 48 hours) and found that echocardiographic measures of LV structure and function were not different at a median duration of follow-up of 8 years between the 2 groups. A similar study also showed no decrease in cardiotoxicity with continuous infusion as opposed to bolus administration, so this practice is no longer recommended for children.[37,38]

Although concomitant radiation therapy is known to potentiate the cardiotoxicity of anthracyclines,[8] similar concern has been raised for other agents such as mitoxantrone, high-dose cyclophosphamide, bleomycin, and vincristine.[25,34,35] Mitoxantrone is an anthraquinone that is used in the treatment of certain childhood leukemias and lymphomas and also disrupts DNA synthesis and repair. Like anthracyclines, it also has a cardiotoxic side effect profile that is dose dependent.[7,27]

Other Risk Factors

Hypertension, diabetes, smoking, dyslipidemia, obesity, and physical inactivity are known risk factors for cardiovascular disease in the general population.[39] Survivors of childhood cancer are not immune to the development of these risk factors, which have been found to increase substantially the risk for cardiac events over therapeutic exposures alone.[40] The Childhood Cancer Survivor Study (CCSS) is a cohort study that follows more than 35,000 survivors of childhood cancer and more than 5000 siblings to assess the development of acute and chronic health conditions. A CCSS report by Meacham and colleagues[41] found that survivors were 1.9 times more likely to report taking medication for hypertension than sibling controls after adjusting for age, ethnicity, and sex. Survivors were also 1.8 times more likely than siblings to report diabetes after adjusting for a number of factors including body mass index and age. Those who have received total body irradiation, abdominal irradiation, and cranial irradiation were at the greatest risk.[42] Similarly, survivors in the CCSS were 1.6 times more likely to be taking medications for dyslipidemia, and were less likely to meet guidelines for physical activity than are their age- and sex-matched controls and siblings.[41,43]

There are a number of potential nonmodifiable risk factors for anthracycline-mediated toxicity that have been described elsewhere including female sex, African American race, younger age at diagnosis, trisomy 21, longer time since treatment, and underlying heart disease or traditional cardiovascular risk factors.[26,28,44] These treatment-related and traditional cardiovascular risk factors do not fully explain the difference in cardiovascular outcomes among survivors, however. To further explain the variation in risk among survivors despite similar treatment exposures, there is ongoing research on the contribution of genetics, particularly variations in genes encoding proteins involved in anthracycline absorption, distribution, metabolism, and elimination.[29,45–47]

SURVEILLANCE

Worldwide, recommendations differ regarding what are considered the highest risk factors and what studies should be performed as part of comprehensive surveillance. There is unanimous agreement, however, that screening should take place in those exposed to anthracyclines, mitoxantrone, radiation affecting the heart, and in the presence of traditional cardiovascular risk factors. Recently, an International Late Effects of Childhood Cancer Guideline Harmonization Group have issued the following consensus surveillance recommendations.[48]

1. Surveillance echocardiography should be lifelong and a minimum of every 5 years.
2. Closer monitoring of survivors during pregnancy is crucial given the increased metabolic demand and volume load on the heart.
3. Cardiology referral is necessary for those with asymptomatic cardiomyopathy.
4. At-risk survivors should be screened regularly for cardiac risk factors (ie, dyslipidemia, diabetes, hypertension, obesity).

The frequency of surveillance may be adjusted based on an individual's risk for the development of cardiovascular disease. Patients exposed to greater than 250 mg/m^2 of anthracyclines or greater than 35 Gy of radiation are felt to be at the greatest risk.[8] A recent international collaboration featuring more than 15,000 long-term childhood cancer survivors from the CCSS and 3 other cohorts has produced an evidence-based risk score algorithm that predicts the development of clinical cardiomyopathy by age 40 with reasonable accuracy and discrimination (Tables 1 and 2; on-line calculator at: www.ccss.stjude.org/chfcalc).[49]

Echocardiography

In addition to careful physical examination and patient history, an echocardiogram is the recommended surveillance modality to assess for changes in ventricular contractility and filling. It is widely available, noninvasive, and does not expose the patient to ionizing radiation. Detailed 2-dimensional (2D) assessment should be performed according to the American College of Cardiology/American Heart Association guidelines for clinical application of echocardiograms (Fig. 1). The most frequently used and most reproducible quantitative assessments of systolic function in this population include the ejection fraction (EF), FS, and wall stress. EF is typically assessed by 2D echocardiography, although the American Society of Echocardiography and the European Association of Cardiovascular Imaging now recommend the inclusion of 3-dimensional echocardiogram to assess these parameters (Fig. 2). When assessing EF in 2D, the recommendation is for Simpson's biplane in addition to M-mode to make this measurement (Fig. 3).[50] To assess diastolic function, the E/A ratio and isovolumic relaxation time are helpful in examining ventricular relaxation.

Surrogates for afterload assessment are end-systolic wall stress, which increases as blood pressure and LV cavity dimension increase and LV wall thickness decreases.[51]

There are also new echocardiographic modalities that have been developed to assess subclinical dysfunction in this population, which offer the promise of greater sensitivity versus more conventional imaging parameters. These include tissue Doppler imaging (Fig. 4) and deformation imaging (strain and strain rate; Fig. 5). In a study of 1820 adult survivors of childhood cancer exposed to anthracyclines, chest irradiation, or both, 28% of the population studied had evidence of cardiac dysfunction by global longitudinal strain, whereas only 6% of the population studied had an abnormal LVEF.[50] In another study of 134 young adult survivors of childhood cancer treated with anthracyclines or mediastinal irradiation, abnormal global longitudinal strain was seen in 18% of patients with a normal LVEF an average of 15 years after diagnosis. Overall, abnormal strain measurements were present in 23% of patients in this study, whereas the FS and EF were abnormal in only 5% and 6%, respectively.[52] Strain and strain rate may detect cardiotoxicity earlier than with quantitative measures of systolic function, such as the EF and SF, but given the cross-sectional design of these studies, it remains unclear what the clinical implications of these measurements are in this population. Although specific recommendations for the use of these modalities exist for adult cancer patients, no such expert consensus statement has yet been published for survivors of childhood cancer.[50]

Cardiac MRI

Although 2D and M-mode echocardiography is the recommended imaging modality, it is limited by patient acoustic windows, poor sensitivity for subtle changes, inadequate reproducibility of measurements, and an inability to quantitatively assess the right ventricle.[53] Cardiac MRI (CMR) is a well-validated tool for the assessment of cardiac structure and function and can provide additional information to fill in these gaps. Additionally, the use of gadolinium-chelated contrast allows for the assessment of myocardial fibrosis, clinical evidence of myocardial cell apoptosis.[54] In a study of 62 long-term survivors of childhood cancer therapy, 79% of patients had either an abnormal or subnormal LVEF (<45% or between 55% and 45%, respectively) and 80% had either abnormal or subnormal right ventricular EF. The LVEF was significantly lower than reference values in all age groups and the LV end-diastolic and end-systolic

Table 1
Childhood cancer survivor CHF risk scores

Characteristic	Simple Model[a]	Standard Model	Heart Dose Model
Sex			
Male	0	0	0
Female	1	1	1
Age at diagnosis (y)			
<5	1	2	2
5–9	0	1	1
10–14	0	0	1
≥15	0	0	0
Anthracycline (mg/m^2)			
None	0	0	0
Any	3	—	—
<100	—	1	2
100–249	—	3	3
≥250	—	4	4
Chest/heart radiation (Gy)[b]			
None	0	0	0
Any	3	—	—
<5	—	0	0
5–14	—	2	1
15–34	—	2	3
≥35	—	4	4
Cohort (no. cases/overall cohort size)			
CCSS (285/13,060)[c]			
AUC	0.71	0.74	0.76
C-statistic	0.72	0.76	0.77
Netherlands (26/1362)			
AUC	0.74	0.81	0.74
C-statistic	0.75	0.80	0.78
Wilms tumor (48/6760)			
AUC	0.76	0.72	—
C-statistic	0.79	0.82	—
St. Jude (19/1695)			
AUC	0.63[d]	0.68	—
C-statistic	0.63[d]	0.68[d]	—

Risk scores 0, 1, 2, 3, and 4, correspond to relative risks of less than 1.3, 1.3 to 1.9, 2.0 to 2.9, 3.0 to 4.9, and 5.0 or greater, respectively.

Abbreviations: AUC, area under the curve; CCSS, Childhood Cancer Survivor Study; CHF, congestive heart failure.

[a] Anthracycline and radiotherapy exposures classified as yes/no only.

[b] Simple model, patients who received only radiation scatter from adjacent fields classified as unexposed; standard model, scatter from adjacent fields classified as less than 5 Gy; heart dose model, exposures based on heart-specific dosimetry.

[c] Training dataset, with estimates reflecting within the CCSS cohort cross-validation.

[d] Estimate is significantly different (*P*<.05) from the corresponding CCSS estimate.

From Chow EJ, Chen Y, Kremer LC, et al. Individual prediction of heart failure among childhood cancer survivors. J Clin Oncol 2015;33(5):397; with permission.

Table 2
Classification of CHF risk scores into risk groups

	Risk Group	Risk Score[a]	Cumulative Incidence (95% CI)[b,c]
Siblings	—	—	0.3 (0.1–0.5)
Simple model	Low	<3	0.5 (0.2–0.8)
	Moderate	3–4	3.1 (2.5–3.7)
	High	≥5	9.2 (6.8–11.6)
Standard model	Low	<3	0.5 (0.2–0.8)
	Moderate	3–5[d]	2.4 (1.8–3.0)
	High	≥6	11.7 (8.8–14.5)
Heart dose model	Low	<3	0.5 (0.2–0.7)
	Moderate	3–5[d]	2.3 (1.7–2.9)
	High	6–8	7.8 (5.9–9.7)
	Very high	≥9	23.7 (14.5–32.9)

Abbreviations: CCSS, Childhood Cancer Survivor Study; CI, confidence interval; CHF, congestive heart failure.

[a] Per Table 1.

[b] At age 40 years.

[c] Comparisons are versus the immediate preceding group (eg, moderate vs low risk group, high vs moderate risk group).

[d] Survivors with total risk score = 3 under the standard and heart dose models without both anthracycline and chest/heart radiation exposures are classified as low risk; the cumulative incidence of CHF at age 40 years among these individuals was 0.2%.

From Chow EJ, Chen Y, Kremer LC, et al. Individual prediction of heart failure among childhood cancer survivors. J Clin Oncol 2015;33(5):398; with permission.

volumes were significantly greater than reference data. Interestingly, however, none of the patients showed late gadolinium enhancement, although diffuse fibrosis was nulled out to highlight focal fibrosis.[55] Another study of 114 adult survivors exposed to anthracyclines or radiation compared

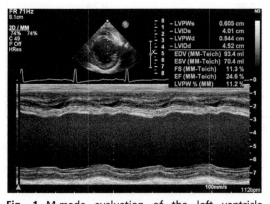

Fig. 1. M-mode evaluation of the left ventricle showing reduced shortening fraction (FS) of 11.3% and ejection fraction (EF) of 24.6%. EDV, end-diastolic volume; ESV, end-systolic volume; LVIDd, left ventricular internal dimension at diastole; LVIDs, left ventricular internal dimension at systole; LVPW%, fractional thickening of the left ventricular posterior wall; LVPWd, left ventricular posterior wall at diastole; LVPWs, left ventricular posterior wall at systole.

echocardiogram with CMR and found no difference in the mean EF from 3D echocardiogram with CMR, whereas 2D echocardiograms had on average 5% higher EF when compared with MRI. Relative to CMR, 2D echocardiography also had higher false-negative rates. Additionally, volume measurements were lower with echocardiography compared with CMR and cardiac mass was overestimated.[53] Despite this, echocardiography remains the main screening tool given greater ease and availability, and lower cost over CMR.

Radionuclide Angiography

Radionuclide cardiac angiography, often referred to as a MUGA or multiple gated acquisition scan, can also assess ventricular function.[56,57] When compared with 2D echocardiography, it has been shown to more accurately and reproducibly predict EF, allowing for detection of very subtle changes over serial studies.[58] Its use was widespread at one time, but has now largely being replaced by echocardiography because of its many limitations, which include associated radiation. Its sensitivity has been decreased over time because changes in image acquisition, which are meant to limit radiation exposure, limit resolution as well. Additionally, it provides no information about the right heart, valvular disease, pericardial disease, or diastolic function.[50]

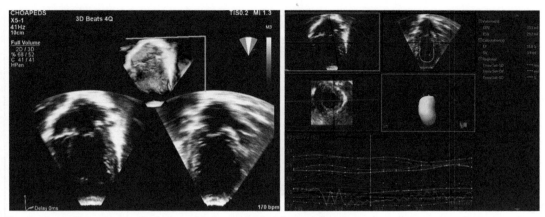

Fig. 2. Three-dimensional calculation of left ventricular ejection fraction.

Stress Echocardiography and Exercise Testing

Exercise testing in adult survivors of childhood cancer therapy have shown that survivors are at increased risk for LV dysfunction and impaired exercise capacity than controls. In a 2015 study of 138 adult survivors, there was a significantly decreased percent predicted Vo_{2max} in asymptomatic anthracycline-treated adult survivors when compared with controls, in a dose-dependent manner.[59] Another study using exercise echocardiography to examine functional changes showed preserved exercise aerobic capacity at peak exercise in asymptomatic adolescent survivors but significant differences in resting parameters including a significantly higher resting heart rate and lower E/A ratio in

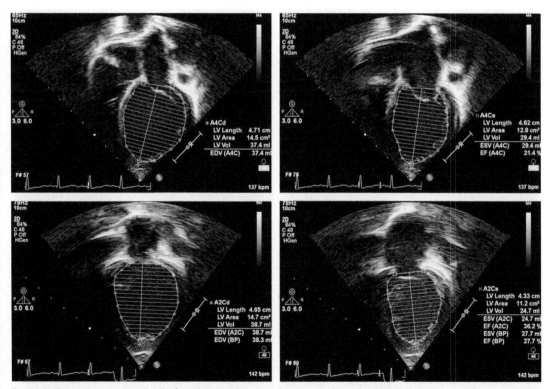

Fig. 3. Biplane Simpson method of evaluating ejection fraction (EF) in the apical 4- and 2-chamber views. This shows a reduced biplane EF of 27.7%. (*Top left*) Apical 4-chamber dimension in diastole. (*Top right*) Apical 4-chamber dimension in systole. (*Bottom left*) Apical 2-chamber in diastole. (*Bottom right*) Apical 2-chamber in systole.

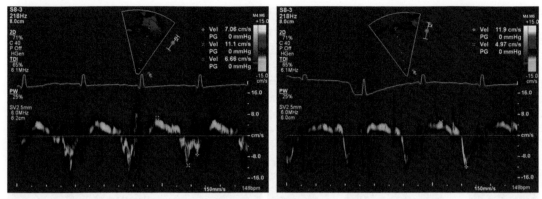

Fig. 4. Tissue Doppler evaluation of contractility by sampling the lateral mitral annulus (*left*) and the septal mitral annulus (*right*). Systolic and diastolic myocardial velocities are measured.

higher risk survivors.[60] With longer time since therapy, significant differences in systolic function have been detected at peak exercise, despite the absence of reported symptoms.[61]

Blood Biomarkers

Various serum biomarkers have been studied as a way to detect subclinical cardiac dysfunction and monitor progression of dysfunction in patients treated with anthracyclines.[62] Cardiac troponin T and I have been shown to correlate with acute coronary injury and cardiac ischemia in adults and have also been used to monitor acute anthracycline-related toxicity.[62,63] A 2012 study by Lipshultz and colleagues[63] found that baseline cardiac troponin T levels were similar in children

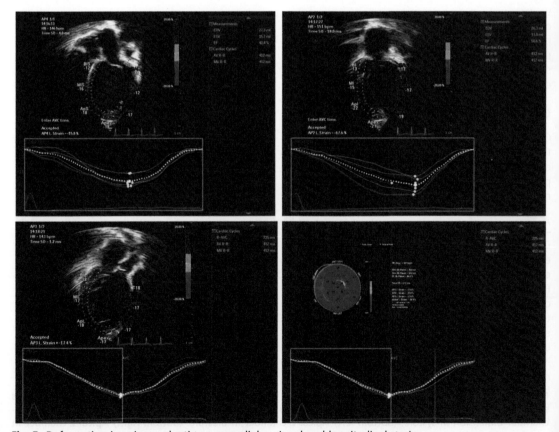

Fig. 5. Deformation imaging evaluating myocardial regional and longitudinal strain.

with high-risk acute lymphoblastic leukemia receiving either doxorubicin or doxorubicin combined with dexrazoxane (DRZ), but were significantly different after treatment, with increases in 47% of the doxorubicin group and only 13% in the combined therapy group. Elevation in cardiac troponin T in the first 90 days of treatment was then associated with abnormally reduced LV mass and LV end-diastolic posterior wall thickness 4 years after treatment. In a study of adults with aggressive malignancies requiring high-dose chemotherapy, those with an elevation in troponin I had a more marked and longer lasting decline in LVEF after treatment.[64] Nevertheless, routine use of troponins has not been adopted owing to insufficient evidence demonstrating that troponin elevation alone is predictive of future cardiotoxicity.

The natriuretic peptides B-type natriuretic peptide (BNP) and N-terminal pro-BNP are released in response to myocardial wall stress and have a well-established role in the detection of cardiac dysfunction and after the progression of congestive heart failure.[62] However, the routine use of BNP in asymptomatic survivors of childhood cancer treatment has not been incorporated into guidelines.[48] In 1 large study examining late cardiotoxicity in pediatric survivors, although BNP values were significantly higher in those with cardiac dysfunction as measured by echocardiography, there was great variation in the BNP levels, precluding definition of a cutoff level with sufficient sensitivity and specificity to identify those with cardiac dysfunction.[65]

CARDIOPROTECTIVE STRATEGIES

Once cardiac dysfunction has been identified, there are limited therapeutic interventions. At present, a number of studies have evaluated different preventative strategies mostly in adults, but with mixed results.

Primary Cardioprotection

DRZ is a bisdioxopiperazine compound similar to ethylene diamine tetra-acetic acid. DRZ is the only cardioprotective agent approved by the US Food and Drug Administration for use with anthracyclines. It is thought to affect the configuration of topoisomerase 2β by binding to its ATP-binding sites, preventing anthracycline from binding and limiting its mechanism of cardiotoxicity.[66] As an iron chelator, it may also decrease oxygen free radical formation. However, other iron chelators have not demonstrated a comparable cardioprotective effect.[67] An early randomized controlled trial of doxorubicin with DRZ compared with doxorubicin alone showed a significantly decreased

risk of subclinical cardiotoxicity (22% vs 67%; $P<.01$) despite higher doses of anthracyclines in the DRZ-treated group and a smaller decrease in LVEF per equivalent dose of anthracycline (1.0% vs 2.7%; $P = .02$).[68] As mentioned, DRZ has also been associated with a significant reduction of troponin T during and soon after doxorubicin exposure among pediatric leukemia survivors.[69] Subsequent studies have shown that, among pediatric survivors 3 to 5 years after treatment, those treated with doxorubicin with DRZ may have reduced pathologic LV remodeling (as measured by wall thickness to dimension ratios) compared with those who received doxorubicin alone.[70,71] However, overall, its use in pediatric patients has been limited owing to concerns about long-term cardioprotective efficacy and the possible induction of second cancers.[72,73] However, multiple studies have not shown DRZ to be associated with a significantly increased rate of secondary neoplasms.[70,71,74]

Liposomal encapsulation is another strategy that has been adopted, which may modify tissue distribution and pharmacokinetics without hopefully compromising therapeutic effect.[75] However, these formulations are costlier and have not been approved by the US Food and Drug Administration for use in children in the United States, so also have not been widely used to date.

Secondary Cardioprotection

Because contractile dysfunction is often irreversible after diagnosis, the use of medications like angiotensin-converting-enzyme inhibitors has been studied for their possible cardioprotective effect.[21] In 1 study, 114 adult patients (mean age, 45 years) receiving chemotherapy who showed an increase in troponin I with initiation of chemotherapy were divided into a control or enalapril group starting 1 month after the initiation of therapy and continuing for 1 year. Cardinale and colleagues[76] found a significant decrease in the LVEF by more than 10% to an abnormal range and an increase in end-systolic and end-diastolic LV volumes for the control group. They also found a significantly higher number of cardiac events in the control versus the enalapril group. In a similar study of 40 adults with Hodgkin's lymphoma, compared with controls, those given valsartan, an angiotensin II receptor blocker, had significantly less changes in QTc, LV end-diastolic diameter, and BNP during chemotherapy, but these changes also normalized in controls by the end of treatment as well.[77]

In a retrospective study, 18 childhood cancer survivors treated with enalapril demonstrated improvement in LV dimension, afterload, FS, and mass in the first 6 years of therapy but no improvement and even a decrease was seen in the 6- to 10-year follow-up period. Those with congestive heart failure at the start of enalapril therapy either died or went on to cardiac transplantation by the end of 6 years.[78]

Carvedilol is a nonselective beta-adrenergic receptor (β-blocker) antagonist and alpha receptor antagonist shown to improve morbidity and mortality in heart failure with a reduced LVEF and has been shown to have potent antioxidant properties.[79,80] Carvedilol and its metabolites prevent lipid peroxidation and antioxidant depletion, and impede the formation of reactive oxygen free radicals.[81,82] For these reasons, a number of studies have examined whether carvedilol can act as a cardioprotectant for patients receiving cardiotoxic therapies.

In a study of adults receiving chemotherapy from 2006, patients (mean age, 48 years) for whom anthracyclines were planned were randomized to receive once daily carvedilol for 6 months or placebo. In the placebo group, there was a significant decline in LVEF from 69% to 52% after treatment, increased systolic and diastolic diameters, and a decline in both E velocities and E/A ratios.[83] A 2013 study with 90 adult patients diagnosed with leukemia or undergoing hematopoietic stem cell transplantation randomized to receive either carvedilol and enalapril or placebo followed patients with echocardiography and CMR to evaluate change in cardiac function. The authors found that LVEF was decreased significantly, although not substantially (−3.1% by echocardiography and −3.4% by CMR) in controls. They also found that the treatment group had a significantly decreased risk of combined death and heart failure.[84] Similar studies using strain imaging to assess subclinical cardiotoxicity showed a significant decrease in systolic strain imaging in the control group.[85]

Despite numerous adult and ex vivo studies demonstrating the beneficial effects of carvedilol in prevention of anthracycline-mediated cardiotoxicity, there have not been many controlled studies in the pediatric population. In a randomized trial involving 50 children who received doxorubicin, one-half were treated with carvedilol 5 days before each dose of chemotherapy and were followed with echocardiographic measurements including EF, SF, and peak systolic 2D strain as measurements of systolic function and pulsed tissue Doppler to assess diastolic function. The authors found that there was a significant improvement in FS and 2D strain in the carvedilol group after therapy compared with baseline, whereas the doxorubicin only group had worsening of both parameters 1 week after the completion of therapy. They also measured troponin I and lactate dehydrogenase and found that carvedilol pretreatment inhibited the increase in troponin I and lactate dehydrogenase seen with doxorubicin. However, this study only followed patients for about 1 month.[86]

Other agents have been proposed to mitigate the harmful effects of cancer therapies on the heart without great evidence to support their routine use. N-Acetyl cysteine has been proposed because of its antioxidant effect as a promoter of intracellular glutathione synthesis; however, it did not show a cardioprotective benefit when given with doxorubicin in a randomized trial, and caused significant nausea.[87] Coenzyme Q10 was studied in 1 very small trial and although the coenzyme Q10 treatment group was found to have less of a decrease in the LV FS, they were also exposed to lower doses of anthracyclines than were the control group, making conclusions very difficult to draw.[88] Phenethylamines, the combination of vitamin E, vitamin C, L-carnitine, and amifostine, have also been studied, although there are no randomized controlled trials demonstrating a decreased rate of congestive heart failure with any of these agents.[89]

TREATMENT CONSIDERATIONS

The recent recommendations for cardiomyopathy surveillance for survivors of childhood cancer strongly recommend cardiology consultation for individuals with abnormal cardiac function detected during surveillance.[48] Once referred to the cardiologist, however, there are few evidence-based guidelines to drive treatment, because there are few randomized controlled trials examining the effects of medical therapies on clinical and subclinical cardiac dysfunction in survivors of childhood cancers.[90] Therefore, the treatment of congestive heart failure in this population is often adapted from treatment used for other cardiomyopathies or adapted from adult studies.[91] There is only 1 randomized, controlled trial examining the effect of enalapril on childhood cancer survivors with asymptomatic cardiac dysfunction. This study randomized 135 long-term survivors of childhood cancer with at least 1 cardiac abnormality identified after anthracycline exposure to either enalapril or placebo. The endpoints were maximal cardiac index on exercise testing and LV end-systolic wall stress. The authors found no difference in the rate of change of maximal cardiac index over time between the 2 groups, but a reduction in LV end-systolic wall stress over time in the enalapril group both in the first year and throughout the study period. However, nearly one-quarter of the patients in the enalapril group experienced dizziness or hypotension, leading the authors to conclude that clinicians should weigh the possible benefits of this therapy against these known side effects.[92]

In a 2010 study of adults with anthracycline-induced cardiomyopathy, defined as an LVEF of less than or equal to 45%, 201 patients were started on enalapril with or without carvedilol at the detection of LVEF impairment and followed serially thereafter with echocardiography. The patients were considered responders, partial responders, and nonresponders based on their recovery in LVEF. The authors found that about 42% of patients responded with complete normalization of LVEF, 13% had some improvement, and 45% no improvement at all. Responders had a significantly shorter time to heart failure treatment and a lower rate of cardiac events than nonresponders. The percentage of responders progressively decreased as the time to heart failure treatment increased with no complete responders with time to heart failure of greater than 6 months.[93]

While we await more evidence for the treatment of these patients, it is reasonable to adapt recommendations from the International Society for Heart and Lung Transplantation guidelines for the management of heart failure in children, which mirror the adult American Heart Association/American College of Cardiology recommendations. These guidelines separate patients into classes ranging from A to D, with A being those with increased risk of developing heart failure but normal cardiac function and chamber size and D being those with end-stage heart failure despite maximal medical therapy.[94] By definition, all survivors exposed to cardiotoxic chemotherapy are class A or greater. These guidelines make recommendations for both structural and nonstructural heart disease and systolic and diastolic dysfunction. Diastolic dysfunction is characterized by impaired ventricular filling and diastolic heart failure is clinical heart failure with preserved systolic function and may be from impaired relaxation or increased myocardial stiffness.

For the treatment of systolic dysfunction, the guidelines recommend the following goal-directed therapies: (1) diuretics to achieve a clinically euvolemic state if the dysfunction causes fluid retention (class I recommendation), (2) angiotensin-converting-enzyme inhibitors for the treatment of symptomatic LV dysfunction (class I recommendation) or asymptomatic LV dysfunction unless there is a specific contraindication (class IIa recommendation), (3) beta blockers to treat LV systolic dysfunction with or without symptoms (class IIa recommendation), (4) aldosterone receptor antagonists to treat LV dysfunction (class I recommendation), and (5) low-dose digoxin for symptomatic heart failure to provide symptom relief (class IIa recommendation).

Although diastolic dysfunction can be seen in anthracycline-induced cardiomyopathy, the literature remains mixed with regard to its predictability for the development of clinically significant cardiomyopathy when seen in the absence of systolic dysfunction. Additionally, the medical management of diastolic dysfunction is very limited. The only class I recommendation from the International Society for Heart and Lung Transplantation guidelines is the use of diuretics to establish a euvolemic state.[94]

Limitations on Physical Activity

Programs designed to promote physical activity in patients and survivors of childhood cancer generally increased cardiopulmonary fitness, improved muscle strength and flexibility, reduced fatigue, and improved physical function.[95] For this reason, the guidelines for cardiomyopathy surveillance for survivors of childhood cancer strongly recommend regular exercise for survivors treated with anthracyclines or chest radiation who have normal cardiac function. Because the American Heart Association and the European Society of Cardiology recommend limits on those with asymptomatic cardiac dysfunction, consultation with a cardiologist is recommended for those with asymptomatic dysfunction.[48] Owing to anecdotal reports of cardiac deterioration with intense isometric exercise in childhood cancer survivors, as well as extrapolation from other cardiomyopathies, most clinicians restrict patients from intense static isometric activities that rapidly increase cardiac afterload ("burst exertion"), such as power weight lifting. In patients with dilated cardiomyopathy, restrictive cardiomyopathy and infiltrative cardiac myopathies, which incorporates the phenotypes of survivors with cardiac dysfunction, the American Heart Association and the American College of Cardiology recommend restriction from competition in most competitive sports, with the possible exception of low-intensity (class 1A sports) for the time being.[96,97] However, which activities to specifically restrict and what parameters are considered "safe" in this population remain controversial and require further research.

SUMMARY

Although tremendous advances in pediatric cancer treatment have improved the survival of many children, they remain at increased risk of early morbidity and mortality with cardiovascular disease as a leading cause of death. Heightened awareness in providers with increased surveillance and improvement in cardiovascular imaging modalities have led to earlier detection of cardiac dysfunction, but the outcomes remain poor once this dysfunction has developed. A great deal of work remains to be done to refine screening and identify high-risk patients more precisely, and to develop more evidence-based strategies for effective primary and secondary cardioprotection and treatment.

REFERENCES

1. Howlader N, Noone AM, Krapcho M, et al, editors. SEER cancer statistics review, 1975–2013. Bethesda (MD): National Cancer Institute; 2016. Based on November 2015 SEER data submission, posted to the SEER web site. Available at: http://seer.cancer.gov/csr/1975_2013/.
2. Phillips SM, Padgett LS, Leisenring WM, et al. Survivors of childhood cancer in the United States: prevalence and burden of morbidity. Cancer Epidemiol Biomarkers Prev 2015;24(4):653–63.
3. Robison LL, Hudson MM. Survivors of childhood and adolescent cancer: life-long risks and responsibilities. Nat Rev Cancer 2014;14(1):61–70.
4. Oeffinger KC, Mertens AC, Sklar CA. Chronic health conditions in adult survivors of childhood cancer. N Engl J Med 2006;355(15):1572–82.
5. Mertens AC, Liu Q, Neglia JP, et al. Cause-specific late mortality among 5-year survivors of childhood cancer: the Childhood Cancer Survivor Study. J Natl Cancer Inst 2008;100(19):1368–79.
6. Mertens AC, Yasui Y, Neglia JP, et al. Late mortality experience in five-year survivors of childhood and adolescent cancer: the Childhood Cancer Survivor Study. J Clin Oncol 2001;19(13):3163–72.
7. Floyd JD, Nguyen DT, Lobins RL, et al. Cardiotoxicity of cancer therapy. J Clin Oncol 2005;23(30):7685–96.
8. Mulrooney DA, Yeazel MW, Kawashima T, et al. Cardiac outcomes in a cohort of adult survivors of childhood and adolescent cancer: retrospective analysis of the Childhood Cancer Survivor Study cohort. BMJ 2009;339:b4606.
9. Hudson MM, Ness KK, Gurney JG, et al. Clinical ascertainment of health outcomes among adults treated for childhood cancer: a report from the St. Jude lifetime cohort study. JAMA 2013;309(22):2371–81.
10. Mulrooney DA, Armstrong GT, Huang S, et al. Cardiac outcomes in adult survivors of childhood cancer exposed to cardiotoxic therapy: a cross-sectional study. Ann Intern Med 2016;164(2):93–101.
11. Adams MJ, Hardenbergh PH, Constine LS, et al. Radiation-associated cardiovascular disease. Crit Rev Oncol Hematol 2003;45(1):55–75.
12. Tukenova M, Guibout C, Oberlin O, et al. Role of cancer treatment in long-term overall and cardiovascular mortality after childhood cancer. J Clin Oncol 2010;28(8):1308–15.
13. Konings AW, Hardonk MJ, Wieringa RA, et al. Initial events in radiation induced atheromatosis I. Activation of lysosomal enzymes. Strahlentherapie 1975;150(4):444–8.
14. Konings AW, Smit Sibinga CT, Aarnoudse MW, et al. Initial events in radiation-induced atheromatosis. II. Damage to intimal cells. Strahlentherapie 1978;154(11):795–800.
15. Robert J, Fajardo LF, Constine LS, et al. Radiation injury to the heart. Int J Radiat Oncol Biol Phys 1995;31(July 1994):1205–11.
16. Hatoum OA, Otterson MF, Kopelman D, et al. Radiation induces endothelial dysfunction in murine intestinal arterioles via enhanced production of reactive oxygen species. Arterioscler Thromb Vasc Biol 2006;26(2):287–94.
17. Hayashi T, Kusunoki Y, Hakoda M, et al. Radiation dose-dependent increases in inflammatory response markers in A-bomb survivors. Int J Radiat Biol 2003;79(2):129–36.
18. Chello M, Mastroroberto P, Romano R, et al. Changes in the proportion of types I and III collagen in the left ventricular wall of patients with post-irradiative pericarditis. Cardiovasc Surg 1996;4(2):222–6.
19. Orzan F, Brusca A, Gaita F, et al. Associated cardiac lesions in patients with radiation-induced complete heart block. Int J Cardiol 1993;39(2):151–6.
20. Gewirtz DA. A critical evaluation of the mechanisms of action proposed for the antitumor effects of the anthracycline antibiotics adriamycin and daunorubicin. Biochem Pharmacol 1999;57(7):724–41.
21. Sawyer DB, Peng X, Chen B, et al. Mechanisms of anthracycline cardiac injury: can we identify strategies for cardioprotection? Prog Cardiovasc Dis 2010;53(2):105–13.
22. Ewer MS, Ali MK, Mackay B, et al. A comparison of cardiac biopsy grades and ejection fraction estimations in patients receiving adriamycin. J Clin Oncol 1984;2(2):112–7.
23. Arola OJ, Saraste A, Pulkki K, et al. Acute doxorubicin cardiotoxicity involves cardiomyocyte apoptosis. Cancer Res 2000;60(7):1789–92.
24. Lipshultz SE, Colan SD, Gelber RD, et al. Late cardiac effects of doxorubicin therapy for acute lymphoblastic leukemia in childhood. N Engl J Med 1990;324(12):808–15.

25. Adams MJ, Lipshultz SE. Pathophysiology of anthra-cycline- and radiation-associated cardiomyopa-thies: implications for screening and prevention. Pediatr Blood Cancer 2005;44(7):600–6.

26. Krischer JP, Epstein S, Cuthbertson DD, et al. Clin-ical cardiotoxicity following anthracycline treatment for childhood cancer: the pediatric oncology group experience. J Clin Oncol 1997;15(4):1544–52.

27. Yeh ETH, Tong AT, Lenihan DJ, et al. Cardiovascular complications of cancer therapy: diagnosis, patho-genesis, and management. Circulation 2004; 109(25):3122–31.

28. Lipshultz SE, Lipsitz SR, Sallan SE, et al. Chronic progressive cardiac dysfunction years after doxoru-bicin therapy for childhood acute lymphoblastic leu-kemia. J Clin Oncol 2005;23(12):2629–36.

29. Blanco JG, Sun C-L, Landier W, et al. Anthracycline-related cardiomyopathy after childhood cancer: role of polymorphisms in carbonyl reductase genes — a report from the children's oncology group. J Clin Oncol 2012;30(13):1415–21.

30. Swain SM, Whaley FS, Ewer MS. Congestive heart failure in patients treated with doxorubicin: a retro-spective analysis of three trials. Cancer 2003; 97(11):2869–79.

31. van Dalen EC, Michiels EM, Caron HN, et al. Different anthracycline derivates for reducing cardi-otoxicity in cancer patients. Cochrane Database Syst Rev 2006;(4):CD005006.

32. Feijen EAM, Leisenring WM, Stratton KL, et al. Equivalence ratio for daunorubicin to doxorubicin in relation to late heart failure in survivors of child-hood cancer. J Clin Oncol 2015;33(32):3774–80.

33. Smith LA, Cornelius VR, Plummer CJ, et al. Cardio-toxicity of anthracycline agents for the treatment of cancer: systematic review and meta-analysis of randomised controlled trials. BMC Cancer 2010; 10:337.

34. Wouters KA, Kremer LCM, Miller TL, et al. Protecting against anthracycline-induced myocardial damage: a review of the most promising strategies. Br J Hae-matol 2005;131:561–78.

35. Barry E, Alvarez JA, Scully RE, et al. Anthracycline-induced cardiotoxicity: course, pathophysiology, prevention and management. Expert Opin Pharmac-other 2007;8(8):1039–58.

36. Lipshultz SE. Doxorubicin administration by contin-uous infusion is not cardioprotective: the Dana-Farber 91-01 acute lymphoblastic leukemia protocol. J Clin Oncol 2002;20(6):1677–82.

37. Levitt GA, Dorup I, Sorensen K, et al. Does anthracy-cline administration by infusion in children affect late cardiotoxicity? Br J Haematol 2004;124(4):463–8.

38. Ewer MS, Ewer SM. Cardiotoxicity of anticancer treatments: what the cardiologist needs to know. Nat Rev Cardiol 2010;7(10):564–75.

39. Berry JD, Dyer A, Cai X, et al. Lifetime risks of car-diovascular disease. N Engl J Med 2012;366(4):321–9.

40. Armstrong GT, Oeffinger KC, Chen Y, et al. Modifi-able risk factors and major cardiac events among adult survivors of childhood cancer. J Clin Oncol 2013;31(29):3673–80.

41. Meacham LR, Chow EJ, Ness KK, et al. Cardiovas-cular risk factors in adult survivors of pediatric can-cer–a report from the Childhood Cancer Survivor Study. Cancer Epidemiol Biomarkers Prev 2010; 19(1):170–81.

42. Meacham LR, Sklar CA, Li S, et al. Diabetes mellitus in long-term survivors of childhood cancer: increased risk associated with radiation therapy a report for the Childhood Cancer Survivor Study (CCSS). Arch Intern Med 2009;169(15):1381–8.

43. Ness KK, Leisenring WM, Huang S, et al. Predictors of inactive lifestyle among adult survivors of child-hood cancer: a report from the Childhood Cancer Survivor Study. Cancer 2009;115(9):1984–94.

44. Lipshultz SE, Alvarez JA, Scully RE. Anthracycline associated cardiotoxicity in survivors of childhood cancer. Heart 2008;94(4):525–33.

45. Leger KJ, Cushing-Haugen K, Hansen JA, et al. Clinical and genetic determinants of cardiomyopa-thy risk among hematopoietic cell transplantation survivors. Biol Blood Marrow Transplant 2015; 22(6):1094–101.

46. Wojnowski L, Kulle B, Schirmer M, et al. NAD(P)H oxidase and multidrug resistance protein genetic polymorphisms are associated with doxorubicin-induced cardiotoxicity. Circulation 2005;112(24):3754–62.

47. Rajic V, Aplenc R, Debeljak M, et al. Influence of the polymorphism in candidate genes on late cardiac damage in patients treated due to acute leukemia in childhood. Leuk Lymphoma 2009;50(10):1693–8.

48. Armenian SH, Hudson MM, Mulder RL, et al. Recom-mendations for cardiomyopathy surveillance for sur-vivors of childhood cancer: a report from the International Late Effects of Childhood Cancer Guideline Harmonization Group. Lancet Oncol 2015;16(3):e123–36.

49. Chow EJ, Chen Y, Kremer LC, et al. Individual pre-diction of heart failure among childhood cancer sur-vivors. J Clin Oncol 2015;33(5):394–402.

50. Plana JC, Galderisi M, Barac A, et al. Expert consensus for multimodality imaging evaluation of adult patients during and after cancer therapy: a report from the American Society of Echocardiogra-phy and the European Association of Cardiovascu-lar Imaging. J Am Soc Echocardiogr 2014;27(9):911–39.

51. Kremer LCM, van der Pal HJH, Offringa M, et al. Fre-quency and risk factors of subclinical cardiotoxicity

after anthracycline therapy in children: a systematic review. Ann Oncol 2002;13:819–29.

52. Yu AF, Raikhelkar J, Zabor EC, et al. Two-dimensional speckle tracking echocardiography detects subclinical left ventricular systolic dysfunction among adult survivors of childhood, adolescent, and young adult cancer. Biomed Res Int 2016; 2016:9363951.

53. Armstrong GT, Plana JC, Zhang N, et al. Screening adult survivors of childhood cancer for cardiomyopathy: comparison of echocardiography and cardiac magnetic resonance imaging. J Clin Oncol 2012; 30(23):2876–84.

54. Wu E, Judd RM, Vargas JD, et al. Visualization of presence, location, and transmural extent of healed Q-wave and non-Q-wave myocardial infarction. Lancet 2001;357:21–8.

55. Ylanen K, Poutanen T, Savikurki-Heikkila P, et al. Cardiac magnetic resonance imaging in the evaluation of the late effects of anthracyclines among long-term survivors of childhood cancer. J Am Coll Cardiol 2013;61(14):1539–47.

56. Agarwala S, Kumar R, Bhatnagar V, et al. High incidence of adriamycin cardiotoxicity in children even at low cumulative doses: role of radionuclide cardiac angiography. J Pediatr Surg 2000;35(12): 1786–9.

57. Palmeri ST, Bonow RO, Myers CE, et al. Prospective evaluation of doxorubicin cardiotoxicity by rest and exercise radionuclide angiography. Am J Cardiol 1986;58(7):607–13.

58. Bellenger NG, Burgess MI, Ray SG, et al. Comparison of left ventricular ejection fraction and volumes in heart failure by echocardiography, radionuclide ventriculography and cardiovascular magnetic resonance; are they interchangeable? Eur Heart J 2000; 21(16):1387–96.

59. Christiansen JR, Kanellopoulos A, Lund MB, et al. Impaired exercise capacity and left ventricular function in long-term adult survivors of childhood acute lymphoblastic leukemia. Pediatr Blood Cancer 2015;62(8):1437–43.

60. Ryerson AB, Border WL, Wasilewski-Masker K, et al. Assessing anthracycline-treated childhood cancer survivors with advanced stress echocardiography. Pediatr Blood Cancer 2015;62(3):502–8.

61. Jarfelt M, Kujacic V, Holmgren D, et al. Exercise echocardiography reveals subclinical cardiac dysfunction in young adult survivors of childhood acute lymphoblastic leukemia. Pediatr Blood Cancer 2007;49(6):835–40.

62. Braunwald E. Biomarkers in heart failure. N Engl J Med 2008;358:2148–59.

63. Lipshultz SE, Miller TL, Scully RE, et al. Changes in cardiac biomarkers during doxorubicin treatment of pediatric patients with high-risk acute lymphoblastic leukemia: associations with long-term echocardiographic outcomes. J Clin Oncol 2012; 30(10):1042–9.

64. Cardinale D, Sandri MT, Martinoni A, et al. Left ventricular dysfunction predicted by early troponin I release after high-dose chemotherapy. J Am Coll Cardiol 2000;36(2):517–22.

65. Aggarwal S, Pettersen MD, Bhambhani K, et al. B-type natriuretic peptide as a marker for cardiac dysfunction in anthracycline-treated children. Pediatr Blood Cancer 2007;49:812–6.

66. Lyu YL, Kerrigan JE, Lin CP, et al. Topoisomerase IIbeta mediated DNA double-strand breaks: implications in doxorubicin cardiotoxicity and prevention by dexrazoxane. Cancer Res 2007;67(18): 8839–46.

67. Vejpongsa P, Yeh ETH. Topoisomerase 2β: a promising molecular target for primary prevention of anthracycline-induced cardiotoxicity. Clin Pharmacol Ther 2014;95(1):45–52.

68. Wexler LH, Andrich MP, Venzon D, et al. Randomized trial of the cardioprotective agent ICRF-187 in pediatric sarcoma patients treated with doxorubicin. J Clin Oncol 1996;14(2):362–72.

69. Lipshultz SE, Rifai N, Dalton VM, et al. The effect of dexrazoxane on myocardial injury in doxorubicin-treated children with acute lymphoblastic leukemia. N Engl J Med 2004;351(2):145–53.

70. Lipshultz SE, Scully RE, Lipsitz SR, et al. Assessment of dexrazoxane as a cardioprotectant in doxorubicin-treated children with high-risk acute lymphoblastic leukaemia: long-term follow-up of a prospective, randomised, multicentre trial. Lancet Oncol 2010;11(10):950–61.

71. Chow EJ, Asselin BL, Schwartz CL, et al. Late mortality after dexrazoxane treatment: a report from the children's oncology group. J Clin Oncol 2015; 33(24):2639–45.

72. Walker DM, Fisher BT, Seif AE, et al. Dexrazoxane use in pediatric patients with acute lymphoblastic or myeloid leukemia from 1999 and 2009: analysis of a national cohort of patients in the pediatric health information systems database. Pediatr Blood Cancer 2013;60(4):616–20.

73. Tebbi CK, London WB, Friedman D, et al. Dexrazoxane-associated risk for acute myeloid leukemia/myelodysplastic syndrome and other secondary malignancies in pediatric Hodgkin's disease. J Clin Oncol 2007;25(5):493–500.

74. Barry EV, Vrooman LM, Dahlberg SE, et al. Absence of secondary malignant neoplasms in children with high-risk acute lymphoblastic leukemia treated with dexrazoxane. J Clin Oncol 2008;26(7):1106–11.

75. Gabizon AA. Stealth liposomes and tumor targeting: one step further in the quest for the magic bullet. Clin Cancer Res 2001;7:223–5.

76. Cardinale D, Colombo A, Sandri MT, et al. Prevention of high-dose chemotherapy – induced

cardiotoxicity in high-risk patients by angiotensin-converting enzyme inhibition. Circulation 2006;114: 2474–81.

77. Nakamae H, Tsumura K, Terada Y, et al. Notable effects of angiotensin II receptor blocker, valsartan, on acute cardiotoxic changes after standard chemotherapy with cyclophosphamide, doxorubicin, vincristine, and prednisolone. Cancer 2005; 104(11):2492–8.

78. Lipshultz SE, Lipsitz SR, Sallan SE, et al. Long-term enalapril therapy for left ventricular dysfunction in doxorubicin-treated survivors of childhood cancer. J Clin Oncol 2002;20(23):4517–22.

79. Dulin B, Abraham WT. Pharmacology of carvedilol. Am J Cardiol 2004;93(9A):3B–6B.

80. Packer M, Fowler MB, Roecker EB, et al. Effect of carvedilol on the morbidity of patients with severe chronic heart failure: results of the carvedilol prospective randomized cumulative survival (COPERNICUS) study. Circulation 2002;106(17):2194–9.

81. Feuerstein G, Yue TL, Ruffolo RR. Carvedilol update: a multiple action antihypertensive agent with antioxidant activity and the potential for myocardial and vascular protection. Drugs Today 1993;29(6): 401–19.

82. Noguchi N, Nishino K, Niki E. Antioxidant action of the antihypertensive drug, carvedilol, against lipid peroxidation. Biochem Pharmacol 2000;59(9): 1069–76.

83. Kalay N, Basar E, Ozdogru I, et al. Protective effects of carvedilol against anthracycline-induced cardiomyopathy. J Am Coll Cardiol 2006;48(11):2258–62.

84. Bosch X, Morales-ruiz M, Esteve J. Enalapril and carvedilol for preventing chemotherapy-induced left ventricular systolic dysfunction in patients with malignant hemopathies. J Am Coll Cardiol 2013; 61(23):2355–62.

85. Elitok A, Oz F, Cizgici AY, et al. Effect of carvedilol on silent anthracycline-induced cardiotoxicity assessed by strain imaging: a prospective randomized controlled study with six-month follow-up. Cardiol J 2014;21(5):509–15.

86. El-shitany NA, Tolba OA, El-shanshory MR. Protective effect of carvedilol on adriamycin-induced left ventricular dysfunction in children with acute lymphoblastic leukemia. J Card Fail 2012;18(8): 607–13.

87. Myers C, Bonow R, Palmeri S, et al. A randomized controlled trial assessing the prevention of doxorubicin cardiomyopathy by N-acetylcysteine. Semin Oncol 1983;10(1 Suppl 1):53–5.

88. Iarussi D, Auricchio U, Agretto A, et al. Protective effect of coenzyme Q10 on anthracyclines cardiotoxicity: control study in children with acute lymphoblastic leukemia and non-Hodgkin lymphoma. Mol Aspects Med 1994;15(Suppl):s207–12.

89. vanDalen EC, Caron HB, Dickinson HO, et al. Cardioprotective interventions for cancer patients receiving anthracyclines. Cochrane Database Syst Rev 2011;(6):CD003917.

90. Sieswerda E, van Dalen EC, Postma A, et al. Medical interventions for treating anthracycline-induced symptomatic and asymptomatic cardiotoxicity during and after treatment for childhood cancer. Cochrane Database Syst Rev 2011;(9):CD008011.

91. Kay JD, Colan SD, Graham TP Jr. Congestive heart failure in pediatric patients. Am Heart J 2001;142(5): 923–8.

92. Silber JH, Cnaan A, Clark BJ, et al. Enalapril to prevent cardiac function decline in long-term survivors of pediatric cancer exposed to anthracyclines. J Clin Oncol 2004;22(5):820–8.

93. Cardinale D, Colombo A, Lamantia G, et al. Anthracycline-induced cardiomyopathy: clinical relevance and response to pharmacologic therapy. J Am Coll Cardiol 2010;55(3):213–20.

94. Kirk R, Dipchand AI, Rosenthal DN, et al. The international society for heart and lung transplantation guidelines for the management of pediatric heart failure: executive summary. J Heart Lung Transplant 2014;33(9):888–909.

95. Huang T-T, Ness KK. Exercise interventions in children with cancer: a review. Int J Pediatr 2011; 2011:1–11.

96. Maron BJ, Chaitman BR, Ackerman MJ, et al. Recommendations for physical activity and recreational sports participation for young patients with genetic cardiovascular diseases. Circulation 2004;109(22): 2807–16.

97. Maron BJ, Udelson JE, Bonow RO, et al. AHA/ACC scientific statement eligibility and disqualification recommendations for competitive athletes with cardiovascular abnormalities: and other cardiomyopathies, and myocarditis and American College of Cardiology. J Am Coll Cardiol 2015;66:273–81.

Advanced Heart Failure Therapies for Cancer Therapeutics–Related Cardiac Dysfunction

CrossMark

Christopher M. Bianco, DO, Sadeer G. Al-Kindi, MD,
Guilherme H. Oliveira, MD*

KEYWORDS

- Heart failure • Right ventricular failure • Chemotherapy-induced cardiomyopathy
- Cancer therapeutics–related cardiac dysfunction • Anthracyclines
- Mechanical circulatory support devices • Heart transplant • Cardiac resynchronization therapy

KEY POINTS

- Cancer survivors who undergo advanced therapies for heart failure (HF) are predominantly young women with low prevalence of traditional cardiovascular comorbidities.
- Valvular disease is common especially among patients with chest radiation and may require surgical intervention.
- Mechanical circulatory support (MCS) is safe in carefully selected patients with chemotherapy-induced cardiomyopathy (CCMP).
- Careful assessment of right ventricular (RV) function should be performed in patients with CCMP given the high rates of RV failure in patients undergoing left ventricular assist device (LVAD) implantation.
- Orthotopic heart transplant (OHT) in patients with CCMP is associated with comparable outcomes to other causes of HF.

INTRODUCTION

Over the past decade, evolving cancer treatments have resulted in improved overall survival. It is estimated that there are approximately 15 million cancer survivors in the United States today and this number is expected to reach 20 million by 2026.[1] Thus, many cancer survivors in the current era die from noncancer causes, such as cardiovascular diseases.[2–4]

Although novel cancer therapies are increasingly used, anthracyclines remain the cornerstone of cancer treatment, especially in hematologic malignancies, sarcomas, and breast cancer. Anthracyclines have long been known to predictably cause cardiotoxicity, which may progress to long-term HF.[5] In addition, new targeted therapies (namely, human epidermal growth factor receptor 2 antagonists as well as other tyrosine kinase inhibitors) have also been associated with HF.[6] Thus, unsurprisingly, many cancer survivors are living with and dying from progressive HF.

Moreover, other treatment modalities, such as radiation, further increase this risk through direct

Disclosures: The authors have no conflicts of interest to disclose.
Onco-Cardiology Program, Advanced Heart Failure & Transplantation Center, Harrington Heart & Vascular Institute, University Hospitals Cleveland Medical Center, Case Western Reserve University School of Medicine, 11100 Euclid Avenue, Cleveland, OH 44106, USA
* Corresponding author. University Hospitals, Case Western Reserve University School of Medicine, 11100 Euclid Avenue, Lakeside 3012, Cleveland, OH 44106.
E-mail address: guilherme.oliveira@uhhospitals.org

Heart Failure Clin 13 (2017) 327–336
http://dx.doi.org/10.1016/j.hfc.2016.12.005
1551-7136/17/© 2016 Elsevier Inc. All rights reserved.

myocardial effects, valvulopathy, and accelerated vascular disease.[7] Therefore, 2 main types of cardio-myopathies that result from the cardiotoxic effects of cancer therapies are recognized: CCMP and radiotherapy-induced cardiomyopathy (RT-CMP), collectively known as cancer therapeutics–related cardiac dysfunction (CTRCD).[8] Comorbid cardio-vascular diseases in cancer survivors confer poorer survival, and patients with HF from chemotherapy have one of the worst prognoses of all forms of HF.[9]

Recently, oncocardiology has emerged as a multidisciplinary practice to mitigate the risk of cardiovascular disease in cancer patients through prevention and early interventions.[10,11] Given the complexity of antineoplastic therapies and extent of comorbid conditions in these patients, advanced HF treatment in this population requires special considerations. This article reviews the epidemiology, pathophysiology, and available treatment modalities for cancer survivors who develop advanced HF in the era of device thera-pies and heart transplantation.

EPIDEMIOLOGY OF ADVANCED HEART FAILURE IN CANCER SURVIVORS

The exact number of patients with advanced HF among cancer survivors is not known. Data extrap-olated from large registries for advanced HF (eg, Interagency Registry for Mechanically Assisted Circulatory Support [INTERMACS] and United Network for Organ Sharing [UNOS]) can, however, reveal the approximate contribution of CTRCD to the overall advanced HF population. For example, in INTERMACS, CCMP was the primary diagnosis in 75 (2%) of 3812 patients implanted between 2006 and 2011 in the United States.[12] In UNOS, CCMP accounted for 453 (0.8%) of 51,765 patients who underwent primary heart transplantation be-tween 1987 and 2011.[13] RT-CMP, on the other hand, is much rarer. For example, in UNOS, RT-CMP was diagnosed in 87 (0.2%) of 45,041 adults who underwent transplantation (2000–2015).[14] Similarly, of 297 patients who underwent heart transplant at Mayo Clinic from 1992 to 2010, only 12 (4%) had history of radiation therapy.[15] These numbers most likely represent an underestimation of the general pool of patients with CTRCD with end-stage HF, because only a small fraction of these patients are eligible for or have access to du-rable mechanical support or transplant.

DEMOGRAPHICS AND CLINICAL CHARACTERISTICS

Large registries have revealed certain unique characteristics of patients with advanced CTRCD. These patients are younger (mean age 44–53 years) and overwhelmingly women (62%–72%), contrary to nonischemic cardiomy-opathy (NICM) and ischemic cardiomyopathy (ICM), which are more prevalent in older and male patients.

For example, in a review of the INTERMACS reg-istry for MCS, the CCMP cohort was predomi-nantly female (CCMP 72% vs NICM 24% vs ICM 13%; $P<.0001$). The CCMP patients were signifi-cantly younger than those receiving MCS for ICM (mean age 53 vs 60 years old; $P<.001$) but of similar age to other forms of NICM (53 vs 51 years old; $P = .41$). Lower body mass index was noted in the CCMP group (CCMP 26.0 vs NICM 28.9; $P<.0001$ vs ICM 28.0; $P = .0019$). Comorbid con-ditions were favorable in the CCMP group with less frequent prevalence of diabetes (CCMP 25% vs NICM 31%; $P = .29$ vs ICM 46%; $P = .0004$), coronary disease (CCMP 0% vs NICM 16%; $P = .0002$ vs ICM 100%; $P<.0001$), previous alcohol abuse (CCMP 5% vs NICM 16%; $P = .01$ vs ICM 18%; $P = .01$), or smoking history (CCMP 1% vs NICM 12%; $P = .01$ vs ICM 15%; $P = .0016$). Therapies prior to MCS implantation were variable in that CCMP patients were more likely to be receiving angiotensin-converting enzyme inhibitors (CCMP 68% vs NICM 53%; $P = .02$ vs ICM 51%; $P = .01$), yet they were less likely to be implanted with an ICD (CCMP 66% vs NICM 77%; $P = .03$ vs ICM 77%; $P = .03$).

Corroborated by data from the transplantation registries, it is clear that patients with CTRCD with advanced HF have lower prevalence of comorbidities, such as hypertension, diabetes, obesity, and ischemic heart disease. There also seems to be lower utilization of implantable defi-brillators (ICDs), probably due to acuity and severity of HF presentation, not allowing time for optimal medical therapy and defibrillator implanta-tion, but this remains speculative. A majority of patients in these registries are breast and hemato-logic cancers survivors, for whom anthracyclines are most commonly given. Table 1 summarizes the demographics and clinical characteristics of these patients.

HEART FAILURE PATHOPHYSIOLOGY AND RIGHT VENTRICULAR INVOLVEMENT

HF caused by cardiotoxicity of drugs is believed to be a global myocardial process. Therefore, it is intuitive to imagine that both the left and right ven-tricles are equally affected. Because the RV con-tains less muscle mass and consequently less contractile reserve, it stands to reason that the toxic effects of chemotherapy should be felt in

Table 1
Characteristics of cancer survivors in the advanced heart failure registries

	Orthotopic Heart Transplant for Chemotherapy-Induced Cardiomyopathy— United Network for Organ Sharing	Mechanical Circulatory Support for Chemotherapy-Induced Cardiomyopathy— Interagency Registry for Mechanically Assisted Circulatory Support	Othotopic Heart Transplant for Restrictive Cardiomyopathy —United Network for Organ Sharing
Number of patients	453	75	87
Percentage of overall population	0.8%	2%	0.2%
Age	44	53	49.1
Female	66%	72%	62%
White/Caucasian	74%	64%	85%
BMI	—	26	26
DM	8%	25%	—
Inotropes	48%	89%	24%
IABP	—	32%	2.3%
ICD	—	66%	40%
Cardiac Index	—	2.0	—
Ventilator	—	9%	2%
Creatinine	—	1.4	1.2
mPAP	30.6	—	30.7
Previous malignancy			
Breast	24%	52%	—
Hematologic	17%	33%	—
Other/unknown	58.6%	15%	—

the RV first. Accordingly, there are data confirming that RV involvement may indeed occur prior to left ventricular involvement. Decreases in tricuspid annular plane systolic excursion and RV fractional area change have been observed after only 2 cycles of doxorubicin in patients undergoing breast cancer treatment.[16] At 1 year, greater RV than left ventricular impairment has been demonstrated on cardiac MRI in patients undergoing doxorubicin and trastuzumab therapy.[17] Furthermore, concomitant RV failure at time of diagnosis is associated with a lower likelihood of left ventricle functional recovery.[18] On long-term follow up, Ylanen and colleagues[19] found that a majority of survivors of childhood cancer with anthracycline exposure demonstrated signs of biventricular dysfunction and that reductions in RV function were more common than left ventricle function.

Recognition of the high incidence of RV dysfunction in CCMP is paramount in management and planning for advanced therapies. INTERMACS registry data show that surrogate hemodynamic markers of RV dysfunction, including elevated right atrial pressure, lower pulmonary artery systolic pressure, and elevated central venous pressure to pulmonary capillary wedge pressure ratio as well as moderate to severe tricuspid regurgitation were significantly more common preoperatively in CCMP patients undergoing MCS than those with other forms of cardiomyopathy (Table 2). Not surprisingly, the same analysis showed that nearly 20% of patients with CCMP undergoing durable LVAD implantation required either concomitant or subsequent implantation of RV assist devices (RVADs). This occurrence was significantly more frequent in CCMP patients than in either ischemic or other nonischemic HF patients (CCMP 19% vs ICM 6% vs NICM 11%; $P = .006$). Also, CCMP patients receiving LVADs commonly require concomitant tricuspid valve repair, likely related to significant underlying functional tricuspid regurgitation associated with a dilated, dysfunctional RV.[12] Similarly, when analyzing the UNOS database, the authors found that CCMP patients listed for heart transplantation were twice as likely to require biventricular support

Table 2
Comparison of right ventricular function parameters before MCSD implantation between chemotherapy-induced cardiomyopathy, nonischemic cardiomyopathy, and ischemic cardiomyopathy

Parameter	Chemotherapy-Induced Cardiomyopathy (n = 75)	Nonischemic Cardiomyopathy (n = 2392)	Ischemic Cardiomyopathy (n = 1345)
RAP (mm Hg)	16.5	13.5	12.5
Systolic PAP (mm Hg)	44	49	51
Diastolic PAP (mm Hg)	25	26	25
Mean PCWP (mm Hg)	24.1	25	24.4
RAP/PCWP	0.68	0.54	0.51
PVR (wood units)	2.4	2.9	2.7
TR (moderate to severe)	62%	43%	49%

Abbreviations: PAP, pulmonary artery pressure; PCWP, pulmonary capillary wedge pressure; PVR, pulmonary vascular resistance; RAP, right atrial pressure; TR, tricuspid regurgitation.

before transplant than those with other forms of NICM (5.6% vs 2.3%; P = .0021).[20]

Because biventricular mechanical support is associated with poorer overall outcomes, it is important to thoroughly interrogate RV function before LVAD implantation and plan accordingly. How to best evaluate RV function in these patients is still debatable and beyond the scope of this article.

ADVANCED HEART FAILURE THERAPIES FOR CHEMOTHERAPY-INDUCED CARDIOMYOPATHY AND RADIOTHERAPY-INDUCED CARDIOMYOPATHY

Unfortunately, many cancer survivors with American College of Cardiology/American Heart Association advanced stage C or stage D HF are either ineligible or do not have access to advanced HF therapies. In addition, the efficacy of available therapeutic modalities for advanced HF in cancer survivors is largely unknown because cancer patients are either excluded or underrepresented in randomized clinical trials. Thus, a majority of data regarding safety and efficacy of these treatments are available through single-center series or large national registries. This review specifically addresses ICDs, cardiac resynchronization therapy (CRT), durable MCS, and heart transplantation.

IMPLANTABLE DEFIBRILLATORS AND CARDIAC RESYNCHRONIZATION THERAPY

ICDs have clearly decreased mortality in a subset of patients with systolic HF and are currently recommended in guidelines regardless of underlying HF etiology.[21] In registry analyses, it seems that patients with advanced CTRCD are less likely to receive ICDs than those with other HF causes. For example, only 66% of CCMP patients in INTERMACS had ICDs compared with 77% of others. Similarly, only 40% of patients with RT-CMP had ICDs compared with 46% of other RCMs in the UNOS registry.

Similarly, CRT also seems used in CCMP. In a recent retrospective review of 272 patients with cancer and HF who met eligibility criteria for CRT, only 58 (21%) had CRT.[22]

Few case series have reported on the efficacy of CRT in CCMP. Ajijola and colleagues[23] reported 4 patients with CCMP and prolonged QRS (129–171 ms) refractory to medical therapy who received CRT with improvement in New York Heart Association (NYHA) class, 6-minute walk test, Minnesota Living with Heart Failure Questionnaire score, mean left ventricular ejection fraction, and ventricular diameters at 6 months. Rickard and colleagues[24] retrospectively reviewed outcomes of CRT in 18 patients with CCMP in comparison to nonischemic patients. CCMP patients were more likely to be female and have narrower QRS; less frequent atrial fibrillation and hypertension; and a history of breast cancer, lymphoma, sarcoma, and chest irradiation. After a mean of 9 months, patients with CCMP had equivalent benefit from CRT to other nonischemic HF patients, reflected by improvement in all echocardiographic parameters, including mean left ventricular ejection fraction (mean 19% to 27%), left ventricular end-diastolic diameter (mean of 6.0 to 5.6 cm), mitral regurgitation severity (from mean of 4.3 to 3.1), and NYHA class (from mean of 2.9 to 2.4).

The common theme of ICD and CRT underutilization requires attention. Although this observation may reflect the late diagnosis and acute presentation of CCMP, it is still concerning that a high percentage of CCMP patients do not receive appropriate prophylaxis for sudden cardiac death. It is possible that patients with a diagnosis of CCMP, because they are younger, may have a long period of undiagnosed and oligosymptomatic cardiomyopathy, until they present acutely with HF. This may explain the clinical impression that anthracyclines cause late cardiomyopathy. More likely, the cardiomyopathy exists and is established shortly (within 1 year) after completion of therapy, but patients remain asymptomatic or compensated for several years, even decades, until they present with catastrophic HF. It is possible that, with widespread establishment of oncocardiology programs and closer surveillance and screening of cancer patients and survivors, fewer patients will remain with cardiomyopathies that are untreated and undiagnosed. Therefore, it is important to emphasize the need for active echocardiographic screening of cancer survivors who received cardiotoxic therapy for early detection and treatment of impaired ventricular function.

Although promising, the role of CRT in treatment of CCMP remains unknown. Because of its rarity, CCMP is likely not well represented in large clinical trials, such as Multicenter Automatic Defibrillator Implantation Trial (MADIT) and MADIT with Cardiac Resynchronization Therapy. The ongoing MADIT—Chemotherapy-Induced Cardiomyopathy study (ClinicalTrials.gov Identifier: NCT02164721), designed to prospectively evaluate the role of resynchronization CCMP patients who meet current guidelines, will likely indicate the value of CRT-D in this population.

MECHANICAL CIRCULATORY SUPPORT

The first reported series of durable ventricular assist device use in patients with CCMP was published by Musci and colleagues[25] more than 20 years ago. A relative paucity of data existed until INTERMACS registry data were reported in 2014. These registry data demonstrated that approximately 2% of LVADs were implanted for CCMP between 2006 and 2011.

Apart from the unique cohort demographics, described previously, there were no differences in NYHA functional class or INTERMACS profile nor inotrope use, ventilatory support, or intra-aortic balloon pump use between CCMP and other causes. Left ventricular ejection fraction and indexed left ventricular end-diastolic diameter were also similar between groups. Significantly, more CCMP patients were implanted as destination therapy (DT) (CCMP 33% vs NICM 14%; $P<.0001$ vs ICM 23%; $P = .03$).

CCMP patients treated with MCS had survival similar to that of ICM and other NICM patients with 1-year, 2-year, and 3-year survival rates of 73%, 63%, and 47%, respectively (Fig. 1). No survival differences existed between the bridge-to-transplant (BTT) and DT cohorts. Although survival was similar, CCMP patients were more likely to experience need for other concomitant cardiac surgeries (CCMP 48% vs NICM 36.5%; $P = .003$ vs ICM 36%; $P = .04$) as well as increased bleeding rates (CCMP 52% vs NICM 38% vs ICM 43%; $P = .0001$) and failure to wean from cardiopulmonary bypass (CCMP 5% vs NICM 2%; $P = .01$ vs ICM 2%; $P = .04$). Approximately half of CCMP patients required concomitant tricuspid repair in comparison with approximately one-third in the other cardiomyopathy groups. Almost one-fifth of CCMP patients required subsequent or concomitant RV support, which was significantly higher than in other forms of cardiomyopathy (CCMP 19% vs NICM 11% vs ICM 6%; $P = .006$) (Table 3).

Patients requiring biventricular support had higher mortality than those with LVAD alone ($P = .0007$) and one-third of those with post-LVAD failure requiring RVAD support died in the early postoperative period.[12] Data not specific to CCMP suggest that planned biventricular assist device insertion improves survival compared with delayed conversion of LVADs to biventricular assist devices in those with suspected high risk for post-LVAD RV failure.[26] Perhaps upfront biventricular support in CCMP with RV dysfunction may lead to improved outcomes in the future. Transplant data from the International Society for Heart & Lung Transplantation (ISHLT) registry between 2002 and 2008 demonstrated the utility of LVAD use as BTT in the CCMP population. Although the rates of RVAD support were overall lower (5.6%) than that seen in the INTERMACS registry (19%), CCMP patients in the ISHLT registry were twice as likely as NICM patients to require an RVAD before transplant (5.6% vs 2.3%; $P = .0021$). Given the biventricular nature of CCMP, the total artificial heart seems an attractive option, although its use in CCMP has been restricted to 1 case report.[9] Currently, total artificial heart is only approved for BTT, although a DT trial is ongoing (ClinicalTrials.gov NCT02232659). Significant RV dysfunction is common in CCMP and has important implications for MCS surgical planning.

Theoretic concerns related to smaller patient size and interactions with potential previous chest

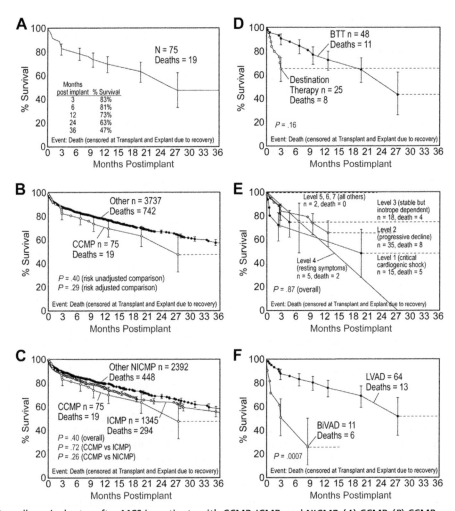

Fig. 1. Overall survival rates after MCS in patients with CCMP, ICMP, and NICMP. (*A*) CCMP. (*B*) CCMP versus (ICMP and NICMP) adult primary implants. (*C*) CCMP versus ICMP versus NICMP adult primary implants. (*D*) CCMP patients by device strategy. (*E*) CCMP patient profile. (*F*) CCMP by device side. BiVAD, biventricular assist device. (*From* Oliveira GH, Dupont M, Naftel D, et al. Increased need for right ventricular support in patients with chemotherapy-induced cardiomyopathy undergoing mechanical circulatory support: outcomes from the INTER-MACS Registry (Interagency Registry for Mechanically Assisted Circulatory Support). J Am Coll Cardiol 2014;63:246; with permission.)

radiotherapy have been raised in CTRCD patients undergoing MCS.[27,28] To date, no significant data directly substantiating either concern for MCS in CCMP have been reported. Stunted growth is not uncommon in childhood cancer survivors[29]; however, the advent of centrifugal pumps implanted in the pericardium allow for safe implantation at very small body surface area.[30] Even total artificial heart has been successfully implanted in patients with small body surface area using preoperative 3D-CT modeling technology.[31] Mediastinal radiation has been associated with increased perioperative morbidity and poorer long-term survival after cardiac surgery[32,33]; however, few durable MCS implantations were included in the reported literature. Intuitively, surgical difficulties and the

potential for bleeding as well as poor wound healing, potential respiratory complications related to previous lung radiation injury, and concomitant valvular disease would all be important considerations prior to ventricular assist device implantation. Despite more frequent need for RVAD support and theoretic concerns related to previous cancer therapies, patients with CCMP experience survival equivalent to that of other cardiomyopathy patients undergoing MCS.

ORTHOTOPIC HEART TRANSPLANTATION

Although medical therapy and mechanical support have improved in recent years, OHT remains the definitive therapy for end-stage HF. Furthermore,

Table 3
Outcomes of patients with chemotherapy-induced cardiomyopathy who underwent mechanical circulatory support implantation compared with nonischemic and ischemic cardiomyopathies

	Chemotherapy-Induced Cardiomyopathy (%)	Nonischemic Cardiomyopathy (%)	Ischemic Cardiomyopathy (%)
Concomitant surgery	48	37	36
Failure to wean from bypass	5	2	2
Need for RVAD	19	11	6
Bleeding at last follow-up	52	38	43
Infections at last follow-up	43	39	40
Neurologic events at last follow-up	15	9	23
Right heart failure events at last follow-up	12	12	10

OHT is ideal given the young age at onset, biventricular nature, and low incidence of pulmonary vascular disease found in CCMP patients. In years previous, OHT for CCMP was limited by concerns over cancer recurrence rates, adverse effects related to previous cancer therapies, and the perception of overall poorer outcomes. The totality of data to date, however, demonstrates excellent survival rates with minimal cancer recurrence post-OHT. Previous listing criteria from 2010 stated that active or recent solid organ or blood malignancy within 5 years was an absolute contraindication to OHT[34]; however, updated ISHLT listing criteria published in 2016 allow for a more nuanced approach to listing for those with a cancer history.[35] The 2016 ISHLT listing criteria suggest collaboration with oncology specialists to stratify each patient as to their risk of tumor recurrence and no arbitrary time period for observation should be used. The amount of time to wait to transplant after neoplasm remission should depend on response to therapy, tumor type, and lack of systemic disease.

The first single-center experiences of few CCMP transplant cases were reported in the late 1980s, but it was not until 2012 when the authors' group[20] and then 2013 when Lenneman and colleagues[13] published work examining hundreds of CCMP transplant patients using large, multicenter registry data. The authors reviewed the ISHLT registry and identified 232 patients who underwent OHT between 2000 and 2008, with CCMP defined as their primary HF cause; these patients outcomes were then compared with 8890 NICM patients who underwent OHT during the same period. The most common pre-OHT malignancies in the CCMP cohort were leukemia or lymphoma in 33%, followed by breast cancer in 31% and sarcomas in 7.5%. The different demographics of those patients compared with other causes highlight the unique patient type encountered in advanced HF secondary to CCMP. Approximately 20% of patients in either group were BTT with LVAD; however, CCMP patients were more than twice as likely to require RVAD before OHT (5.6% vs 2.3%; $P = .0021$). Despite difference in demographics and pre-OHT RVAD use, short-term and long-term survival rates were similar between groups. Survival rates at 1 year, 3 years, and 5 years between CCMP and NICM were, respectively, 86% versus 87%, 79% versus 81%, and 71% versus 74% ($P = .19$) (Fig. 2).

CCMP patients in this registry experienced similar survival outcomes despite significantly longer allograft ischemic times (mean 3.1 vs 2.6 hours; $P<.001$). It was speculated that longer ischemic times were due to difficult recipient dissection related to previous chest radiation or increased RVAD use. Whatever the cause, this finding may have implications in timing between graft harvesting and transplant planning. Allograft rejection in the first year after transplant was significantly lower in patients with CCMP compared with the NICM group (28% vs 38%; $P = .03$), perhaps related to persistent immunosuppression from previous cancer therapies. Although hospitalizations for post-transplant infections were higher in the CCMP group (22% vs 14%; $P = .04$), infections leading to death within the first year post-transplant were no different between the 2 groups (CCMP 12.5% vs NICM 20.4%; $P = .157$). Perhaps the most important finding, aside from comparable post-transplant survival rates, was that only 1 case of cancer recurrence was seen in the CCMP

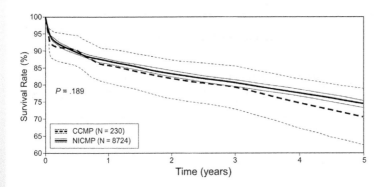

Fig. 2. Survival rates after heart transplantation in CCMP versus NICMP. (*From* Oliveira GH, Hardaway BW, Kucheryavaya AY, et al. Characteristics and survival of patients with chemotherapy-induced cardiomyopathy undergoing heart transplantation. J Heart Lung Transplant 2012;31:808; with permission.)

group, dispelling a long-held fear related to cancer recurrence in CCMP patients after transplant.

The UNOS analysis by Lenneman and colleagues[13] compared outcomes of 435 CCMP transplant recipients against 51,312 OHTs for all other causes of cardiomyopathy between 1987 and 2011. Similar to aforementioned ISHLT registry data, the UNOS registry CCMP patients who received OHT were more likely female (66% vs 25%; P<.001), younger (median age 44 vs 52 years old; P<.001), and of lower body weight (mean 64 vs 72 kg; P<.001) than those with other cardiomyopathies. CCMP patients also had lower cardiac output (3.6 vs 4.2 L/min; P<.001) and were more commonly treated with pre-OHT inotropes (48% vs 39%; P<.001). Unadjusted 10-year OHT survival rates were no different between groups (HR 1.14; (95% CI, 0.94–1.39); P = .198), and in fact the CCMP groups survival was found superior after adjusting for age, gender, and history of malignancy (HR 1.28 [CI, 1.03–1.59]; P = .026). Death due to malignancy was the same between the 2 groups.

Another important observation from both studies was an increasing temporal trend in CCMP referrals and transplants in recent years. Data from the ISHLT registry revealed that almost one-quarter of the CCMP transplants occurred in the final year of the 8-year data set, ranging from 2000 to 2008. Lenneman and colleagues[13] demonstrated a statistically significant increase in percentage of OHTs per year between 1987 and 2011. These findings likely reflect both an increasing appreciation of CCMP as an underlying cause as well as recognition that CCMP patients can undergo successful OHT with outcomes comparable to those with other forms of cardiomyopathy.

Until recently, little was known about the natural history of patients with CCMP on the transplant waitlist. The authors' group recently reported waitlist outcomes on patients between January 2004

and June 2014 using the UNOS database. Median times listed, as well as overall mortality and access to OHT, were no different between those with CCMP compared with NICM. The incidence of fatal cerebrovascular events, although listed, was almost 3-fold higher in the CCMP group (31.4% vs 12.8%; P = .002). It seems that 8.6% of these deaths were due to hemorrhagic events compared with 3% in the NICM group (P = .037).[36] Although increased frequency of cerebrovascular events in cancer patients has been previously appreciated,[37] this finding in listed CCMP patients has not been previously reported.

End-stage HF related to previous cancer therapies, in particular chest radiation, may take on a distinct restrictive phenotype as opposed to the dilated, biventricular phenotype typical of CCMP. Cardiac transplants for restrictive cardiomyopathy (RCM) of any cause are performed less commonly, between 1.4% and 2.5% of OHTs, yet overall outcomes seem comparable to transplants for dilated cardiomyopathies.[38] Few data, with conflicting results, have been published concerning transplant outcomes for those with RCM secondary to radiation therapy (RT-CMP). Although a Mayo Clinic series of 12 patients undergoing OHT for radiation-induced disease showed comparable results to the overall transplant cohort,[15] a slightly larger series of 35 patients transplanted for RCM with a history of previous chest irradiation/chemotherapy demonstrated significantly worse outcomes, with a 1.8-fold increased risk of post-transplant mortality.[38] Using UNOS registry data between 2000 and 2015, the authors' group reported outcomes for 87 adults listed for OHT with a cause of RT-CMP. Overall the RT-CMP cohort made up 0.2% of the total OHT listed population, whereas transplant listing for other causes of RCM made up 2.3%. Patients with RT-CMP were significantly younger and more commonly female as well as more likely to have undergone another previous cardiac surgery compared with both the remaining RCM cohort and the non-RCM cohort. Unfortunately, 6-month post-transplant mortality was significantly higher in the RT-CMP group (RT-CMP 21.2% vs RCM 7.6% vs other 7.8%; $P = .004$). Post-transplant 1-year, 3-year, and 5-year cumulative survival rates were lowest among RT-CMP (76%, 66%, and 58%, respectively), RCM (88%, 79%, and 73%, respectively; $P = .025$ compared with RT-RCM), and other causes (88%, 82%, and 76%, respectively; $P = .012$ compared with RT-RCM).[14] Complicating factors, such as concomitant radiation-induced multiorgan dysfunction, in addition to contemporary radiation doses used in RT-CMP subgroups, remain unknown, and these factors may impact prognosis and outcomes.

OHT remains the definitive therapy for end-stage CCMP. Despite increased need for pre-OHT RVAD, survival rates comparable with other forms of cardiomyopathy have been demonstrated in 2 large multicenter data registries. Transplanted CCMP patients seem to suffer from fewer episodes of early allograft rejection yet are at increased risk of hospitalization for infections. Transplant outcomes for RT-CMP are unfortunately poor. Further study may help elucidate more refined risk stratification methods as well as help define optimal immunosuppressive regimens in this unique transplant cohort.

SUMMARY

CTRCD, which may result from chemotherapy and radiation, is typically a biventricular cardiomyopathy, often manifest with significant RV dysfunction. Advanced CTRCD patients more likely are female, are younger, and have fewer traditional comorbid conditions. Durable MCS represents a viable option for advanced CCMP patients, with survival rates similar to other forms of cardiomyopathy although these patients may require concomitant RV support. Heart transplantation is the definitive therapy for patients with advanced CCMP, and overall excellent outcomes, comparable to those found in other cardiomyopathies can be achieved in properly selected candidates. Patients with RT-CMP have worse post-transplantation survival compared with other causes. Cancer recurrence after transplantation is exceptionally rare in properly selected candidates. Although patients with CCMP may be at risk for unique comorbid events, the overall mortality and access to transplantation are not different than those with other forms of cardiomyopathy. An increasing number of CTRCD patients are referred for advanced therapies and this number is likely to grow in the future given improved cancer survival rates. It is also likely that different forms of CTRCD will arise with the emergence of novel anticancer therapies.

REFERENCES

1. Miller KD, Siegel RL, Lin CC, et al. Cancer treatment and survivorship statistics, 2016. CA Cancer J Clin 2016;66:271–89.
2. Al-Kindi SG, Abu-Zeinah GF, Kim CH, et al. Trends and disparities in cardiovascular mortality among survivors of hodgkin lymphoma. Clin Lymphoma Myeloma Leuk 2015;15:748–52.
3. Venturini M, Michelotti A, Del Mastro L, et al. Multicenter randomized controlled clinical trial to evaluate cardioprotection of dexrazoxane versus no cardioprotection in women receiving epirubicin chemotherapy for advanced breast cancer. J Clin Oncol 1996;14:3112–20.
4. Tukenova M, Guibout C, Oberlin O, et al. Role of cancer treatment in long-term overall and cardiovascular mortality after childhood cancer. J Clin Oncol 2010;28:1308–15.
5. Von Hoff DD, Layard MW, Basa P, et al. Risk factors for doxorubicin-induced congestive heart failure. Ann Intern Med 1979;91:710–7.
6. Keefe DL. Trastuzumab-associated cardiotoxicity. Cancer 2002;95:1592–600.
7. Boivin J-F, Hutchison GB. Coronary heart disease mortality after irradiation for Hodgkin's disease. Cancer 1982;49:2470–5.
8. Plana JC, Galderisi M, Barac A, et al. Expert consensus for multimodality imaging evaluation of adult patients during and after cancer therapy: a report from the American Society of Echocardiography and the European Association of Cardiovascular Imaging. J Am Soc Echocardiogr 2014;27:911–39.
9. Felker GM, Thompson RE, Hare JM, et al. Underlying causes and long-term survival in patients with initially unexplained cardiomyopathy. N Engl J Med 2000;342:1077–84.
10. Al-Kindi SG, Oliveira GH. Prevalence of preexisting cardiovascular disease in patients with different types of cancer: the unmet need for onco-cardiology. Mayo Clin Proc 2015;91(1):81–3.
11. Yeh ET. Onco-cardiology: the time has come. Tex Heart Inst J 2011;38:246–7.
12. Oliveira GH, Dupont M, Naftel D, et al. Increased need for right ventricular support in patients with chemotherapy-induced cardiomyopathy undergoing mechanical circulatory support: outcomes from the INTERMACS Registry (Interagency Registry for Mechanically Assisted Circulatory Support). J Am Coll Cardiol 2014;63:240–8.
13. Lenneman AJ, Wang L, Wigger M, et al. Heart transplant survival outcomes for adriamycin dilated cardiomyopathy. Am J Cardiol 2013;111:609–12.

14. Al-Kindi SG, Oliveira GH. Heart transplantation outcomes in radiation-induced restrictive cardiomyopathy. J Card Fail 2016;22(6):475–8.

15. Saxena P, Joyce LD, Daly RC, et al. Cardiac transplantation for radiation-induced cardiomyopathy: the Mayo Clinic experience. Ann Thorac Surg 2014;98:2115–21.

16. Tanindi A, Demirci U, Tacoy G, et al. Assessment of right ventricular functions during cancer chemotherapy. Eur J Echocardiogr 2011;12:834–40.

17. Grover S, Leong DP, Chakrabarty A, et al. Left and right ventricular effects of anthracycline and trastuzumab chemotherapy: a prospective study using novel cardiac imaging and biochemical markers. Int J Cardiol 2013;168:5465–7.

18. Calleja A, Poulin F, Khorolsky C, et al. Right ventricular dysfunction in patients experiencing cardiotoxicity during breast cancer therapy. J Oncol 2015; 2015:609194.

19. Ylanen K, Poutanen T, Savikurki-Heikkila P, et al. Cardiac magnetic resonance imaging in the evaluation of the late effects of anthracyclines among long-term survivors of childhood cancer. J Am Coll Cardiol 2013;61:1539–47.

20. Oliveira GH, Hardaway BW, Kucheryavaya AY, et al. Characteristics and survival of patients with chemotherapy-induced cardiomyopathy undergoing heart transplantation. J Heart Lung Transplant 2012;31:805–10.

21. Russo AM, Stainback RF, Bailey SR, et al. ACCF/HRS/AHA/ASE/HFSA/SCAI/SCCT/SCMR 2013 appropriate use criteria for implantable cardioverter-defibrillators and cardiac resynchronization therapy: a report of the American College of Cardiology Foundation appropriate use criteria task force, Heart Rhythm Society, American Heart Association, American Society of Echocardiography, Heart Failure Society of America, Society for Cardiovascular Angiography and Interventions, Society of Cardiovascular Computed Tomography, and Society for Cardiovascular Magnetic Resonance. Heart Rhythm 2013;10:e11–58.

22. Fadol AP, Mouhayar E, Fellman B, et al. The use of cardiac resynchronization therapy in cancer patients with heart failure: preliminary findings in a comprehensive cancer center. J Card Fail 2016;22:S57.

23. Ajijola OA, Nandigam KV, Chabner BA, et al. Usefulness of cardiac resynchronization therapy in the management of Doxorubicin-induced cardiomyopathy. Am J Cardiol 2008;101:1371–2.

24. Rickard J, Kumbhani DJ, Baranowski B, et al. Usefulness of cardiac resynchronization therapy in patients with Adriamycin-induced cardiomyopathy. Am J Cardiol 2010;105:522–6.

25. Musci M, Loebe M, Grauhan O, et al. Heart transplantation for doxorubicin-induced congestive heart failure in children and adolescents. Transplant Proc 1997;29:578–9.

26. Fitzpatrick JR 3rd, Frederick JR, Hiesinger W, et al. Early planned institution of biventricular mechanical circulatory support results in improved outcomes compared with delayed conversion of a left ventricular assist device to a biventricular assist device. J Thorac Cardiovasc Surg 2009;137:971–7.

27. Shah S, Nohria A. Advanced heart failure due to cancer therapy. Curr Cardiol Rep 2015;17:16.

28. Ghosh N, Hilton J. Orthotopic heart transplantation and mechanical circulatory support in cancer survivors: challenges and outcomes. J Oncol 2015;2015: 232607.

29. Haddy TB, Mosher RB, Nunez SB, et al. Growth hormone deficiency after chemotherapy for acute lymphoblastic leukemia in children who have not received cranial radiation. Pediatr Blood Cancer 2006;46:258–61.

30. Miera O, Kirk R, Buchholz H, et al. A multicenter study of the HeartWare ventricular assist device in small children. J Heart Lung Transplant 2016;35: 679–81.

31. Moore RA, Madueme PC, Lorts A, et al. Virtual implantation evaluation of the total artificial heart and compatibility: beyond standard fit criteria. J Heart Lung Transplant 2014;33:1180–3.

32. Wu W, Masri A, Popovic ZB, et al. Long-term survival of patients with radiation heart disease undergoing cardiac surgery: a cohort study. Circulation 2013; 127:1476–84.

33. Chang AS, Smedira NG, Chang CL, et al. Cardiac surgery after mediastinal radiation: extent of exposure influences outcome. J Thorac Cardiovasc Surg 2007;133:404–13.

34. Mancini D, Lietz K. Selection of cardiac transplantation candidates in 2010. Circulation 2010;122: 173–83.

35. Mehra MR, Canter CE, Hannan MM, et al. The 2016 International Society for Heart Lung Transplantation listing criteria for heart transplantation: a 10-year update. J Heart Lung Transplant 2016;35:1–23.

36. Mehanna E, Al-Kindi SG, Ige M, et al. Increased risk of cerebrovascular death in patients with chemotherapy-induced cardiomyopathy. J Card Fail 2015;21:S61–2.

37. Schwarzbach CJ, Schaefer A, Ebert A, et al. Stroke and cancer: the importance of cancer-associated hypercoagulation as a possible stroke etiology. Stroke 2012;43:3029–34.

38. DePasquale EC, Nasir K, Jacoby DL. Outcomes of adults with restrictive cardiomyopathy after heart transplantation. J Heart Lung Transplant 2012;31: 1269–75.

Cardiac Dysfunction and Heart Failure in Hematopoietic Cell Transplantation Survivors
Emerging Paradigms in Pathophysiology, Screening, and Prevention

Saro H. Armenian, DO, MPH[a,*], Thomas D. Ryan, MD, PhD[b], Michel G. Khouri, MD[c]

KEYWORDS

- Cardiac dysfunction • Heart failure • Hematopoietic cell transplantation • Survivors
- Pathophysiology • Screening • Prevention

KEY POINTS

- Hematopoietic cell transplantation (HCT) has been increasingly used for curative intent in patients with hematologic and nonhematologic malignancies, resulting in an increasing number of HCT survivors.
- These survivors are at risk for developing serious and sometimes life-threatening complications, including cardiovascular disease (CVD).
- This article provides an overview of CVD in HCT survivors, describing the pathophysiology of disease, emphasizing therapeutic exposures and comorbidities unique to this population.

INTRODUCTION

During the past 4 decades, hematopoietic cell transplantation (HCT) has been increasingly used as a treatment of choice for a large number of hematologic and nonhematologic diseases.[1] Patients who undergo HCT are often exposed to a combination of high-dose chemotherapy, total body irradiation, and immunosuppressive agents.[1] For many, this is in addition to therapeutic exposures (chemotherapy, radiation) they may have received before HCT.[1] Despite the relative intensity of such multimodal therapy, improvements in transplant strategy and clinical care have resulted in an incremental improvement of survival of 10% per decade.[2–4] In fact, among those who survive the first 2 years after HCT, nearly 80% of allogeneic HCT recipients and 70% of autologous HCT recipients are expected to become long-term survivors.[2–4] It is estimated that there are well over 160,000 HCT survivors living in the United States today, and that number is expected to exceed 500,000 by 2030.[5,6]

Disclosure: The authors have no conflicts of interest to disclose.

Funding: Leukemia & Lymphoma Society Scholar in Clinical Research (2315-17), Reducing risk of anthracycline-related heart failure after childhood cancer R01CA196854 (S.H. Armenian).

[a] Division of Outcomes Research, Department of Population Sciences, Comprehensive Cancer Center, City of Hope, 1500 East Duarte Road, Duarte, CA 91010-3000, USA; [b] Department of Cardiology, The Heart Institute, Cincinnati Children's Hospital Medical Center, 3333 Burnet Avenue, Cincinnati, OH 45229-3026, USA; [c] Division of Cardiology, Department of Medicine, Duke University, 2301 Erwin Road, Durham, NC 27710, USA

* Corresponding author.

E-mail address: sarmenian@coh.org

Heart Failure Clin 13 (2017) 337–345

http://dx.doi.org/10.1016/j.hfc.2016.12.008

As a result of improvements in the survival rate, important issues for HCT patients have expanded to include areas relevant to long-term survivorship, such as prevention of adverse health-related outcomes, maintenance of good health, and quality of life.[7] Studies conducted during the past 2 decades have highlighted the substantial burden of morbidity faced by HCT survivors. A report from the Bone Marrow Transplant Survivor Study[8] found that nearly two-thirds will develop a chronic health condition, and approximately 35% will develop a condition that is considered severe or life threatening; compared with sibling controls, they were twice as likely to develop a chronic health condition and nearly 4 times as likely to develop a severe or life-threatening condition. These conditions include subsequent malignancies, endocrine dysfunction, chronic kidney disease, visual impairment, and cardiopulmonary dysfunction.[8–11]

The burden of chronic health conditions is especially high in older HCT survivors, because they are dealing with the interacting effects of the biologic and physiologic changes of aging, the effects of cancer-directed therapy, after effects of cancer, and multiple chronic health conditions that develop over time.[12,13] These biologic changes are postulated to lead to physiologic consequences that can manifest by declines in organ reserve across nearly all organ systems.[12–14] In these survivors, although organ physiologic function generally remains adequate to compensate for activities required for daily living, the decline in reserves can leave HCT survivors vulnerable to premature onset of chronic health conditions, a process akin to accelerated aging.[12–14] For example, a recent report from the Bone Marrow Transplant Survivor Study[15] found that the prevalence of frailty, characterized as self-reported exhaustion, weakness, low physical activity, slow walking speed, and unintentional weight loss, in 18- to 64-year-old subjects was comparable (approximately 10%) with that documented in a community-based elderly (>65 years) population (N = 61,500). The rate of frailty was more than 8-fold higher when compared with sibling controls, with the highest risk seen in survivors transplanted for multiple myeloma, those with lower socioeconomic status, or those with chronic graft versus host disease (GVHD).

CARDIOVASCULAR AGING AND THE BURDEN OF CARDIOVASCULAR MORBIDITY

Among HCT survivors, cardiovascular disease (CVD; eg, heart failure, stroke, myocardial infarction) is a leading cause of non–relapse-related morbidity and mortality.[10] The risk of cardiovascular-related mortality is 2- to 4-fold greater than would be expected for the general population, and the incidence increases with time from HCT.[16,17] However, mortality attributed to CVD underestimates the true burden of CVD after HCT. HCT survivors have a 4-fold greater risk of developing CVD when compared with the general population,[18] adding to the already high burden of chronic health-related conditions in these survivors. Median age at first cardiovascular event such as myocardial infarction or heart failure is 53 years (range, 35–66),[19] which is much lower than would be expected in the general population (67 years).[20] The markedly increased risk of CVD, coupled with the recognition that these complications develop earlier than would be expected in the general population, suggests an accelerated cardiovascular aging phenotype that may be initiated by pre-HCT and HCT-related therapeutic exposures, and worsened by post-HCT complications such as GVHD, comorbidities (eg, hypertension, diabetes), and lifestyle behaviors (eg, physical deconditioning; Fig. 1).

The cardiovascular system has an inherent reserve capacity (cardiovascular reserve capacity) that is maintained by organ systems (cardiac, pulmonary, hematologic, musculoskeletal) that adapt to physiologic and/or pathologic perturbations.[21,22] However, this reserve capacity is finite and injury to 1 or more of the organ systems that maintain its integrity precipitates cardiovascular aging.[21] Moreover, repeated injuries to these systems sustained before, during, or after HCT can deplete cardiovascular reserve capacity, culminating in premature onset of CVD, or even cardiovascular death, among HCT survivors.

In clinical practice, cardiovascular risk is often determined via resting assessment of cardiac left ventricular ejection fraction (LVEF). However, the resting LVEF provides a snapshot of the heart's performance under optimal circumstances, and is a poor prognosticator of future cardiovascular events or mortality in patients undergoing HCT.[9,10] Importantly, the LVEF does not adequately evaluate or reflect cardiovascular reserve capacity, because it provides no information on the functional integrity of other organ systems that maintain cardiovascular reserve.[23–25] Peak oxygen consumption (VO_{2peak}), as derived from cardiopulmonary exercise testing (CPET), has been established as the gold standard measure of cardiovascular reserve, because it represents the integrative capacity with which multiple systems (cardiac, pulmonary, hematologic, musculoskeletal) deliver and use oxygen for ATP resynthesis. The VO_{2peak} is correlated inversely and independently with cardiovascular and all-cause mortality in a range of adult populations,

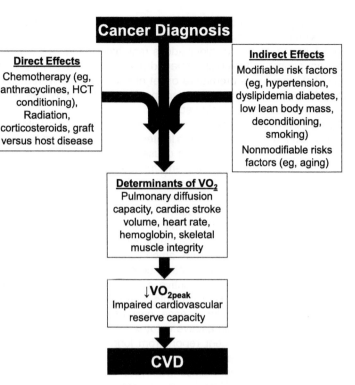

Cancer Diagnosis

Direct Effects
Chemotherapy (eg, anthracyclines, HCT conditioning), Radiation, corticosteroids, graft versus host disease

Indirect Effects
Modifiable risk factors (eg, hypertension, dyslipidemia diabetes, low lean body mass, deconditioning, smoking)
Nonmodifiable risks factors (eg, aging)

Determinants of VO$_2$
Pulmonary diffusion capacity, cardiac stroke volume, heart rate, hemoglobin, skeletal muscle integrity

↓**VO$_{2peak}$**
Impaired cardiovascular reserve capacity

CVD

Fig. 1. Mechanism of decline in cardiovascular reserve capacity, resulting in accelerated cardiovascular aging in hematopoietic cell transplantation (HCT) survivors. CVD, cardiovascular disease.

and has been established as a safe and reliable measure of cardiovascular reserve in CVD prevention trials for breast and lung cancer patients with advanced disease.[26] There is a paucity of information regarding VO$_{2peak}$ in HCT survivors, and how organ-specific perturbations may impact cardiovascular reserve capacity in these survivors. The usefulness of submaximal O$_2$ uptake measurements have emerged as increasingly important in adult heart failure patients, and in some cases seem to be superior to VO$_{2peak}$ in prognostic capabilities.[27] Submaximal indices may be easier to achieve in patients with the physical limitations that can result from treatment in HCT and have relevance to activities of daily living, but have not yet been assessed in survivors of HCT.

To date, there have been 3 pilot studies (sample size range, 21–29)[28–30] that have evaluated the role of CPET in the HCT setting. Two studies[29,30] examined the prognostic usefulness of CPET before HCT, and found that a low VO$_{2peak}$ was associated with an increased risk of nonrelapse mortality, irrespective of pre-HCT prognostic measures such as resting LVEF and 6-minute walk test. A third study[28] examined the feasibility of CPET in 22 patients with multiple myeloma who were a median of 17 months from autologous HCT. In these survivors, the VO$_{2peak}$ was on average 38% less than expected for age-matched sedentary normative values;

27% had a VO$_{2peak}$ of less than 14 mL/kg per minute, which, notably, is the threshold for consideration of referral for cardiac transplantation in patients with heart failure. Larger studies are needed to (1) accurately characterize cardiovascular reserve capacity in HCT survivors, (2) identify specific populations at risk for VO$_{2peak}$ impairment, and (3) describe the organ-specific perturbations that contribute to VO$_{2peak}$ impairment. The information obtained can set the stage for the development of tailored interventions to improve cardiovascular reserve capacity in a population at high risk for CVD. Importantly, these physiologic assessments have to be considered in the context of existing large epidemiologic studies that have identified subsets of HCT survivors who are at an especially high risk of developing cardiovascular complications after HCT. Recognizing the impact of these risk factors on long-term cardiovascular reserve has the potential to facilitate the development of primary (avoidance of certain exposures) or secondary (early screening and intervention) prevention strategies.

CLINICAL AND TREATMENT-RELATED RISK FACTORS FOR CARDIAC COMPLICATIONS

The best described treatment-related cardiac complications in HCT survivors include valvular disease, conduction abnormalities, pericarditis, and cardiomyopathy/heart failure.[10,31] Although the latency for many of these complications can be short (<1 year), survivors can have no symptoms until years after HCT.[10,31] Acute (<1 year from HCT) cardiotoxicity is often owing to exposure to HCT conditioning-related exposures, such as high-dose cyclophosphamide, total body irradiation, or infections complications during post-HCT leukopenia.[31]

The risk of cardiotoxicity associated with high-dose cyclophosphamide is dose dependent, and characterized by cardiac myocyte damage and necrosis.[31] Heart failure can develop within weeks of administration of conditioning therapy, and disease manifestation may be worse among individuals with compromised cardiac function before HCT.[31,32] Decreases in the cumulative dose of cyclophosphamide during the past 2 decades have decreased dramatically the risk of cardiotoxicity in this setting. Total body irradiation, although mostly recognized for its ability to result in endothelial injury, has been known to cause pericarditis in individuals treated without dose fractionation.[10] Last, infectious complications can result from early post-HCT leukopenia or prolonged immunosuppression for management of GVHD.[31] Overwhelming sepsis can lead to cardiopulmonary failure, necessitating circulatory support and intubation, and can be complicated by long-term cardiac or other end-organ dysfunction.[31]

Pre-HCT anthracycline chemotherapy and/or chest radiation therapy are the best-described risk factors for late-occurring (>1 year) cardiotoxicity in HCT survivors.[10,19,33,34] Anthracycline cardiotoxicity is thought to be related to myocardial injury owing to free radicals and intracardiac metabolic derangements.[35] If enough injury occurs, the heart dilates and the chamber walls become thinner, creating a clinical picture similar to de novo dilated cardiomyopathy, and symptomatic heart failure may ensue.[35] For HCT survivors treated with anthracyclines before HCT, additional exposure to potentially cardiotoxic therapies such as high-dose cyclophosphamide used for conditioning, may further compromise cardiomyocyte architecture and function. A recent study[34] found that exposure to cumulative anthracycline dose of 250 mg/m^2 or greater is associated with a 10-fold (odds ratio [OR], 9.9; P<.01) risk of heart failure in HCT survivors, a risk threshold that is markedly lower than conventionally recognized cutoffs (350–450 mg/m^2) in non-HCT cancer populations. Patients who are on either end of the biologic aging spectrum (very young or old) during anthracycline exposure and females have an especially high risk for developing cardiotoxicity.[10,17,33]

In children, damage to the developing heart can cause irreversible tissue damage.[36] On the other hand, older adults may have a reduced capacity to repair damaged healthy heart tissue, resulting in premature onset of heart disease. The mechanism of gender-specific cardiotoxicity has yet to be elucidated.

Unlike chemotherapy-related cardiotoxicity, where injury is limited to the myocardium, radiation exposure can cause impairments across a range of structural and functional cardiac components, including the myocardium, pericardium, valves, conduction system, coronary arteries, and peripheral vasculature.[17,19] A common pathophysiologic pathway seems to be microcirculatory damage, which can cause direct injury to the myocardium or precipitate atherosclerotic plaque buildup that may culminate in coronary artery/ischemic heart disease.[37] Active chronic GVHD, among allogeneic HCT patients, can lead to additional microvascular disease, owing to endothelial infiltration of alloreactive cytotoxic T lymphocytes.[38] Finally, a recent report from long-term HCT survivors[16] found that the cumulative incidence of conduction abnormalities was 10% at 10 years after HCT, significantly higher than the rate (3.5%; P<.01) seen in matched controls. The incidence of conduction disorders as well as other cardiac complications such as valvular disease also increased over time, highlighting the importance of lifelong surveillance for these high-risk populations.

MODIFIABLE CARDIOVASCULAR RISK FACTORS

The incidence of de novo cardiovascular risk factors such as hypertension, diabetes, and dyslipidemia, also increases over time after HCT.[10] In a recent cohort study,[39] the 10-year cumulative incidence of hypertension, diabetes, and dyslipidemia in HCT recipients was 37.7%, 18.1%, and 46.7%, respectively; nearly one-third (32%) had multiple cardiovascular risk factors (compared with 21% in the general population). Overall, HCT survivors have roughly a 2-fold increased risk of developing hypertension (OR, 1.8), diabetes (OR, 2.0), or dyslipidemia (OR, 2.3) as compared with age- and sex-matched controls.[39] For a small subset of HCT survivors, cardiovascular risk factors that develop after HCT may be transient, resolving soon after cessation of immunosuppressive therapy. However, for the vast majority of survivors, cardiovascular risk factors persist even after the discontinuation of immunosuppressive medications.[39,40]

Hypertension has been well-established as an important factor for the development of heart failure in the general population, carrying the highest population-attributable risk for heart failure.[41,42] In animal models, there is evidence that hypertension may accelerate cardiac left ventricular injury after anthracycline exposure.[43] The pathophysiology of heart failure in patients with diabetes is more complex, and can be owing to ischemic heart disease or metabolic derangement from chronic hyperglycemia.[44] In a large cohort study[34] of HCT survivors treated with high-dose ($\geq$250 mg/m^2) anthracyclines, the presence of hypertension was associated with a 35-fold increased risk of heart failure, whereas the risk was nearly 27-fold for survivors who developed diabetes, suggesting that hypertension and diabetes may be critical modifiers of cardiac injury after HCT and these at-risk populations to potentially target for aggressive intervention.

GENETIC SUSCEPTIBILITY

Despite the growing body of literature demonstrating clear associations between clinical risk factors, therapeutic exposures, and heart failure, there is variation in the prevalence and severity of heart failure that is not explained exclusively by these factors alone.[45] Studies have now begun exploring the role of genetic susceptibility in the risk of therapy-related adverse cardiovascular events after HCT. One of the first studies to evaluate the role of genetics identified variants in genes involved in free radical generation (RAC2), anthracycline metabolism (ATP-binding cassette, subfamily C [ABCC2]), and iron homeostasis (hemochromatosis gene [HFE]), as independent predictors of post-HCT heart failure risk.[46] In fact, a combined clinical (anthracycline dose, female sex, chest radiation exposure [yes/no], and hypertension) and genetic (RAC2 [rs13058338], 7508T$\rightarrow$A; HFE [rs1799945], 63C$\rightarrow$G; ABCC2 [rs8187710], 1515G$\rightarrow$A) predictive model performed better (area under the curve [AUC], 0.79) than the clinical (AUC, 0.69) or genetic (AUC, 0.67) models alone.[46] A subsequent study[47] in HCT survivors identified variants in a different set of genes (CELF4, HAS3, and UGT1A6) to be independent modifiers of cardiomyopathy and/or heart failure risk. Additional validation studies are needed before this information can be used as part of clinical decision making. Once these associations are confirmed, this information could form the basis for novel approaches for disease prevention in at-risk survivors of HCT. These would include behavior modification (eg, adoption of a healthy lifestyle, aggressive management of comorbidities such as hypertension), targeted early screening (eg, those with presence of at-risk genotype, treated with higher dose anthracyclines, chest radiation therapy), or early interventions with cardioprotective pharmacologic therapy (eg, angiotensin converting enzyme inhibitors, beta blockers, angiotensin II receptor blockers) to prevent the onset of cardiomyopathy or symptomatic heart failure.

RECOMMENDATIONS FOR THE LONG-TERM MONITORING OF CARDIAC DISEASE AFTER HEMATOPOIETIC CELL TRANSPLANTATION

Recognizing the high burden of serious cardiovascular complications after HCT, a number of recommendations for the long-term health monitoring relevant to survivors of HCT have been developed.[11,48,49] These include guidelines from pediatric oncology groups that address unique HCT exposures to international consensus-based guidelines from HCT-specific professional organizations. Select recommendations for screening, including those issued by the US Preventive Services Task Force for the general population are included in Table 1.

It is important to recognize that oncology- and HCT-specific guidelines often lack the high-quality evidence that is required to inform US Preventive Services Task Force guidelines for the general population. Oncology/HCT guidelines are often based on retrospective observational or self-reported cohort studies focused on describing disease risk factors and incidence rather than optimal screening strategies. That said, given the unique exposures experienced by HCT recipients, many of the recommendations for the general population may be inadequate. As an example, screening for anthracycline-related cardiac dysfunction, for which there are established guidelines in HCT/oncology guidelines, is not discussed in the US Preventive Services Task Force guidelines. Outcomes related to radiation exposure (eg, conduction abnormalities, valvular disease) would also not be covered under established general population guidelines. Therefore, clinicians caring for HCT survivors should evaluate carefully the potential advantage and disadvantages of long-term surveillance strategies in these survivors.

Traditionally, the detection of therapy-related cardiotoxicity has relied on echocardiographic screening using the resting LVEF and/or shortening fraction.[50] However, these parameters are derived from crude ventricular measurements, are load dependent, and have increasingly been recognized as late-occurring changes in myocardial function.[23] By the time changes in LVEF and the shortening fraction are detected, functional

Table 1
Select published recommendations for cardiovascular disease surveillance

Condition (Screening)	General Population: US Preventive Services Task Force[58] [Evidence Grade[a]]	CIBMTR, ASBMT, EBMT, APBMT, BMTSANZ, EMBMT, SBTMO[59]	Children's Oncology Group[60,61] [Evidence Score[b]]
Heart disease (lifestyle factors, eg, diet, physical activity, obesity, tobacco)	Clinicians may choose to selectively counsel patients on initiating behavior changes (diet, physical activity) [grade C]. Obesity screening for all people ≥6 y, and behavioral interventions for those with obesity [grade B]. Screening for tobacco use among adults and promoting tobacco cessation for any users [grade A].	Recommend education and counseling for all survivors.	Same as general population.
Heart disease (electrocardiogram)	Not recommended for screening individuals at low risk for CAD [grade D]. Insufficient evidence for higher risk individuals.	May be indicated for high-risk patients (chest/mediastinal radiotherapy, history of amyloidosis, preexisting cardiovascular disease).	2 y after completing therapy [score 1]
Heart disease (echocardiogram)	Not addressed.	May be indicated for high-risk patients (chest/mediastinal radiotherapy, history of amyloidosis, preexisting cardiovascular disease).	Every 1–5 y depending on age of exposure, cumulative anthracycline dose, and/or chest radiotherapy [score 1]
Heart disease (other markers)	Insufficient evidence for newer biomarkers such as hs-CRP, ankle-brachial index, carotid IMT.	Not addressed.	Not addressed.

Abbreviations: APBMT, Asia-Pacific Blood and Marrow Transplantation Group; ASBMT, American Society for Blood and Marrow Transplantation; SBTMO, Sociedade Brasileira de Transplante de Medula Ossea; BMTSANZ, Bone Marrow Transplant Society of Australia and New Zealand; CAD, coronary heart disease; CIBMTR, Center for International Blood and Marrow Transplant Research; EBMT, European Group for Blood and Marrow Transplantation; EMBMT, East Mediterranean Blood and Marrow Transplantation Group; hs-CRP, high-sensitivity C-reactive protein.

[a] US Preventive Services Task Force evidence grading: (A) high certainty of substantial net benefit—recommended; (B) high certainty of moderate net benefit or moderate certainty of moderate to high net benefit—recommended; (C) moderate certainty of small net benefit—up to clinical judgment; (D) moderate or high certainty of no net benefit or possible harm—Not recommended.

[b] Children's Oncology Group evidence scoring: (1) uniform consensus of high-level evidence; (2A) uniform consensus of high-level evidence; (2B) nonuniform consensus of lower level evidence.

deterioration is essentially irreversible, emphasizing the need for biomarkers that would facilitate identification of cardiac damage at an earlier stage. More sensitive markers of early cardiac dysfunction such as echocardiography-derived myocardial mechanics assessments (eg, strain), tissue Doppler imaging, and 3-dimensional echocardiographic or MRI-derived measures of systolic function have been incorporated into guidelines for the evaluation of patients after cancer therapy.[51,52] The usefulness of these measures has been assessed primarily in patients treated with conventional chemotherapy and have yet to be studied rigorously in HCT. There have been no studies to evaluate the prognostic usefulness of established and/or emerging blood biomarkers of cardiac injury and remodeling (eg, natriuretic peptides, cardiac troponins, ST-2, galectin-3) in HCT survivors. Additional studies are needed to determine the optimal screening modality (imaging, blood biomarkers, or both), as well as timing and frequency of surveillance after HCT.

Smoking cessation and the adoption of a healthy lifestyle should be encouraged strongly for survivors of HCT. In other cancer survivor populations, adherence to lifestyle recommendations has been associated with a reduction in all-cause and CVD-related mortality.[53–55] For example, a recent study[56] of 5-year childhood cancer survivors showed a dose-dependent reduction in CVD risk by duration and intensity of self-reported exercise, suggesting a role for aerobic training for CVD risk reduction in cancer survivors. There are also emerging data among survivors of HCT suggesting that adherence to a healthier lifestyle may attenuate the risk of cardiovascular conditions as well, including a diet richer in fruits and vegetables (associated with lower risk of diabetes and dyslipidemia) and greater physical activity (associated with lower risk of hypertension).[57] Studies are needed to examine systematically the role of lifestyle and behavioral interventions for long-term CVD risk reduction in HCT survivors.

SUMMARY

It is increasingly evident that patients undergoing HCT are at risk for developing CVD. Studies in non-HCT cancer survivors are emerging to demonstrate that early primary or secondary interventions can result in clear CVD risk reduction. There is a compelling need to carry out studies that will improve the long-term cardiovascular health of HCT survivors. These efforts can be facilitated through ongoing collaboration between the hematology and cardiology communities, establishing the next generation of CVD prevention studies in this increasing population of HCT survivors.

REFERENCES

1. Copelan EA. Hematopoietic stem-cell transplantation. N Engl J Med 2006;354(17):1813–26.
2. Wingard JR, Majhail NS, Brazauskas R, et al. Long-term survival and late deaths after allogeneic hematopoietic cell transplantation. J Clin Oncol 2011; 29(16):2230–9.
3. Bhatia S, Francisco L, Carter A, et al. Late mortality after allogeneic hematopoietic cell transplantation and functional status of long-term survivors: report from the Bone Marrow Transplant Survivor Study. Blood 2007;110(10):3784–92.
4. Bhatia S, Robison LL, Francisco L, et al. Late mortality in survivors of autologous hematopoietic-cell transplantation: report from the Bone Marrow Transplant Survivor Study. Blood 2005;105(11):4215–22.
5. Altekruse SF, Kosary CL, Krapcho M. SEER cancer statistics review, 1975–2007. 2010. Available at; http://seer.cancer.gov/csr/1975_2007. Accessed August 15, 2016.
6. Majhail NS, Tao L, Bredeson C, et al. Prevalence of hematopoietic cell transplant survivors in the United States. Biol Blood Marrow Transplant 2013;19(10): 1498–501.
7. Majhail NS, Rizzo JD. Surviving the cure: long term followup of hematopoietic cell transplant recipients. Bone Marrow Transplant 2013;48(9):1145–51.
8. Sun CL, Francisco L, Kawashima T, et al. Prevalence and predictors of chronic health conditions after hematopoietic cell transplantation: a report from the Bone Marrow Transplant Survivor Study. Blood 2010;116(17):3129–39.
9. Sun CL, Kersey JH, Francisco L, et al. Burden of morbidity in 10+ year survivors of hematopoietic cell transplantation: report from the bone marrow transplantation survivor study. Biol Blood Marrow Transplant 2013;19(7):1073–80.
10. Armenian SH, Chow EJ. Cardiovascular disease in survivors of hematopoietic cell transplantation. Cancer 2014;120(4):469–79.
11. Chow EJ, Anderson L, Baker KS, et al. Late effects surveillance recommendations among survivors of childhood hematopoietic cell transplantation: a children's oncology group report. Biol Blood Marrow Transplant 2016;22(5):782–95.
12. Henderson TO, Ness KK, Cohen HJ. Accelerated aging among cancer survivors: from pediatrics to geriatrics. Am Soc Clin Oncol Educ Book 2014;e423–30.
13. Cohen HJ. Keynote comment: cancer survivorship and ageing–a double whammy. Lancet Oncol 2006;7(11):882–3.
14. Campisi J. Aging, cellular senescence, and cancer. Annu Rev Physiol 2013;75:685–705.

15. Arora M, Sun CL, Ness KK, et al. Physiologic frailty in nonelderly hematopoietic cell transplantation patients: results from the Bone Marrow Transplant Survivor Study. JAMA Oncol 2016;2(10):1277–86.

16. Chow EJ, Mueller BA, Baker KS, et al. Cardiovascular hospitalizations and mortality among recipients of hematopoietic stem cell transplantation. Ann Intern Med 2011;155(1):21–32.

17. Chow EJ, Wong K, Lee SJ, et al. Late cardiovascular complications after hematopoietic cell transplantation. Biol Blood Marrow Transplant 2014; 20(6):794–800.

18. Chow EJ, Baker KS, Flowers ME, et al. Influence of metabolic traits and lifestyle factors on cardiovascular disease after hematopoietic cell transplantation. Biol Blood Marrow Transplant 2012;18:S226–7.

19. Armenian SH, Sun CL, Mills G, et al. Predictors of late cardiovascular complications in survivors of hematopoietic cell transplantation. Biol Blood Marrow Transplant 2010;16(8):1138–44.

20. Greenland P, Alpert JS, Beller GA, et al. ACCF/AHA guideline for assessment of cardiovascular risk in asymptomatic adults: a report of the American College of Cardiology Foundation/American Heart Association Task Force on Practice Guidelines. Circulation 2010;122(25):e584–636.

21. Koelwyn GJ, Khouri M, Mackey JR, et al. Running on empty: cardiovascular reserve capacity and late effects of therapy in cancer survivorship. J Clin Oncol 2012;30(36):4458–61.

22. Brilla CG, Maisch B. Regulation of the structural remodelling of the myocardium: from hypertrophy to heart failure. Eur Heart J 1994;15(Suppl D):45–52.

23. Ewer MS, Lenihan DJ. Left ventricular ejection fraction and cardiotoxicity: is our ear really to the ground? J Clin Oncol 2008;26(8):1201–3.

24. Wang TJ, Levy D, Benjamin EJ, et al. The epidemiology of "asymptomatic" left ventricular systolic dysfunction: implications for screening. Ann Intern Med 2003;138(11):907–16.

25. Wang TJ, Evans JC, Benjamin EJ, et al. Natural history of asymptomatic left ventricular systolic dysfunction in the community. Circulation 2003;108(8):977–82.

26. Balady GJ, Arena R, Sietsema K, et al. Clinician's Guide to cardiopulmonary exercise testing in adults: a scientific statement from the American Heart Association. Circulation 2010;122(2):191–225.

27. Malhotra R, Bakken K, D'Elia E, et al. Cardiopulmonary exercise testing in heart failure. JACC Heart Failure 2016;4(8):607–16.

28. Tuchman SA, Lane A, Hornsby WE, et al. Quantitative measures of physical functioning after autologous hematopoietic stem cell transplantation in multiple myeloma: a feasibility study. Clin Lymphoma Myeloma Leuk 2015;15(2):103–9.

29. Wood WA, Deal AM, Reeve BB, et al. Cardiopulmonary fitness in patients undergoing hematopoietic SCT: a pilot study. Bone Marrow Transplant 2013; 48(10):1342–9.

30. Kelsey CR, Scott JM, Lane A, et al. Cardiopulmonary exercise testing prior to myeloablative allo-SCT: a feasibility study. Bone Marrow Transplant 2014; 49(10):1330–6.

31. Armenian SH, Bhatia S. Cardiovascular disease after hematopoietic cell transplantation–lessons learned. Haematologica 2008;93(8):1132–6.

32. Braverman AC, Antin JH, Plappert MT, et al. Cyclophosphamide cardiotoxicity in bone marrow transplantation: a prospective evaluation of new dosing regimens. J Clin Oncol 1991;9(7):1215–23.

33. Armenian SH, Sun CL, Francisco L, et al. Late congestive heart failure after hematopoietic cell transplantation. J Clin Oncol 2008;26(34):5537–43.

34. Armenian SH, Sun CL, Shannon T, et al. Incidence and predictors of congestive heart failure after autologous hematopoietic cell transplantation. Blood 2011;118(23):6023–9.

35. Gianni L, Herman EH, Lipshultz SE, et al. Anthracycline cardiotoxicity: from bench to bedside. J Clin Oncol 2008;26(22):3777–84.

36. Lipshultz SE, Adams MJ, Colan SD, et al. Long-term Cardiovascular toxicity in children, adolescents, and young adults who receive cancer therapy: pathophysiology, course, monitoring, management, prevention, and research directions: a scientific statement from the American Heart Association. Circulation 2013;128(17):1927–95.

37. Lee PJ, Mallik R. Cardiovascular effects of radiation therapy: practical approach to radiation therapy-induced heart disease. Cardiol Rev 2005;13(2): 80–6.

38. Biedermann BC, Sahner S, Gregor M, et al. Endothelial injury mediated by cytotoxic T lymphocytes and loss of microvessels in chronic graft versus host disease. Lancet 2002;359(9323):2078–83.

39. Armenian SH, Sun CL, Vase T, et al. Cardiovascular risk factors in hematopoietic cell transplantation survivors: role in development of subsequent cardiovascular disease. Blood 2012;120(23):4505–12.

40. Baker KS, Ness KK, Steinberger J, et al. Diabetes, hypertension, and cardiovascular events in survivors of hematopoietic cell transplantation: a report from the bone marrow transplantation survivor study. Blood 2007;109(4):1765–72.

41. Hunt SA, Abraham WT, Chin MH, et al. 2009 focused update incorporated into the ACC/AHA 2005 Guidelines for the Diagnosis and Management of Heart Failure in Adults A Report of the American College of Cardiology Foundation/ American Heart Association Task Force on Practice Guidelines Developed in Collaboration With the International Society for Heart and Lung Transplantation. J Am Coll Cardiol 2009;53(15): e1–90.

42. Levy D, Larson MG, Vasan RS, et al. The progression from hypertension to congestive heart failure. JAMA 1996;275(20):1557–62.

43. Herman EH, el-Hage AN, Ferrans VJ, et al. Comparison of the severity of the chronic cardiotoxicity produced by doxorubicin in normotensive and hypertensive rats. Toxicol Appl Pharmacol 1985;78(2):202–14.

44. Giles TD, Sander GE. Diabetes mellitus and heart failure: basic mechanisms, clinical features, and therapeutic considerations. Cardiol Clin 2004;22(4):553–68.

45. Armenian SH, Bhatia S. Chronic health conditions in childhood cancer survivors: is it all treatment-related–or do genetics play a role? J Gen Intern Med 2009;24(Suppl 2):S395–400.

46. Armenian SH, Ding Y, Mills G, et al. Genetic susceptibility to anthracycline-related congestive heart failure in survivors of haematopoietic cell transplantation. Br J Haematol 2013;163(2):205–13.

47. Leger KJ, Cushing-Haugen K, Hansen JA, et al. Clinical and genetic determinants of cardiomyopathy risk among hematopoietic cell transplantation survivors. Biol Blood Marrow Transplant 2016;22(6):1094–101.

48. Rizzo JD, Wingard JR, Tichelli A, et al. Recommended screening and preventive practices for long-term survivors after hematopoietic cell transplantation: joint recommendations of the European Group for Blood and Marrow Transplantation, the Center for International Blood and Marrow Transplant Research, and the American Society of Blood and Marrow Transplantation. Biol Blood Marrow Transplant 2006;12(2):138–51.

49. Majhail NS, Rizzo JD, Lee SJ, et al. Recommended screening and preventive practices for long-term survivors after hematopoietic cell transplantation. Hematol Oncol Stem Cell Ther 2012;5(1):1–30.

50. Yahalom J, Portlock CS. Long-term cardiac and pulmonary complications of cancer therapy. Hematology 2008;22(2):305–18, vii.

51. Plana JC, Galderisi M, Barac A, et al. Expert consensus for multimodality imaging evaluation of adult patients during and after cancer therapy: a report from the American Society of Echocardiography and the European Association of Cardiovascular Imaging. J Am Soc Echocardiogr 2014;27(9):911–39.

52. Zamorano JL, Lancellotti P, Rodriguez Munoz D, et al. 2016 ESC Position Paper on cancer treatments and cardiovascular toxicity developed under the auspices of the ESC Committee for Practice Guidelines: the Task Force for Cancer Treatments and Cardiovascular Toxicity of the European Society of Cardiology (ESC). Eur J Heart Fail 2016;37(36):2768–801.

53. Blanchard CM, Courneya KS, Stein K. Cancer survivors' adherence to lifestyle behavior recommendations and associations with health-related quality of life: results from the American Cancer Society's SCS-II. J Clin Oncol 2008;26(13):2198–204.

54. Inoue-Choi M, Lazovich D, Prizment AE, et al. Adherence to the World Cancer Research Fund/American Institute for Cancer Research recommendations for cancer prevention is associated with better health-related quality of life among elderly female cancer survivors. J Clin Oncol 2013;31(14):1758–66.

55. Mosher CE, Lipkus I, Sloane R, et al. Long-term outcomes of the FRESH START trial: exploring the role of self-efficacy in cancer survivors' maintenance of dietary practices and physical activity. Psychooncology 2013;22(4):876–85.

56. Jones LW, Liu Q, Armstrong GT, et al. Exercise and risk of major cardiovascular events in adult survivors of childhood Hodgkin lymphoma: a report from the childhood cancer survivor study. J Clin Oncol 2014;32(32):3643–50.

57. Chow EJ, Baker KS, Lee SJ, et al. Influence of conventional cardiovascular risk factors and lifestyle characteristics on cardiovascular disease after hematopoietic cell transplantation. J Clin Oncol 2014;32(3):191–8.

58. U.S. Preventive Services Task Force Recommendations. Available at: https://www.uspreventiveservices taskforce.org/BrowseRec/Index. Accessed August 12, 2013.

59. Majhail NS, Rizzo JD, Lee SJ, et al. Recommended screening and preventive practices for long-term survivors after hematopoietic cell transplantation. Biol Blood Marrow Transplant 2012;18(3):348–71.

60. Landier W, Bhatia S, Eshelman DA, et al. Development of risk-based guidelines for pediatric cancer survivors: the children's oncology group long-term follow-up guidelines from the children's oncology group late effects committee and nursing discipline. J Clin Oncol 2004;22(24):4979–90.

61. Shankar SM, Marina N, Hudson MM, et al. Monitoring for cardiovascular disease in survivors of childhood cancer: report from the Cardiovascular Disease Task Force of the Children's Oncology Group. Pediatrics 2008;121(2):e387–396.

How to Develop a Cardio-Oncology Clinic

David Snipelisky, MD, Jae Yoon Park, MD, Amir Lerman, MD, Sharon Mulvagh, MD, Grace Lin, MD, Naveen Pereira, MD, Martin Rodriguez-Porcel, MD, Hector R. Villarraga, MD, Joerg Herrmann, MD*

KEYWORDS

- Cardio-oncology clinics • Cardio-oncology programs • Cardiotoxicity • Multidisciplinary practice

KEY POINTS

- Cardio-oncology is an evolving field and so is its clinical practice service line.
- Three milestones, each with 3 steps, are proposed as a road map to the successful implementation of a cardio-oncology clinic.
- Variant practice models and settings dictate the individual cardio-oncology clinic model.

EVOLUTION OF CARDIO-ONCOLOGY

Cancer and heart disease are the 2 leading causes of death and have been for some time in Western societies but continue to be viewed as 2 separate entities without much interaction. Interestingly, even though the prognosis of some cardiovascular diseases is worse than that of some cancers, the perception has usually been the opposite. Cancer has been perceived as universally fatal, and for this reason, historically, there has been a high acceptance rate of complications and comorbidities.[1–12] On this background, unwanted cardiovascular side effects of cancer therapies were relatively unrecognized until they were noted to be associated with dosing thresholds in patients receiving anthracycline therapy.[13] It was further recognized that an antecedent decline in left ventricular ejection fraction often heralded the clinical presentation of anthracycline-induced heart failure and that recognizing this trend and suspending therapy could potentially avert further asymptomatic or symptomatic loss of cardiac function.[14] Although a comfort level was reached for the management of the cardiotoxicity risk with anthracyclines during the active treatment period, it became apparent that there also was a late presentation of anthracycline cardiotoxicity. An exponential dose-effect relationship was identified and thereby created an opportunity for a cutoff selection of acceptable risk and benefit. This initially was thought to be accomplished at a cumulative dose of 550 mg/m^2 based on therapeutic efficacy and a predicted risk of clinical heart failure of 5% at this level. More than 2 decades later, however, it was recognized that anthracyclines were more cardiotoxic than initially appreciated, and cumulative doses of 450 mg/m^2 already yielded a 5% clinical heart failure risk.[15–17] Furthermore, significant interindividual differences were noted, and recent studies confirm that some patients have significant cardiotoxicity at doses well less than the deflection point of 300 mg/m^2 currently used, for instance, in the US Food and Drug Administration approval label for the cardioprotective agent dexrazoxane.[18]

Although the described evolution of anthracycline cardiotoxicity in itself is compelling, the completely unexpected occurrence of heart failure events in the pivotal trastuzumab metastatic

Conflicts of Interest: J. Herrmann participated in the 2014 and 2016 Ponatinib in CML Cardio-Oncology Advisory Board meeting organized by ARIAD Pharmaceuticals and is a member of the Institute for Cardio-Oncology advisory panel sponsored by Bristol-Myers Squib.
Department of Cardiovascular Diseases, Mayo Clinic, 200 First Street Southwest, Rochester, MN 55905, USA
* Corresponding author.
E-mail address: herrmann.joerg@mayo.edu

Heart Failure Clin 13 (2017) 347–359
http://dx.doi.org/10.1016/j.hfc.2016.12.011

breast cancer trial of 2001 generated the final momentum for greater attention to the cardiovascular care of cancer patients.[19] Development of symptomatic (New York Heart Association class III or IV) heart failure was the most important adverse event and occurred in 27% of patients with combined anthracycline, cyclophosphamide, and trastuzumab therapy (vs 8% in the group with anthracycline and cyclophosphamide). The impact of these findings was tremendous not only for the development of any future trials with HER-2 inhibitors but also for clinical practice leading to the implementation of every-3-month cardiac surveillance protocols for patients on trastuzumab therapy. Moreover, studies evaluating the mechanisms underlying this clinical observation led to completely new discoveries on the significance of HER-2 signaling for the heart.

A second group of targeted therapies, collectively called *tyrosine kinase inhibitors* emerged in the 1990s, similarly with the occurrence of unanticipated cardiovascular side effects that have continued to intrigue ever since. A recent prominent example is ponatinib, a BCR-Abl tyrosine kinase inhibitor used in patients with chronic myeloid leukemia, which has been found to cause adverse vascular events.[20] With anticancer therapeutics being the leading class in drug development and more than 1500 anticancer compounds in clinical trials currently,[21] one may postulate that (unexpected) cardiovascular side effects will continue to emerge. Furthermore, as preclinical screening is not as rigorous as it could be, newer anticancer therapies are poised to continue to create challenges in cardiovascular clinical practice for years to come.[22]

These developments have generated a level of complexity that is unprecedented, requiring familiarity with both the beneficial and the unwanted cardiovascular side effects of an ever-increasing number of chemotherapeutic agents. This fact is compounded by the increasing number of cardiovascular comorbidities or risk factors in the oncologic population presenting for cancer treatments. Such patients have a reduced cardiovascular reserve and require thorough pretreatment assessment, on-treatment management, and posttreatment care that is truly comprehensive and longitudinal.

Based on this escalating level of complexity in the care for cancer patients, a multidisciplinary approach has been enthusiastically embraced in recent years. This team-based approach is very much at odds with the classical 1-provider practice model of the universal physician who manages everything.[23] As a consequence, a multidisciplinary effort is sometimes viewed as fragmentation, not complementation. However, the goal of the cardio-oncology clinics should be to achieve complementation. Although it may be perceived as trivial, the mindset is key to how much any subspecialty is welcomed into the care of cancer patients in any given clinical practice. For the cardiovascular aspects, the integration of specialist care has become known as *cardio-oncology* or *onco-cardiology*. This care model has evolved and has been developed with examples on both sides of the provider equation. There has been a tremendous growth in the presence of cardio-oncology clinics in the United States over the last 5 years (Fig. 1).

In 2014, the American College of Cardiology Early Section on Cardio-Oncology conducted a nationwide online survey of more than 400 adult and pediatric cardiology division chiefs and fellowship program training directors with a response rate of 24%.[24] Of those who responded, and likely skewed to a group more familiar with the topic, the key responses were as follows. Most felt that this service line was important and would improve the care of patients but was largely not well developed. A significant number of participants did not feel confident in providing cardiovascular care to cancer patients and gave mostly an average rating to the understanding of the mutual impact of care on the individual disciplines. At the time of the survey, cardio-oncology activities fell within preoperative consultation services managed by general cardiology in one-third of the centers. Only one-quarter of centers had an established, specialized cardio-oncology service with multiple clinicians, 16% of respondents relied on a single cardiologist with expertise in this area, and 12% had plans to add a cardio-oncology service. Importantly, the following barriers to a cardio-oncology service line were mentioned: lack of national guidelines (44%), lack of funding (44%), limited interest/perceived value (38%), limited infrastructure (36%), and limited educational opportunities (29%). More than 40% of the programs had no formal training in cardio-oncology, whereas an equal number seemed to provide at least an exposure during regular clinical rotations. Only 11% offered lectures in cardio-oncology as part of a core curriculum. Most participants, however, stated that they would likely use educational material for their fellows and staff if those were available.[24] This article aims to address these needs, focusing on the cardio-oncology clinic.

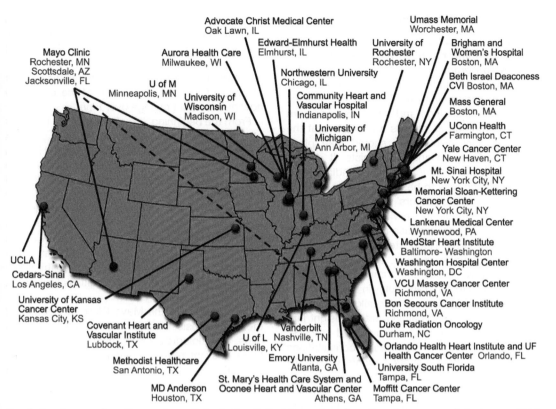

Fig. 1. Landscape of cardio-oncology clinics in the United States based on Google term search in August 2016.

CARDIO-ONCOLOGY CLINIC DEVELOPMENT

Although there is a general notion of benefit and advocacy as outlined above, the case for a cardio-oncology clinic is to be made at any given institution. In essence, there are only 3 broad categories or milestones to the development of cardio-oncology clinics, and all of these need to be successfully in place for a successful service line (Fig. 2). The first category of steps is related to the vision, the second to institutional support, and the third to establishing and growing the successful operation. It is important to emphasize that these are general recommendations, intended to provide an operational framework and that each institution should adapt to their own interest and feasibility.

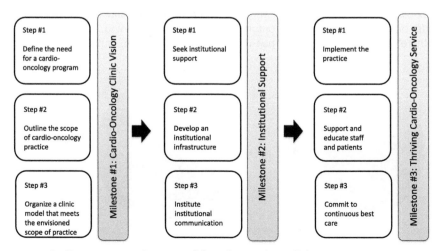

Fig. 2. Key steps and milestones toward a successful cardio-oncology clinic.

First Milestone: the Cardio-Oncology Clinic Vision

Step #1: defining the need for a cardio-oncology program

In the initial development of a cardio-oncology clinic, it is important to understand the specific needs of the institution and what resources are available. Through all phases and starting at the beginning, joint discussions should take place among cardiologists and oncologists. It is truly important to gain a complete understanding of patient needs and how to best deliver care to these patients.[25,26] At the authors' institution, the initial decision was made to provide cardio-oncology e-consultations only because many patients seen at the Mayo Clinic Rochester are referred from different geographic regions, and a model was needed that would guarantee consultative advice within 24 hours to avoid any delay in treatment recommendations. This model also allowed for education of the staff and gaining further insight into the needs and demands on the clinical practice. Intriguingly, although the virtual consultations were in place, many cancer patients would still be referred to various cardiology clinics indicating that face-to-face consultations were very much desired by the patient or the provider. This impression was confirmed by a survey conducted among oncologists and hematologists. Although the need for formal encounters became clear, the specific model to provide this care was not so apparent. One challenge already alluded to was the generation of a clinic model that can provide access on a daily basis rather than restricting access to 1 full or half day per week. Thus, we decided to create 1 consultation appointment per day for cardio-oncology patients that would become available for other patients if not requested in a timely fashion. This model worked well, allowing for availability and flexibility without any additional burden for the provider or institution. However, it outgrew its capacity; therefore, we added a regular half-day weekly clinic. This change was also pursued in an effort to grant the clinic more physical presence and to lay the foundation for an education and training program. Accordingly, it would be our recommendation that specific attention needs to be paid to the dynamic nature of the clinic and how needs might change over time.

From the beginning, it is also important to reflect on the patient population expected to be seen. At the Cardiac Oncology Clinic of the Ottawa Hospital Cancer Center, for instance, the leading population has been breast cancer patients (nearly 60%) and the leading reasons for referral have been a decline in cardiac function, cardiomyopathy, or heart failure (>40%).[27] These data matched well our initial experience; however, since the institution of the half-day clinic, the referral pattern has changed at our institution and is now evenly split into thirds between breast cancer, hematologic malignancies, and other cancers (Fig. 3).

Interestingly, at the Mayo Clinic in Rochester, the amyloidosis clinic is staffed by hematologists, cardiologists, and nephrologists; thus, there has not been a need to refer this patient population to the cardio-oncology clinic. This might not be and has not been the case for other institutions. It, therefore, needs to be defined which patients and disease patterns oncologists and hematologists would like to refer to a clinic with additional cardiovascular specialist care. Clearly, this action will define demands on practice, education, and staffing.

Step #2: outlining the scope of cardio-oncology practice

Referral population and cancer types are the leading factors that determine the cardiovascular disease spectrum to be encountered and addressed. Indeed, it is important to draw attention to this subject and to set the expectations from the beginning. For instance, risk assessment, mitigation, or management of trastuzumab

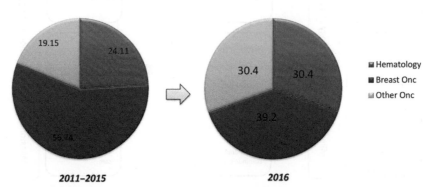

2011–2015   *2016*

Fig. 3. Change in referral population to the cardio-oncology clinic at the Mayo Clinic Rochester over time.

cardiotoxicity is a classic example of what to expect and to address with a high level of proficiency in a cardio-oncology care at a primary breast cancer center. This action, however, will likely not be the prime expectation at a primary hematologic malignancy center, where other drugs might relate to cardiotoxicity. In fact, numerous other challenges may coexist such as vascular toxicities. The same might be true for centers preferentially providing care for gastrointestinal malignancies and renal cell carcinomas, for which vascular endothelial growth factor receptor pathway inhibitors are used and hypertension and QTc prolongation often become important topics. Because the spectrum of cardio-oncology is truly broad, the specific scope of practice should be envisioned upfront for the cardio-oncology clinic to be optimally prepared to address the clinical needs and to meet its expectations.

Conversations need to take place among cardiologists and oncologists on this matter early on, and these discussions should take into account the initiation of a cardio-oncology clinic and evaluate its progression. As the clinic progresses, expansion should be done carefully and slowly, as this type of subspecialty clinic is different to many others. A multidisciplinary approach is key, and continued discussion among all subspecialists remains important throughout.[23] Additionally, both oncologists and cardiologists should discuss ancillary services that may be offered, including palliative care resources, rehabilitation, and family support. The concept of such a specialized clinic should stem from the need to provide timely and complete care for patients.[25,26]

Step #3: organizing a clinic model that meets the envisioned scope of practice

Once the needs and scope of practice are defined, the best-suited staffing model can be outlined. Although cardio-oncology clinics have been primarily staffed by cardiologists,[28] this is by no means a set rule, and cardio-oncology clinics can be and have been staffed by either cardiologists or oncologists, as long as the provider is well versed in cardio-oncology. An oncologist/hematologist may take this aspect of care on and consult with cardiologists on demand. Other institutions may prefer to staff this clinic by oncologists and cardiologists, without one subspecialty being dominant. Such design needs to be consistent with the underlying needs of the program and resources available, as each design brings forth different pros and cons and implications for practice (Fig. 4). Institutions may also consider including nurses, nurse practitioners, physician assistants, and pharmacists. This activity likely will depend on the patient volume and the overall integration of the clinic into patient care. Finally, one may add that the specific clinic models could be envisioned as interacting with centers of

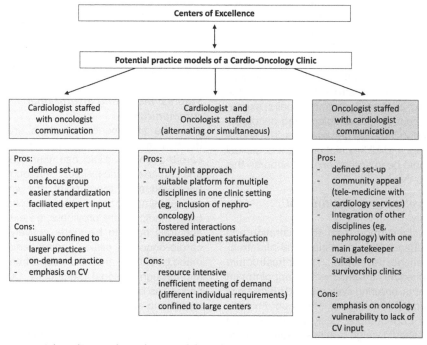

Fig. 4. Three potential cardio-oncology clinic models with potential supplementation by centers of excellence.

excellence. Although not in wide use yet, this may, indeed, be an attractive venue, especially for nonacademic centers.

Importantly, most of the cardio-oncology clinics have started at academic centers,[28] despite the fact that most malignancies are being treated in the community setting. Building adequate infrastructure and developing resources for this type of practice should be an important initiative in the future as further outlined below. The third, oncologist-driven model might be appealing for this setting with expansion of virtual or Web-based consultations, possibly in the context of a larger affiliated care network.

Second Milestone: The Institutional Support for the Cardio-Oncology Clinic

Step #1: seeking institutional support

Once the need, the scope, and the shape of the cardio-oncology clinic are defined, the next milestone is to secure institutional support. For decades, oncologists and hematologists have managed all aspects of the care of cancer patients, and this mindset may need to be addressed. Furthermore, implementing a new clinic includes far more than physicians interested in this field. These providers would have less time for other tasks, and their work (effort) allocations will require reassessment. Additional staffing for appointment coordinators, desk staff, nurses, nurse practitioners, and pharmacists may be required. It thereby becomes an investment for the institution, and from an administrative perspective, one would like to see a cardio-oncology unit be well justified, planned, and presented, which is why the first milestone is so important and cannot be emphasized enough. In addition to support from the hospital administration, there needs to be strong support from the leadership (eg, division/department chairs, executive committees) of the cardiology and oncology/hematology divisions and departments. The scope is far reaching, and all key stakeholders of clinical practice should be in agreement and endorse this clinic for it to thrive.

Step #2: developing an institutional infrastructure

With the crucial support from administration and departmental leadership, an institutional infrastructure can then be developed. This infrastructure includes schedule arrangements, appointment referral patterns, ordering systems, and triage algorithms. Operation managers, staff coordinators, appointment coordinators, desk attendants, and many others should weigh in at this stage to create the best possible practice flow. Input from cardiology and oncology specialties is required in this process, and once the direction of work flow is clear, this input needs to become very concrete. Again, having a clear concept of the clinical model is of utmost importance. Would the oncology/hematology division/department refer or defer to the cardiology department? Who would have access to the calendars? Who would have scheduling privileges? Are there triage algorithms to be followed (Fig. 5)? How can the process be streamlined? In this context, the physical location of the cardio-oncology clinic itself needs to be well thought through. Should it be in a cancer center or in the cardiology center? Both settings have their own pros and cons outlined in a recent review (Table 1).[29] As mentioned earlier, one particular logistic challenge often is to provide timely consultations. Ideally, a cardio-oncology service line would be available 24/7, but this is often not practical, at least not at primary noncancer centers and in the early stages of the clinic when the infrastructure is still developing and the number of specialists may still be small. It is also a question whether the service line should be strictly outpatient or also inpatient, whether it should be combined with the general inpatient or outpatient cardiology consultation service. The benefit may be the gradual infiltration of practice over time and engagement and education of multiple providers. The disadvantage would be reduced specialization given the context of greater generalization. Either way, a key point is that an infrastructure should be laid that will be absolutely functional, fully operational, and rewarding. For this, it is advisable to start with a volume/scope that is comfortably manageable from all aspects of care rather than overcommitting and not meeting expectations at the end.

Step #3: instituting institutional communication

After the aforementioned steps are taken and the infrastructure is approved and in place, the cardio-oncology clinic can then be announced and made accessible. Although possibly perceived as a moot point, the importance of announcement cannot be overemphasized. Typically, medical care providers are extremely busy and thus need to be made actively aware of a cardio-oncology clinic. Announcements can be made by E-mail, at division/department meetings, and through personal interactions. Our own experience has been that the former 2 require multiple repetitions and personal interactions but far surpass all other means of communication. Accordingly, it might be best to cooperate with one specific provider or provider group and allow for

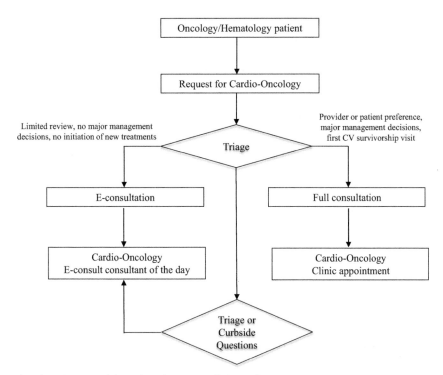

Fig. 5. Example of a triage model used at the Mayo Clinic Rochester.

future expansion. The personal note is key, and it is about establishing a working relationship. In addition, presentations at multidisciplinary grand rounds and division/department meetings, which introduce the concept, need, and goals of the cardio-oncology practice, are very effective in educating all colleagues about this emerging discipline.

Third Milestone: the Thriving Cardio-Oncology Service

Step #1: implementing the practice
The first day of practice is always exciting, and the goal is to maintain this momentum. With all of the prior steps being taken, the referral of patients should be adequately set up. The key next step is then to refine the clinical practice and meet the provider and patient needs. This refinement may entail development of best practice patterns, standardization of care, and communication models with the referring providers.

Regarding the latter, each clinic should ensure that clinical data regarding treatments and diagnostic studies are shared efficiently among all providers involved in the care system. A system for exchange of such information should be set up and easily accessible. Many institutions have a shared electronic medical record that allows for this, yet in some circumstances in which a shared medical record system does not yet exist, it will be crucial for providers to decide on how to share information efficiently. Medication records should be updated, and each clinic must have personnel to ensure this takes place. Both cardiac and oncologic medication regimens can be very dynamic and, considering patients are generally on numerous medications, it should not be left up to the patient to share this information among providers. Providers in cardio-oncology clinics should also have scheduled time set aside to allow for communication among all teams involved in the care of a specific patient, especially considering that compromises may need to be made in the extent of treatment, or discontinuation of treatment, and well-thought out management plans should be entertained and discussed based on patients' wishes.[25,26]

Another important aspect is the standardization of clinical processes and care.[25] Algorithms that are based on expert consensus are often embraced, and most of these are available for the topics initially of greatest concerns such as cardio-toxicity, QTc prolongation, and hypertension but less so for others such as vascular toxicity.[7] Although not to be mistaken as a program to be executed without reflection, these efforts pursue the goal that regardless of circumstances, patients referred to the cardio-oncology unit will receive the same and highest possible

Table 1
Pros and cons of a cardio-oncology clinic location

	Cardio-Oncology Clinic in Cardiovascular Center	Cardio-Oncology Clinic in Cancer Center
Pros	• Support staff that are familiar with the spectrum of cardiovascular disease • Patient and provider proximity to cardiovascular services such as ECG and echocardiography services	• Easy patient access to cardio-oncology • Capacity for more comprehensive patient care • Improved contact with the oncologists for immediate questions, consultations, and tumor board opinions, and a generally more inclusive care of the cancer patient
Cons	• Loss of exclusivity to the special needs of the cancer patient • Lack of awareness by the oncologists about a special cardiology service dedicated to serving their patients • Less spontaneous consultations and interactions between oncologists and serving cardiologist(s), which may hamper the evolution of a comprehensive service	• Limited access to cardiovascular studies such as ECG, echocardiography, and stress tests (depending on size and funding in institution) • Less availability of staff trained in performing ECGs/other cardiac studies, and can answer cardiac questions/educate patients on cardiac care
Circumvent the cons	• The cardiologist should be proactive in fostering relationships with the oncologist and the oncology team • Attendance and contribution to tumor board conferences and oncology grand rounds with the goal of integrating the cardio-oncologist into the day-to-day practices of the oncology team • Additional training of the cardiology clinic staff, including knowledge of common chemotherapies with relevance to cardiovascular health, need for more frequent monitoring, and psychosocial needs of the cancer patient	• ECG and possibly echocardiography machine(s)/services in the cancer center to effect more efficient cardiovascular diagnosis and care of these patients • Institute effective transportation between the cardiac imaging center and oncology clinic • Train oncology staff in cardiovascular care and assistance (including performing ECGs)

Abbreviation: ECG, electrocardiogram.

From Okwuosa TM, Barac A. Burgeoning cardio-oncology programs: challenges and opportunities for early career cardiologists/faculty directors. J Am Coll Cardiol 2015;66(10):1196; with permission.

standard of care. Not surprisingly for a relatively new area, most of the "standard process of care," whether related to surveillance or treatment efficacy, are based on expert consensus, rather than randomized clinical trials. We are not advocating that we should wait for randomized, controlled trials, as patients cannot wait, but we should be careful in the implementation of these recommendations and consider them within the broader scope of care, including comorbidities and costs. Regarding costs of care, some recommendations may not be as relevant, whereas others (eg, imaging) may significantly alter the cost/benefit ratio.

Meetings with all providers engaged in the clinic are advisable to reach a consensus on institutional practice. Again, the team approach

cannot be overemphasized, and it might be furthermore advisable to have a team of different cardiovascular specialists. Our cardio-oncology group practice, for instance, integrates cardiovascular specialists in echocardiography, nuclear imaging, vascular interventions, and advanced heart failure therapy. This mosaic approach combines the best of many disciplines and generates novel ideas and well-balanced approaches to the field.

Step #2: supporting and educating staff and patients

Given the existing near vacuum in cardio-oncology practice, there is a need for a continuous support structure and education. Indeed, the educational aspect of a cardio-oncology clinic is another feature that differentiates this subspecialty clinic from general cardiology and hematology/oncology clinics. As discussed, most guidelines for the treatment of cardiac dysfunction in cancer patients evolved from expert consensus and a limited number of studies, many of which being retrospective reviews or limited prospective trials. Additionally, training programs have limited opportunities for trainees to gain additional experience in cardio-oncology. Therefore, it is important to establish educational opportunities for all health care team members involved.

It is also recommended that each cardio-oncology clinic schedules regular sessions to discuss difficult cases and enables teaching opportunities to arise from these sessions. All team members involved in the care of these patients should be engaged and discussions should reflect on not only the medical management but other aspects including quality of life and patient perception. Opportunities for attending formal seminars and symposiums should be available, particularly considering cardio-oncology is still evolving and management paradigms are continuously changing.

Education and support also needs to be considered for patients with readily available resources. Cardio-oncology clinics should provide opportunities for patients to learn more about their disease processes and how cardiovascular and oncologic treatments can affect each other. Teaching material, including educational Web sites and pamphlets, should be made available. Clinics can also consider individual and group sessions for patients and community events. There are several practical measures to support a cardio-oncology clinic at any given institution as summarized in Table 2.[29]

Step #3: committing to continuous best care

The most important aspect and primary reason for creating a cardio-oncology clinic is to offer an integrated multidisciplinary approach to care.[23] Continued communication needs to take place among all parties involved in a patient's care (Fig. 6). A cardio-oncology clinic thrives on optimal coordination of care and should allow for continued conversations to take place that will put the needs of the patients first. It needs to be a priority to ensure that all systems within the clinic support both the oncologic and cardiovascular practices, and discussions among all parties involved can help tailor this approach (see Fig. 6). True engagement is a prerequisite, and it pertains to the cardiologists to have a strong interest in providing the best care and to commit to lifelong learning and the oncologists/hematologists to

identify needs and opportunities and to engage in the dialogue. Cardio-oncology was born out of the need for communication as patients were declaring themselves with unanticipated heart failure presentations. It has since then evolved and will continue to do so. Accordingly, there needs to be a commitment to move the borders and to further advance the care for the best of the patients.

CARDIO-ONCOLOGY: THE ROAD AHEAD

Cardio-oncology has gained momentum, and the number of cardio-oncology clinics is increasing in the United States and globally. This dynamic by itself should help foster the development of additional clinics across the globe. As outlined herein, for this line of service to succeed long-term, it is to be planned carefully from the beginning. Despite the global trend, critics might argue that there is no proof of its value and, especially, cost effectiveness; that it might lose interest over time; and that the scope of work is temporary and changing with new drug developments and improvements in radiation techniques. Accordingly, one may argue that cardio-oncology is a "trendy" discipline that will be present only for the time being.

The road ahead should, therefore, include assessments of the value of the cardio-oncology service line, which can be done by various means and outcome variables. Positive results would strengthen the case for this service line. Even more so then, there needs to be further development of the infrastructure and assistance for institutions planning to add this line of service, especially easier access for community practices and smaller institutions. Moreover, there needs to be further consensus on how these patients are best managed, and once defined, outcomes assessments will become readily available.

One particular area in need pertains to survivorship. Although several position papers have outlined algorithms for the surveillance and management of cancer patients during therapy, the recommendations are less clear for the cardiovascular care after completion of therapy. One exception is the recommendations on the monitoring of patients after radiation therapy, which were initially outlined by an expert panel of the European Association of Cardiovascular Imaging and the American Society of Echocardiography and then extended to also include vascular toxicity by a Society for Cardiac Angiography and Interventions expert panel.[30,31] Various recommendations for childhood cancer survivors have been given, and an international harmonization attempt has been

Table 2
Measures to facilitate a cardio-oncology service line

Process Measures	Methods
Creating awareness	• Educating and establishing cognizance of the necessity for cardio-oncology within the entire hospital, including other physicians,[a] physician extenders,[b] nurses, and administrative staff, including the hospital leaders and decision makers • May involve multiple presentations on the necessity for and embodiment of cardio-oncology at different forums, including hospital grand rounds, various administrative committees, and hospital symposia • The onco-cardiologist should be prepared to attend (and even seek) meetings with leadership and be prepared with relevant highlights on what necessitates this field
Patient education	• Seminars, community events, symposia • Informs patients to be attentive to the downstream effects of their cancer therapy • Patients are generally interested in learning how to care for their health and may seek out the onco-cardiologist especially for this reason
Hospital staff education	• Includes teaching and providing educational materials on cardio-oncology; cardiovascular risks of cancer therapeutic agents; diagnoses, management, and treatment; when to refer to cardio-oncology; and updates in the published data • Lectures on various cardio-oncology topics should be provided to medical trainees and house staff[c]
Organizing a comprehensive program	• Should involve exchange of patient information with discussions and updates on change in clinical status[d]
Input at oncology forums	• Includes tumor board conferences and oncology grand rounds • Makes for more comprehensive decision making on cancer therapies and overall patient care; oncologists value this sort of input
Providing evidence of growth	• Eventually necessary to convince administration of the need for cardio-oncology[e] • Alerts administration to the need for resources or the fact that already provided resources are being applied in a constructive manner
Providing outcome data	• Providing data on better patient outcomes as a result of the establishment of a cardio-oncology clinic would provide the ultimate driving force for establishment and growth of the program

[a] Oncologists, cardiologists, primary care physicians.
[b] Nurse practitioners/physician assistants.
[c] Including medical students, residents, fellows, other cardiologists, oncologists, general practitioners, and medical support staff including oncology nurses, nurse practitioners, and physician assistants.
[d] Should include the onco-cardiologist, the oncologist, and their support staff, particularly the nurses, nurse practitioners and physician assistants, pharmacist, social services (psychosocial oncology, case managers, and social workers), rehabilitation services (such as cardiac rehabilitation, physical therapy), nutritionist, and palliative care; creation of algorithms for patient education, management, and referrals with special cancer programs such as the cancer survivorship clinic. In turn, attendance at these tumor board conferences and oncology grand rounds helps provide some perspective with respect to patient management from an oncology standpoint, while informing the onco-cardiologist on (previously unknown) characteristics of existing cancer therapies in addition to expectations for newer ones.
[e] Demonstration of growth of cardiovascular services, such as echocardiography or cardiac magnetic resonance imaging referrals, linked to cardio-oncology is generally encouraging to any institution.
From Okwuosa TM, Akhter N, Williams KA, et al. Building a cardio-oncology program in a small to medium-sized, non-primary cancer center, academic hospital in the USA: challenges and pitfalls. Future Cardiol 2015;11:1–8; with permission.

pursued but not necessarily with universal acceptance. It remains a question in general how these patients are to be followed as they transition from pediatric to adult care. Triaging patients early into cardio-oncology programs may address this need and any gaps in care for these patients. It has been recommended that cancer patients who received higher anthracycline and radiation exposure or the combination of the 2 and those planning competitive sports or pregnancy should

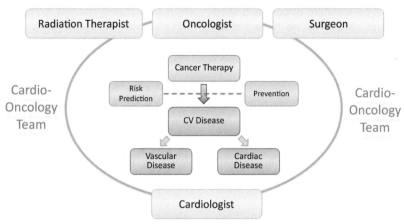

Fig. 6. Multidisciplinary nature of the cardio-oncology care team.

be seen by a cardiologist. However, as cardio-oncology clinics are taking shape, so may their role in survivorship care. In fact, formal recommendations in this regard are expected to be released soon with endorsement of the American Society of Clinical Oncology.

Another area in which cardio-oncology clinics and the field in general need to grow relates to the entire spectrum of cardiovascular diseases. There has been a focus on cardiotoxicity but vascular toxicity, arrhythmias, and valvular heart and pericardial disease are also daily realities. These are areas in need of definition, even more so than the aspect of cardiotoxicity, which also still requires refinement. Accordingly, although the initial impetus came from cases of cardiomyopathy and heart failure, the road ahead is not a single path without cross-roads and intersections. A broad perspective and development of the field and its clinics needs to be kept in mind and fostered. Ideally, this should also include facilitating research in this area.

As alluded to above, there is a need to further develop training of those engaging in the cardio-oncology practice. The International Cardiooncology Society and Canadian Cardiac Oncology Network outlined a proposal that defines the disciplines and goals of training and structure of the fellowship program. Although intended for those in training, this document also provides an excellent proficiency outline for anyone engaged in this practice. At the current time, details regarding proficiency milestones, qualification, and recertification requirements are yet evolving, and the following key questions remain. Should there be a unique credentialing process or should cardio-oncology become a requirement within fellowship training? If its own unique training program, should it be within cardiology or oncology or both?

Finally, as minute as it might be perceived, reimbursement is an important aspect of health care, and questions have been raised regarding how cardio-oncology consultations, subsequent care, and unique testing would be reimbursed or if claims might get denied. In this context, it is important to point out that specialist care such as heart failure consultations are reimbursed even if the patient was already seen by a general cardiologist; the same seems to be applicable to cardio-oncology. Serial echocardiograms have been rated as "appropriate" for monitoring of cardiotoxicity during chemotherapy in the American Society of Echocardiography Appropriate Use Criteria document. Further emergence of guidelines, consensus and position papers should only be helpful in this regard.

SUMMARY

Cardio-oncology has evolved much over the last decade and is expected to continue to do so even more in the upcoming years. Formal organizations and committees have been created and recognize the dynamic nature of this field. Ongoing clinical research will help providers continue to deliver the best care possible to patients with cardiac manifestations of oncologic treatment. With recognition for the need and continual addition of cardio-oncology clinics, patients should, increasingly, receive optimal care to prevent the onset and progression of cardiovascular toxicities. Even more, from a training perspective, emphasis has been given to formalization of training programs within cardio-oncology, as current resources for trainees can be limited.[29] As such, cardio-oncology will continue to progress and, ultimately, optimize the clinical care of cancer patients. What will the cardio-oncology clinic look like in 2020? Will it be standard of care and will it have a standard of care? Will we have cardio-oncology board certified providers? It will be exciting to see this discipline evolve to a mature subspecialty.

REFERENCES

1. Ky B, Vejpongsa P, Yeh ET, et al. Emerging paradigms in cardiomyopathies associated with cancer therapies. Circ Res 2013;113:754–64.
2. Nolan MT, Lowenthal RM, Venn A, et al. Chemotherapy-related cardiomyopathy: a neglected aspect of cancer survivorship. Intern Med J 2014;44:939–50.
3. Cardinale D, Colombo A, Lamantia G, et al. Cardio-oncology: a new medical issue. Ecancermedicalscience 2008;2:126.
4. Ewer M, Ewer SM. Cardiotoxicity of anticancer treatments. Nat Rev Cardiol 2015;12:620.
5. Ewer M, Ewer SM. Cardiotoxicity of anticancer treatments: what the cardiologist needs to know. Nat Rev Cardiol 2010;7:564–75.
6. Yeh ET, Bickford CL. Cardiovascular complications of cancer therapy: incidence, pathogenesis, diagnosis, and management. J Am Coll Cardiol 2009; 53:2231–47.
7. Herrmann J, Lerman A, Sandhu NP, et al. Evaluation and management of patients with heart disease and cancer: cardio-oncology. Mayo Clin Proc 2014;89: 1287–306.
8. Herrmann JLA. An update on cardio-oncology. Trends Cardiovasc Med 2014;24:285–95.
9. Yeh ET, Chang HM. Oncocardiology - past, present, and future: a review. JAMA Cardiol 2016. [Epub ahead of print].
10. Albini A, Pennesi G, Donatelli F, et al. Cardiotoxicity of anticancer drugs: the need for cardio-oncology and cardio-oncological prevention. J Natl Cancer Inst 2010;102:14–25.
11. Eschenhagen T, Force T, Ewer MS, et al. Cardiovascular side effects of cancer therapies: a position statement fromthe Heart Failure Association of the European Society of Cardiology. Eur J Heart Fail 2011;13:1–10.
12. Plana JC, Galderisi M, Barac A, et al. Expert consensus for multimodality imaging evaluation of adult patients during and after cancer therapy: a report from the American Society of Echocardiography and the European Association of Cardiovascular Imaging. J Am Soc Echocardiogr 2014;27:911–39.
13. Lefrak EA, Pitha J, Rosenheim S, et al. A clinicopathologic analysis of adriamycin cardiotoxicity. Cancer 1973;32:302–14.
14. Alexander J, Dainiak N, Berger HJ, et al. Serial assessment of doxorubicin cardiotoxicity with quantiative radionuclide angiocardiography. N Engl J Med 1979;300:278–83.
15. Ewer MS, Von Hoff DD, Benjamin RS. A historical perspective of anthracycline cardiotoxicity. Heart Fail Clin 2011;7:363–72.
16. Von Hoff DD, Layard MW, Basa P, et al. Risk factors for doxorubicin-induced congestive heart failure. Ann Intern Med 1979;91:710–7.
17. Swain SM, Whaley FS, Ewer MS. Congestive heart failure in patients treated with doxorubicin: a retrospective analysis of three trials. Cancer 2003;97: 2869–79.
18. Nysom K, Holm K, Lipsitz SR, et al. Relationship between cumulative anthracycline dose and late cardiotoxicity in childhood acute lymphoblastic leukemia. J Clin Oncol 1998;16(2):545–50.
19. Slamon DJ, Leyland-Jones B, Shak S, et al. Use of chemotherapy plus a monoclonal antibody against HER2 for metastatic breast cancer that overexpresses HER2. N Engl J Med 2001;344:783–92.
20. Herrmann J. Tyrosine kinase inhibitors and vascular toxicity: impetus for a classification system? Curr Oncol Rep 2016;18:33.
21. Moses H 3rd, Matheson DH, Cairns-Smith S, et al. The anatomy of medical research: US and international comparisons. JAMA 2015;313:174–89.
22. Ferri N, Siegl P, Corsini A, et al. Drug attrition during pre-clinical and clinical development: understanding and managing drug-induced cardiotoxicity. Pharmacol Ther 2013;138:470–84.
23. Fleissig AJV, Catt S, Fallowfield L. Multidisciplinary teams in cancer care: are they effective in the UK? Lancet Oncol 2006;7:935–43.
24. Barac A, Murtagh G, Carver JR, et al. Cardiovascular health of patients with cancer and cancer survivors: a roadmap to the next level. J Am Coll Cardiol 2015;65: 2739–46.
25. Barros-Gomes S, Herrmann J, Mulvagh SL, et al. Rationale for setting up a cardio-oncology unit: our experience at Mayo Clinic. Cardiooncology 2016;2:1–9.
26. Gujral DM, Manisty C, Lloyd G, et al. Organisation & models of cardio-oncology clinics. Int J Cardiol 2016;214:381–2.
27. Sulpher J, Mathur S, Graham N, et al. Clinical experience of patients referred to a multidisciplinary Cardiac Oncology Clinic: an observational study. J Oncol 2015;2015:671232.
28. Sulpher J, Mathur S, Lenihan D, et al. An international survey of health care providers involved in the management of cancer patients exposed to cardiotoxic therapy. J Oncol 2015;2015:391848.
29. Okwuosa T, Barac A. Burgeoning cardio-oncology programs: challenges and opportunities for early career cardiologists/faculty directors. J Am Coll Cardiol 2015;66:1193–7.
30. Lancellotti P, Nkomo VT, Badano LP, et al. Expert consensus for multi-modality imaging evaluation of cardiovascular complications of radiotherapy in adults: a report from the European Association of

Cardiovascular Imaging and the American Society of Echocardiography. J Am Soc Echocardiogr 2013;26:1013–32.

31. Iliescu C, Grines CL, Herrmann J, et al. SCAI expert consensus statement: Evaluation, management, and special considerations of cardio-oncology patients in the cardiac catheterization laboratory (Endorsed by the Cardiological Society of India, and Sociedad Latino Americana de Cardiologia Intervencionista). Catheter Cardiovasc Interv 2016;87:895–9.

How to Develop a Cardio-oncology Fellowship

Michelle N. Johnson, MD, MPH[a],*, Richard Steingart, MD[a], Joseph Carver, MD[b]

KEYWORDS

- Cardio-oncology • Fellowship • Cardiovascular disease • Cancer therapeutics

KEY POINTS

- The areas of knowledge required to manage cardiovascular disease in patients with cancer and cancer survivors include specific cardiovascular complications directly related to oncologic therapies and the impact of cancer and its therapies on existing or potential cardiovascular comorbidities, including atherosclerosis, valvular disease, and myocardial disease.
- The cardio-oncology training milieu, the selection process for cardio-oncology trainees, and the cardio-oncology training curriculum must emphasize consultation, education, and research skills.
- Robust fellowship programs are best supported by high-volume centers that can provide a critical mass of patient clinician exposures.
- To date, cardio-oncology fellowships have been pursued and completed by cardiologists and internists but future training models would also include programs designed for oncologists, family medicine specialists, and physician extenders.
- The curriculum for cardio-oncology should be structured with core competency-based goals in a manner that is in keeping with the Accreditation Council for Graduate Medical Education and American College of Cardiology's Core Cardiovascular Training Statements directives. These milestones/goals can best be accomplished through a 1-year immersion fellowship with a combination of inpatient and outpatient exposure.

Management of cardiovascular disease in patients with cancer and cancer survivors requires particular clinical expertise; skills that are central to cardio-oncology.[1] The areas of knowledge required include (1) specific cardiovascular complications directly related to oncologic therapies (eg, hypertension associated with vascular endothelial growth factor (VEGF) signaling pathway inhibitors, left ventricular dysfunction caused by anthracyclines, radiation-related vascular disease) and (2) the impact of cancer and its therapies on existing or potential cardiovascular comorbidities, including atherosclerosis, valvular disease, and myocardial disease.[2] The past decade has seen rapid expansion of cancer therapeutics, many of which have potential cardiotoxicity. In addition,

the conversion of many cancers to chronic conditions, rather than uniformly fatal diseases, has produced an ever-expanding population of patients with cancer at high risk for cardiovascular diseases that require specialized knowledge of treating physicians. Thus, there is a compelling need for enhanced cardio-oncology training.

Historically, oncologists were the predominant long-term providers for patients with cardiovascular comorbidities during active cancer treatment, as well as for survivors. With advances in cardiovascular medicine (drugs, devices, interventions) leading to greatly improved survival in recent years, it is unrealistic to expect that practicing oncologists could provide state-of-the-art care of their patients' cardiovascular disease. In 2014

[a] Department of Medicine, Memorial Sloan-Kettering Cancer Center, 1275 York Avenue, New York, NY 10021, USA; [b] Department of Medicine, Abramson Cancer Center, University of Pennsylvania, 3400 Civic Center Boulevard, Philadelphia, PA 19104, USA
* Corresponding author.
E-mail address: johnsom1@mskcc.org

Heart Failure Clin 13 (2017) 361–366
http://dx.doi.org/10.1016/j.hfc.2016.12.012
1551-7136/17/© 2016 Elsevier Inc. All rights reserved.

there were 14 million cancer patients in the United States and estimates are that there will be more than a 20% increase in cancer rates by 2020 caused by the aging of the population.[3] The number of cancer survivors is also increasing, with predictions forecasting approximately 21 million cancer survivors by 2024.[4–6] Significant comorbidities in cancer survivors include heart failure and diabetes and, as they age, there is increased incidence of comorbidities such as atrial fibrillation and hypertension.[4,7,8] Medical management in survivors will require increasing skills in these areas. Thus it becomes imperative that there is the development of the discipline of cardio-oncology.[9,10]

There is a severe staffing shortage anticipated in oncology services, with decreasing numbers of practicing oncologists in the setting of increased rates of cancer.[11,12] This dynamic will require that more of the cardiovascular conditions related to cancer and its treatments be treated by advanced practice practitioners, internists, family medicine physicians, geriatricians, and cardiologists. Patients with particularly complex cardiovascular problems related to cancer and its treatments will require care by cardio-oncology experts.

In a recent survey of adult and pediatric cardiology division chiefs and fellowship directors, 52% agreed that a cardio-oncology service or dedicated clinician would improve the care of patients with cancer.[10] Cardio-oncology fellowship training develops this coterie of clinicians. Such fellowships are designed to offer a tertiary level of training beyond cardiovascular diseases fellowships.[13] This additional training is necessary because at present more than 40% of cardiovascular training programs report having no formal training in cardio-oncology, and only 11% included lectures on cardio-oncology as part of the core curriculum.[10] The authors support the proposal put forth by the International Cardioncology Society and Canadian Cardiac Oncology Network whereby cardio-oncology fellowship graduates will serve as a small group of experts who provide a resource for all the providers in the community involved in the management of patients with cancer.[13] Community providers will continue to provide almost all of the cardiovascular care for patients with cancer. The cardio-oncologist will be a consultant, educator, and researcher. In addition, cardio-oncology subspecialists will facilitate collaboration between cardiologists and oncologists in the clinical and research arenas. Therefore, the cardio-oncology training milieu, the selection process for cardio-oncology trainees, and the cardio-oncology training curriculum must emphasize consultation, education, and research skills.

Since the 1990s, the number of cardio-oncology training programs in the United States has grown. Successful training programs share several characteristics. Robust fellowship programs are best supported by high-volume centers that can provide a critical mass of patient clinician exposures. This exposure should occur with both inpatients and outpatients to include those issues unique to outpatient cardio-oncology. Note that cardio-oncology clinics are found only in approximately half of the international comprehensive cancer centers despite data suggesting that the presence of these clinics is related to more intensive monitoring for cardiotoxicity as well as long-term monitoring for complications related to radiotherapy.[9] Cardiology and oncology trainees should have an opportunity to rotate through an established cardio-oncology clinic to ensure the broadest exposure as well as to allow them to go on to establish new clinics in centers of need.

To date cardio-oncology fellowships have been pursued and completed by cardiologists and internists but future training models would also include programs designed for oncologists, family medicine specialists, and physician extenders. The authors have considered offering cardio-oncology fellowship positions to board-eligible or board-certified oncologists, but have found that our emphasis on cardiovascular testing, such as electrocardiograms, stress testing, echocardiography, has so far been a challenge. Although we continue to consider the value of tailoring the curriculum to physicians with oncology backgrounds, this article assumes that cardio-oncology fellowship trainees are usually board-certified cardiologists or internists aspiring to become cardiologists.

CURRICULUM

The curriculum for cardio-oncology should be structured with core competency-based goals in a manner that is in keeping with the Accreditation Council for Graduate Medical Education and American College of Cardiology's Core Cardiovascular Training Statements directives.[14] These milestones/goals can best be accomplished through a 1-year immersion fellowship with a combination of inpatient and outpatient exposure. As a guide for the recommended number of patient-fellow interactions, a proposal of a minimum of 100 unique patient visits has been put forth as a requirement for sufficient exposure.[13] The competencies should also be weighted based on the clinical background of the trainee.

Specifics of a curriculum for aspiring cardio-oncologists include sufficient exposure to allow fulfillment of competencies in the subject areas shown in Table 1.

These subject areas include core competencies covered during general internal medicine and cardiology training in addition to more extensive exposures to and understanding of cardiac complications of cancer and cancer therapy.[14,15] Training should stress management of cardiovascular issues before and during oncologic treatment, strategies for preventing or minimizing cardiovascular complications during oncologic treatment, and early detection of cardiovascular complications through the use of biomarkers and cardiac imaging modalities. An understanding of the mechanism of action of various anticancer treatments, basic understanding of tumor biology and disease progression, and treatment of common malignancies are core requirements.

The surveillance of survivors, screening for particular susceptibilities to cardiovascular sequelae, and assistance in management of subsequent malignancies are among the competencies that are not covered in any depth in medicine residence or cardiology fellowship training.[8,16,17] There is not much attention given to this domain in cardiology or internal medicine training. An in-depth understanding of surveillance in cancer survivors, as well as a mastery of the best methods to screen for cardiotoxicity after completing cancer treatment, is critical. A comprehensive appreciation of the emerging role of aggressive cardiovascular risk factor modification in this population is also vital.[8]

Fellows in cardio-oncology training should have opportunities to engage in supervised research. The degree of involvement in research could vary with the career trajectories of trainees. Opportunities for research are vital, because it is anticipated that a firm commitment to disciplined clinical research will be a tenet of training. Research modules are most efficient when they are stand-alone periods of time that afford complete immersion, and allow trainees to be exempt from clinical responsibilities. As part of the research deliverables, trainees should be expected to present at national meetings, and contribute to the medical literature in the form of submitted work for publications in major journals. Such activities should be required even among those planning clinical careers, in an effort to sustain their lifetime commitment to learning and helping to shape the best clinical practice of cardio-oncology.

FACULTY

The presence of faculty dedicated to the mission of cardio-oncology and academic training is essential for a successful cardio-oncology

---

Table 1
Subject areas

• Communication/coordination with patient, primary care physician, oncologist, and radiologists	• Arterial and venous thromboembolism
• Cardiac tumors: primary and metastatic	• Treatment-induced pulmonary hypertension
• Pericardial disease	• Evaluation before stem cell transplant
• Preoperative evaluation in patients with cancer: surgery, endoscopic and interventional radiology therapies	• Cardiotoxicity associated with cancer therapy strategies for preventing adverse effects of cardiotoxic drugs. Examples include anthracyclines, trastuzumab, and other anti–HER-2 therapies; VEGF signaling pathway inhibitors and tyrosine kinase inhibitors; fluorouracil
• Evaluation and treatment of the cardiovascular system of patients before, during, and after cancer therapy	• Surveillance in cancer survivors: hypertension, hyperlipidemia, anticoagulation, metabolic syndrome
• Management of congestive heart failure	• Cardiac effects of radiotherapy
• Management of acute coronary syndromes	• Carcinoid
• Appropriate use of elective and urgent interventional cardiovascular procedures	• Treatment of autonomic dysfunction
• Management of treatment-induced/treatment-related hypertension	• Amyloid
• Management of complex arrhythmias	

Abbreviation: anti–HER-2, human epidermal growth factor receptor 2.

fellowship program. Faculty with expertise in consultative medicine as well as the various cardiac subspecialties, such as echocardiography, nuclear cardiology, and advance cardiac imaging (including cardiac MRI and computed tomography angiography), is desired. The current practice of cardio-oncology is reliant on cardiac imaging, and, as such, fellowship programs should be based in institutions that provide direct access to high-quality cardiac imagers who understand the importance of technical reproducibility and accuracy. Echocardiographers must be adept at assessment of global and longitudinal strain.[18–20] Cardiac MRI readers must be able to interpret changes in tissue characterization and their impact on patients with cancer.[21,22] Such exposure is necessary to allow trainees to learn the proper applications of the different imaging modalities.

It is also desirable to have access to faculty who possess expertise in advanced heart failure management as well as electrophysiology. This access can be provided either at the home institution or through established extrainstitutional sources for subspecialty consultation. Interaction with these faculty members should allow fellows to develop a comprehensive understanding of the role of advanced heart failure management in patients with cancer, the role of cardiac implantable devices, and management of complex arrhythmias in oncologic patients.

In order to have the broadest exposure for the fellowship, it is preferable to have access to faculty in interventional cardiology and cardiothoracic surgery, who have experience in patients receiving oncologic treatment. This access is important to ensure that trainees have exposure to the complex decision making that is required surrounding revascularization and valve repair/replacement. These faculty need to be adept at understanding the implications for antiplatelet agents in the setting of ongoing oncologic treatment, and the impact of past exposure to radiation treatment on methods of revascularization in order to maximize the safety of the major oncologic surgery that is contemplated.

MULTIDISCIPLINARY MANAGEMENT

The practice of cardio-oncology is a primary example of the multidisciplinary management of patients. Fellows in cardio-oncology must have the opportunity to attend and participate in clinical conferences focusing on patient management decisions in which oncologists, radiologists, radiation oncologists, and oncologic surgeons collectively determine the best course of action

for particular patients with cancer. Through this team approach, the goals of safest oncologic care and minimizing unnecessary interruptions in treatment can be best achieved. In the role of the cardiovascular consultant, the fellow must develop an appreciation for the role as a facilitator for best possible oncologic treatment, while bearing a heightened sensitivity for cardiac sequelae and helping to mitigate possible cardiac toxicities. Using a multidisciplinary approach, fellows gain an appreciation for the importance of timely thorough consultations, as well as prompt analysis of cardiac testing and recommendations as they affect ongoing oncologic care.

In addition to multidisciplinary conferences, it is also beneficial to have trainees rotate through oncology subspecialty outpatient clinics so that they can be become more aware of the issues faced by oncologists. Understanding the magnitude of the risks and benefits of different cancer therapeutics and their potential cardiovascular risks is a critical equation that must be computed by effective cardiologists. This exposure is important to allow cardio-oncology consultants to be able to contribute to discussions on goals of care and to weigh in the balance oncologic disease and prevention or mitigation of cardiovascular disease.

INSTITUTIONAL SUPPORT

Institutional support must come in the form of both financial and philosophic support. Fellowship programs that are most effective operate in environments in which there is an institutional commitment to high-quality care. How this translates may vary on an institution to institution basis but should include a commitment to personnel, marketing, and providing state-of-the-art cardiac imaging to keep current with the emerging role of advanced imaging techniques such as strain imaging and cardiac MRI in detecting cardiotoxicity. The research component of the fellowship requires availability of a solid research infrastructure with opportunities for clinical or bench science research in cardio-oncology. Research mentorship should be readily identifiable for fellowship trainees along with informatics support, biostatistical support, and access to research databases.

In terms of a stepwise approach to the development of an institutional presence for cardio-oncology fellowship training, champions must be identified in both cardiology and oncology. An institution would become a preferred site by having a comprehensive approach and commitment to treatment of patients with cancer.

CHALLENGES

There are concerted efforts being made by the International Cardioncology Society and the Canadian Cardiac Oncology Network to advocate for further development of this subspecialty.[13] In response to knowledge gaps and needs identified by the practicing cardio-oncology community, the American College of Cardiology has created a Cardio-Oncology Council with task-oriented working groups to address the major components such as practice requirements, and the curriculum in research.

The next steps in the development of this discipline will include randomized clinical trials, standardization of goals and definitions, and development of clinical practice guidelines based on results of clinical trials. Maturation of the field will require care standardization, performance metrics, along with defining competency. It is not the current short-term expectation that cardio-oncology fellowship training will culminate in board certification, although this is a long-term goal. The last subspecialty areas that developed board certification did so after development of consensus guidelines, core competencies, as well as means of assessing adequacy of training. Cardio-oncology is not yet this developed. In addition, proposals for further specialization must always balance perceived benefits with known and unforeseen costs.[23]

Going forward the training available during cardiology fellowship must continue to be enhanced, as well as the opportunities for pediatricians, family practice physicians, and internists to get exposure in cardio-oncology. The field must continue to be inclusive rather than exclusive to meet the cardio-oncology shortage that exists. Such efforts will have to include mechanisms for exchange of knowledge outside of traditional training venues, such as on-line chat rooms, in addition to the established case-based conferences and presence in national meetings. Cardio-oncology will continue to grow and more clinicians and clinician-scientists who are well versed in this subject area will continue to be required.

Because the potential patient population is rapidly expanding and a dedicated trained cardio-oncology workforce is currently limited, and even with the establishment of training programs will continue to be limited for the next 5–10 years, training programs must also prepare to train a lower level of professionals (generalists, general cardiologists, pediatricians, allied health professionals) to deliver screening and first-line care to this population with knowledge of how to use biomarkers and cardiac imaging and with recommendations about when to refer to cardio-oncology. The level of training is more than a cardiology rotation and less than a dedicated year's immersion in cardio-oncology training.

In addition, because oncology treatment continues to rapidly evolve and as new cardiovascular imaging techniques and knowledge emerge, training programs must also develop a program of ongoing continuing medical education and refresher courses in cardio-oncology.

REFERENCES

1. Yusuf SW, Razeghi P, Yeh ET. The diagnosis and management of cardiovascular disease in cancer patients. Curr Probl Cardiol 2008;33(4):163–96.
2. Yeh ET, Bickford CL. Cardiovascular complications of cancer therapy: incidence, pathogenesis, diagnosis, and management. J Am Coll Cardiol 2009; 53(24):2231–47.
3. CDC. Available at: http://www.cdc.gov/cancer/dcpc/research/articles/cancer_2020.htm. Accessed August 15, 2016.
4. Bluethmann SM, Mariotto AB, Rowland JH. Anticipating the "silver tsunami": prevalence trajectories and comorbidity burden among older cancer survivors in the United States. Cancer Epidemiol Biomarkers Prev 2016;25(7):1029–36.
5. DeSantis CE, Lin CC, Mariotto AB, et al. Cancer treatment and survivorship statistics, 2014. CA Cancer J Clin 2014;64(4):252–71.
6. Siegel R, DeSantis C, Virgo K, et al. Cancer treatment and survivorship statistics, 2012. CA Cancer J Clin 2012;62(4):220–41.
7. de Moor JS, Mariotto AB, Parry C, et al. Cancer survivors in the United States: prevalence across the survivorship trajectory and implications for care. Cancer Epidemiol Biomarkers Prev 2013;22(4):561–70.
8. Oeffinger KC, Mertens AC, Sklar CA, et al. Chronic health conditions in adult survivors of childhood cancer. N Engl J Med 2006;355(15):1572–82.
9. Gujral DM, Lloyd G, Bhattacharyya S. Provision and clinical utility of cardio-oncology services for detection of cardiac toxicity in cancer patients. J Am Coll Cardiol 2016;67(12):1499–500.
10. Barac A, Murtagh G, Carver JR, et al. Cardiovascular health of patients with cancer and cancer survivors: a roadmap to the next level. J Am Coll Cardiol 2015;65(25):2739–46.
11. Erikson C, Salsberg E, Forte G, et al. Future supply and demand for oncologists: challenges to assuring access to oncology services. J Oncol Pract 2007; 3(2):79–86.
12. Yang W, Williams JH, Hogan PF, et al. Projected supply of and demand for oncologists and radiation

oncologists through 2025: an aging, better-insured population will result in shortage. J Oncol Pract 2014;10(1):39–45.

13. Lenihan DJ, Hartlage G, DeCara J, et al. Cardio-oncology training: a proposal from the International Cardioncology Society and Canadian Cardiac Oncology Network for a new multidisciplinary specialty. J Card Fail 2016;22(6):465–71.

14. Fuster V, Halperin JL, Williams ES, et al. COCATS 4 Task Force 1: training in ambulatory, consultative, and longitudinal cardiovascular care. J Am Coll Cardiol 2015;65(17):1734–53.

15. Gillebert TC, Brooks N, Fontes-Carvalho R, et al. ESC core curriculum for the general cardiologist (2013). Eur Heart J 2013;34(30):2381–411.

16. Chow EJ, Chen Y, Kremer LC, et al. Individual prediction of heart failure among childhood cancer survivors. J Clin Oncol 2015;33(5):394–402.

17. Phillips SM, Padgett LS, Leisenring WM, et al. Survivors of childhood cancer in the United States: prevalence and burden of morbidity. Cancer Epidemiol Biomarkers Prev 2015;24(4):653–63.

18. Pepe A, Pizzino F, Gargiulo P, et al. Cardiovascular imaging in the diagnosis and monitoring of cardiotoxicity: cardiovascular magnetic resonance and nuclear cardiology. J Cardiovasc Med (Hagerstown) 2016;17(Suppl 1):S45–54.

19. Thavendiranathan P, Poulin F, Lim KD, et al. Use of myocardial strain imaging by echocardiography for the early detection of cardiotoxicity in patients during and after cancer chemotherapy: a systematic review. J Am Coll Cardiol 2014;63(25 Pt A): 2751–68.

20. Yamada A, Luis SA, Sathianathan D, et al. Reproducibility of regional and global longitudinal strains derived from two-dimensional speckle-tracking and Doppler tissue imaging between expert and novice readers during quantitative dobutamine stress echocardiography. J Am Soc Echocardiogr 2014;27(8): 880–7.

21. Thavendiranathan P, Wintersperger BJ, Flamm SD, et al. Cardiac MRI in the assessment of cardiac injury and toxicity from cancer chemotherapy: a systematic review. Circ Cardiovasc Imaging 2013;6(6): 1080–91.

22. Pizzino F, Vizzari G, Qamar R, et al. Multimodality Imaging in cardiooncology. J Oncol 2015;2015: 263950.

23. Blackwell T, Cassel C, Duffy FD, et al. Final Report of the Committee on Recognizing New and Emerging Disciplines in Internal Medicine (NEDIM)-2. American Board of Internal Medicine; 2006. Available at: http://www.abim.org/pdf/nedim-2-report. pdf. Accessed January 8, 2017.

Cardio-oncology Related to Heart Failure
Common Risk Factors Between Cancer and Cardiovascular Disease

Anne Blaes, MD, MS[a],*, Anna Prizment, PhD[b],
Ryan J. Koene, MD[c], Suma Konety, MD, MS[d]

KEYWORDS

- Cardiooncology • Risk factors • Cancer • Heart disease • Risk

KEY POINTS

- There is a growing body of evidence that suggests cancer and cardiovascular disease have shared biological mechanisms.
- There are several shared risk factors for both cancer and cardiovascular disease: age, gender, obesity, diabetes mellitus, physical activity, diet, and tobacco use.
- Although inflammation seems to play a major role in both diseases, other common mechanisms have been described, including the role of hyperglycemia, hyperinsulinemia, and insulinlike growth factor 1 (IGF-1).
- Controlling cardiac risk factors may also improve cancer incidence and outcomes.
- Further collaboration between oncology and cardiology needs to occur as part of not only primary prevention but also secondary prevention.

Cardiovascular disease and cancer are 2 of the largest contributors to death in the United States. Currently, there are more than 15 million individuals with a history of cardiovascular disease and 14 million with a history of cancer.[1] This number is only expected to rise as the population in the United States ages and advances in the management of both cardiovascular disease and cancer are made. There is a growing body of evidence that suggests cancer and cardiovascular disease share a biological mechanism. In the complex process of carcinogenesis, cells go through several genetic "hits" before the full neoplastic phenotype of growth, invasion, and metastasis occurs. This process of malignant transformation can be divided into the following: initiation (irreversible step), promotion (stimulation of the growth of initiated cells), and progression (development of a more aggressive phenotype of promoted cells).[2] Similarly, the pathogenesis of cardiovascular

Disclosure: No author has any financial or commercial conflicts of interest.
Funding: A. Prizment was supported by the National Center for Advancing Translational Sciences of the National Institute of Health (NIH)Award Number UL1 TR000114. A. Blaes was supported by the Building Interdisciplinary Research Careers in Women's Health (NIH #K12-HD055887).
[a] Division of Hematology and Oncology, University of Minnesota, 420 Delaware Street, Southeast, MMC 480, Minneapolis, MN 55455, USA; [b] School of Public Health, University of Minnesota, 1300 South 2nd Street, 7525A, Minneapolis, MN 55454, USA; [c] Division of Cardiology, University of Minnesota, 420 Delaware Street, Southeast, MMC 480, Minneapolis, MN 55455, USA; [d] Division of Cardiology, University of Minnesota, 420 Delaware Street, Southeast, MMC 508, Minneapolis, MN 55455, USA
* Corresponding author.
E-mail address: Blaes004@umn.eu

disease is a multistep process. Although inflammation seems to play a major role in both diseases, other mechanisms have also been described, including the role of hyperglycemia, hyperinsulinemia, and IGF-1.[3] Gaining a better understanding of these shared mechanisms is vital. This review explores the risk factors common to cardiovascular disease and cancer, focusing on the epidemiologic studies that have been completed as well as how underlying cardiovascular disease affects cancer and cancer treatments.

MECHANISMS COMMON TO CANCER AND CARDIOVASCULAR DISEASE
Inflammation and Cancer

The connection between inflammation and cancer has long been established. Initially in the nineteenth century, Virchow appreciated the presence of leukocytes within neoplastic tissue. From his work, speculations arose as to whether cancer started in inflammatory sites. Further work demonstrated the associations between some chronic infections and cancers, that is, human papillomavirus and cervical cancer,[4] *Helicobacter pylori*, and stomach cancer,[5] Epstein-Barr virus and cancers.[6,7] Nonhealing wounds of the skin can develop into squamous cell carcinomas. There is also an association between chronic inflammatory diseases and cancer, that is, systemic sclerosis and cancer,[8] celiac disease, and small bowel lymphomas.[9] Approximately 10% to 20% of cancers arise at the site of chronic inflammation.[10] Through time, it has been appreciated that inflammation in the tumor microenvironment promotes malignant transformation and carcinogenesis. The presence of signaling between immune cells is required for tumor growth. There have been suggestions that stopping this inflammation with the use of anti-inflammatory medication actually delays cancer growth. For example, the use of aspirin, a cyclooxygenase 2 inhibitor, prevents the growth of primary and secondary polyps.[11] Similarly, aspirin use may be preventative for lung, esophagus, and stomach cancer.[12] There is ongoing research that perhaps statins, a cholesterol-lowering agent, may decrease inflammation and result in improvements in cancer outcomes.[3]

Inflammation and Cardiovascular Disease

Atherosclerotic disease, initially thought a lipid storage disease, is now known to be well-characterized by inflammation. Many risk factors for cardiovascular disease (hypertension, tobacco use, hyperlipidemia, and insulin resistance) trigger atherosclerosis through the promotion of adhesion of endothelial cells and the stimulation of leukocyte attachment to blood vessel walls that normally resist attachment.[3,13] With hyperlipidemia, excess lipoproteins accumulate in the subendothelial space, leading to oxidation and uptake by monocytes and macrophages.[14] Similarly with hypertension, there is oxidative stress on blood vessel walls. Elevations in inflammatory biomarkers, such as the C-reactive protein (CRP), have been associated with both primary and secondary cardiovascular events.[15–17] There are ongoing investigations looking at immunotherapy for the reduction in cardiovascular events. For example, an inhibitor of interleukin (IL)-1B, a proinflammatory cytokine involved in atherosclerosis and the regulation of CRP, is currently being studied for its effects on reduction in cardiovascular disease events in the Canakinumab Anti-inflammatory Thrombosis Outcomes Study (CANTOS) trial (NCT01327846) as well as its effects on vascular endothelial function (NCT02272946). Additional trials are also ongoing looking at the effects of statins and its effects on a reduction in inflammation.

Although diabetes, smoking, and obesity contribute to inflammation, there are a variety of other mechanisms that may also result in the shared risk factors between cancer and cardiovascular disease. These mechanisms are discussed.

SHARED RISK FACTORS FOR CANCER AND CARDIOVASCULAR DISEASE

There are many potential risk factors (modifiable and nonmodifiable) common to both cancer and cardiovascular disease, include aging, gender, obesity, diabetes mellitus, physical activity, diet, and smoking.

Age

The incidence of most cancers increases with advancing age. In developed countries, 78% of all newly diagnosed cancers occurs in individuals over the age of 55 years.[18] Similarly, cardiovascular risk increases with advancing age. Although 4.3% of individuals ages 18 to 44 years have heart disease, this prevalence increases to 12% for those ages 45 to 64 years, 24.6% for those ages 65 to 74 years, and 35% in those over the age of 75 years.[19]

Gender

Although certain cancers are gender-specific (cervix, testicular, uterine, and prostate), overall, cancer occurs more frequently in men. Similarly, men have a higher risk of developing cardiovascular disease.[19,20]

Obesity

According to epidemiologic data, 20% of all cancers are considered weight related.[21,22] According to the American Institute of Cancer Research and the World Cancer Research Fund, there is a link between obesity and many cancers, including esophageal adenocarcinoma, pancreatic, liver, colorectal, postmenopausal breast cancer, endometrial, and kidney cancers (Fig. 1).[23,24] It also seems that among those with a higher body mass index (BMI), cancer risk is higher. For those with a BMI between 27.5 kg/m^2 and 29.9 kg/m^2, the risk of cancer increases by 12% whereas those with a BMI greater than 40 kg/m^2 have a 70% increased risk[25] of cancer compared with those with a normal BMI. Similarly, in a large meta-analysis by Renehan and colleagues,[26] a 5-kg/m^2 increase in BMI was strongly associated with the risk of esophageal adenocarcinoma (relative risk [RR] 1.52, $P<.001$), thyroid cancer (RR 1.33, $P = .02$), colon cancer (RR 1.24, $P<.001$), and kidney cancer (RR 1.24, $P<.0001$) in men and endometrial cancer (RR 1.59, $P<.0001$), gallbladder cancer (RR 1.59, $P = .04$), esophageal adenocarcinoma (RR 1.51, $P<.0001$), and kidney cancer (RR 1.34, $P<.0001$) in women. On the contrary, dramatic weight loss from gastric bypass surgery is associated with reduced cancer mortality by approximately 60%.[27,28] These data suggest that promoting healthy weight change in adults can have important health benefits and outcomes from a cancer perspective.

Obesity has been associated with an increased risk of cardiovascular disease as outlined by the Framingham data.[29] The age-adjusted RR for cardiovascular disease is higher for those who are overweight (men RR 1.21 [1.05–1.40]; women RR 1.20 [1.03–1.41]) or obese (men RR 1.46 [1.20–1.77]; women RR 1.64 [1.37–1.98]). Obesity has been associated with a proinflammatory state, a prothrombotic state, insulin resistance, and atherogenic dyslipidemia.[30,31] Obesity causes an increase in cardiac output and hence overall cardiac workload to meet the metabolic demands of the expanded adipose tissue. Obesity has been linked to several cardiovascular changes, including hyperdynamic circulation, structural changes, sleep apnea, and overt heart failure.[32] This combination of factors leads to a concentric left ventricular hypertrophy and cardiovascular effects, even without associated hypertension.[33]

Biologically, there are plausible overlapping mechanisms associating the inflammatory state of obesity with both cardiovascular disease and cancer (Box 1). Elevated levels of IGF-1, found in obesity and the metabolic syndrome, are associated in preclinical models with tumor growth.[34,35] IGF-1 and its effects are discussed later.[36–41] Elevated estrogen levels are commonly seen in obesity; elevated estrogen levels are associated with breast and endometrial cancers. Biologically, estrogen is associated with tumor proliferation. Higher levels of IL-6, produced by adipose tissue, have been associated with hypertension and hepatic production of CRP, known to be associated with cardiovascular disease. From a cancer perspective, IL-6 has been shown to inhibit cancer cell apoptosis, stimulate angiogenesis, and play a role in drug resistance and tumor progression.[42,43] Leptin, thought to be related to cardiovascular disease,[44] has been associated with obesity and tumor growth and invasion. It has been associated with hepatocellular carcinoma, prostate cancer, and ovarian cancer. Leptin seems to up-regulate the expression of cyclin D1 and Mcl-1 to stimulate cell growth by activating the PI3K/Akt and MEK/ERK1/2 pathways in ovarian cancer.[45,46]

Diabetes

In 2010, the American Diabetes Association issued a statement linking diabetes to colon, liver, endometrial, pancreas, and bladder cancers (see Fig. 1).[20] There are also concerns about its association with leukemia, kidney cancer, and esophageal cancer. Although some inclusion criteria in this analysis were debated,[47] a recent review of meta-analyses of observational studies provided a significant amount of evidence to support this association of type 2 diabetes mellitus with cancer.[48]

Diabetes mellitus affects large and small vessels in the vasculature system and has long been associated with cardiovascular disease. The pathophysiology is likely multifaceted. Insulin resistance leads to dyslipidemia and abnormalities in lipoproteins through oxidative stress, glycolysis, and triglyceride enhancement. Endothelial function, an early marker for atherosclerosis, is stimulated by hyperglycemia induced free radical damage.[13] With higher levels of glucose, IGF-1 stimulates the migration and proliferation of smooth muscle cells, a part of early cardiovascular disease development.[20]

From a biological perspective, hyperglycemia, hyperinsulinemia, and the role of IGF-1 all likely contribute to the underlying biological link between cancer, cardiovascular disease, and diabetes mellitus. Many cancers, such as breast cancer, overexpress the insulin receptor.[49] IGF-1 promotes cell proliferation by stimulating cancer cell proliferation and metastasis; this seems

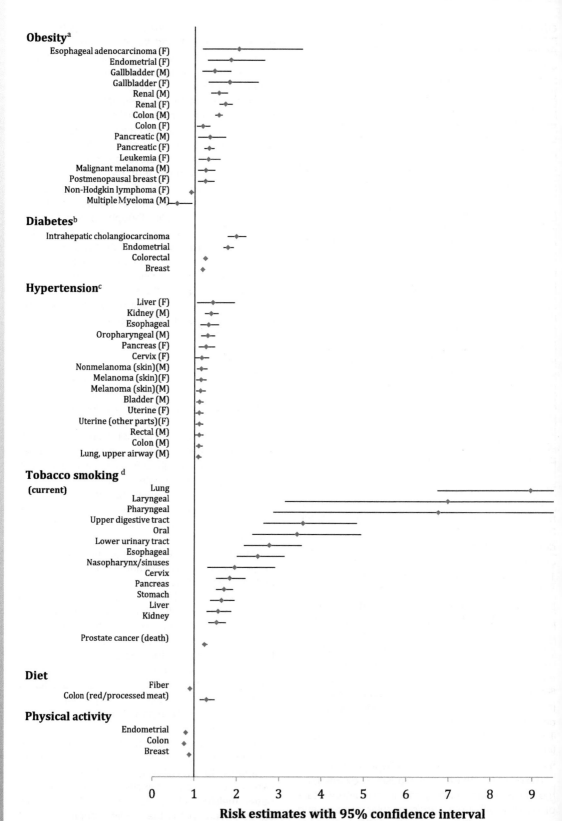

Fig. 1. Modifiable cardiac risk factors with their estimated cancer risk. Figure limited to only the positive and/or negative associations using the most recently published meta-analysis or prospective cohort study investigating

evident even in cells in which the IGF receptors are deficient.[49,50] Multiple signaling pathways are activated after insulin receptors or IGF-1 receptors interact with their ligands. This complex pathway leads to proliferation, protection from apoptotic stimuli, invasion, and metastasis. Additionally, hyperglycemia allows IGF-1 to stimulate vascular smooth muscle proliferation and migration. This mechanism furthers cancer growth and metastasis[51]; the smooth muscle proliferation and migration is also a hallmark of atherosclerosis pathophysiology.[52]

Separate from the direct effects of insulin on cancer cells, it has been theorized that hyperinsulinemia may promote carcinogenesis indirectly through IGF-1.[53] Insulin reduces the hepatic production of IGF-binding protein, resulting in higher levels of IGF-1.[54] IGF-1 has more potent antiapoptotic activities than insulin. It may act as a growth stimulus. Current cancer clinical trials are examining inhibitors of IGF-1.[55] Although insulin reduces the hepatic production of IGF-binding protein, it also reduces blood levels of sex hormone–binding globulin, leading to increases in bioavailable estrogen in both men and women. Although this increase in sex hormones may explain the increased risk of premenopausal breast cancer and endometrial cancer seen among those with hyperinsulinemia,[21] it does not explain a positive association between hyperinsulinemia and the cardiovascular system, because estrogen has a beneficial effect in cardiovascular disease. Higher levels of IGF have also been associated with colon and prostate cancer.

Tobacco Use

Tobacco usage, in particular cigarette smoking, is a heavily weighted risk factor for multiple types of cancers (see **Fig. 1**), including lung cancer, esophageal cancer, and pancreas cancer.[56] The American Cancer Society estimates that smoking is responsible for 30% of all cancer-related deaths in the United States. Although rates of tobacco use are decreasing in the United States and Canada, trends continue to increase globally, according to the World Health Organization's Global Report on Trends in Prevalence of Tobacco Use 2015.[57]

Cigarette smoking contributes to all stages of atherosclerosis, including stroke, myocardial infarction, hypertension, and aortic aneurysms; it has also been associated with approximately one-third of all first myocardial infarctions worldwide.[56] By decreasing nitric oxide, causing vasomotor dysfunction, increasing oxidative stress, and contributing to endothelial damage, tobacco use contributes to atherosclerosis.[58]

Biologically, tobacco smoke produces several irritants, carcinogens, proinflammatory stimuli, and oxidizing agents. These processes affect signaling found in both tobacco-related and cardiovascular disease. Nicotine has also been found directly related to the pathogenesis of both cardiovascular disease and cancer by inhibiting apoptosis and increasing angiogenesis.[58]

Hypertension

Hypertension has a particularly strong association with kidney cancers.[59,60] Also, in the Metabolic Syndrome and Cancer Project,[34] hypertension was positively correlated to total incident cancer (hazard ratio [HR] per 10–mm Hg increment: 1.07) and to cancers of the oropharynx, colon, rectum, lung, bladder, kidney, and melanoma in men and to cancers of the liver, pancreas, cervix, uterus, and melanoma in women.

Hypertension contributes to cardiovascular disease through various mechanisms, including its direct hemodynamic consequences, neurohormonal activation, autonomic influences, oxidative stress, and inflammation. These mechanisms may also be related to cancer and cancerous growth. In hypertension, vascular endothelial growth factor (VEGF) increases. VEGF is needed for tumors to induce new blood vessel formation. Angiotensin II, increased in hypertension,

the associations between a cardiac risk factor and various cancer sites; hyperlipidemia was excluded from the figure due to inconclusive evidence that it is associated with cancer risk. All cancer estimates were reported as a RR except where noted. [a] Risk for BMI greater than 30 kg/m². [b] Note, there were several additional positive (bladder, esophageal, extrahepatic cholangiocarcinoma, gallbladder, gastric, hepatocellular carcinoma, kidney, leukemia, multiple myeloma, non-Hodgkin lymphoma, ovarian cancer, and pancreatic cancer) and negative (lung and prostate) associations by fixed effects models, but the authors did not deem these positive associations because their 95% prediction intervals included the null value. [c] Prospective observational cohort; Cox regression was used to calculate HRs of cancer per 10–mm Hg increments of mid–blood pressure. [d] Only cancer sites with sufficient evidence of carcinogenicity related to tobacco exposure in humans were considered in the meta-analysis. (*From* Koene RJ, Prizment AE, Blaes A, et al. Shared risk factors in cardiovascular disease and cancer. Circulation 2016;133(11):1106; with permission.)

Box 1
Biological mediators linking obesity, cancer, and cardiovascular disease

1. IGF-1
2. Estrogen
3. IL-6
4. Leptin
5. Adiponectin

---

stimulates VEGF production.[61] Additionally further oxidative stress on blood vessel walls in the tumor microenvironment may further carcinogenesis.

Hyperlipidemia

Animal models have predicted that a high cholesterol diet may lead to colon polyps. It has been hypothesized that chronic saturated fat with increased cholesterol intake leads to an increase in hepatic bile acids and promotes carcinogenesis.[62–64] Other studies suggest there may also be an association between hyperlipidemia and breast cancer.[65,66] The cholesterol metabolite 27-hydroxycholesterol is similar to estradiol. Studies suggest that 27-hydroxycholesterol behaves as an endogenous selective estrogen receptor modulator. Similar to estradiol, 27-hydroxycholesterol, behaving as a partial agonist, positively regulates gene transcription and cell proliferation in cellular models of breast cancer and, as a result, may influence the pathology of breast cancer.[67] Several recent studies suggest there are improved cancer outcomes in those on cholesterol-lowering agents; these are discussed later.

In cardiovascular disease, the link between hyperlipidemia and cardiovascular disease has long been established. Excess lipoproteins in hyperlipidemia accumulate in the subendothelial space. This accumulation leads to oxidation, and further uptake by monocytes and macrophages causing further inflammation, thus promoting carcinogenesis.

Diet

Diet has been linked to both cancer and cardiovascular disease in both direct and indirect ways. There are direct carcinogens in foods, such as aflatoxins and nitrosamines. Aflatoxins can cause liver cancer. Nitrosamines, produced from nitrates and added to processed meat for conservation, are genotoxic substances that can act directly on DNA, causing point mutations, deletions, and insertions. Additionally, dietary fats found primarily in beef and dairy products can lead to inflammation and increases in carcinogenic bile acids and nitrosamines. In animal species as well as in human case-control studies, nitrosamines have been associated with gastric cancer and esophageal cancer.[68] In contrast, the Mediterranean-style diet, focused on high amounts of fruits, vegetables, whole grains, and unsaturated fats, has been associated with an approximately 10% decrease in cancer mortality.[69] It has been linked to a decrease in the incidence of many cancers, in particular gastric cancer and colon cancer.[70–73] It is hypothesized that the Mediterranean diet results in a decrease in inflammatory cytokines and, as result, a decrease in cancer incidence. The beneficial role of fruits and vegetables on cancer incidence is thought to be a result of the high levels of polyphenols. Polyphenols seem to affect several metabolic pathways, including mitogen-activated protein kinases, phosphatidylinositol 3-kinases, IGF-1, nuclear factor κB, and reactive oxygen species, leading to reductions in both cardiovascular disease and cancer.[74]

Finally, a Mediterranean-style diet indirectly reduces cancer risk by improving intermediaries associated with cancer, such as obesity, hyperlipidemia, hyperinsulinemia, and inflammation (discussed previously).

Diet and nutrition have long been associated with cardiovascular disease. Based on several previously published articles, there is an increased risk of cardiovascular disease associated with high content of saturated fats, red meat, sugar, and processed food.[71,75–78] In contrast, the Dietary Approaches to Stop Hypertension (DASH) diet and a Mediterranean-style diet focused on high amounts of fruits, vegetables, whole grains, and unsaturated fats are associated with better cardiovascular outcomes. The Mediterranean diet has been linked to approximately one-third fewer cardiovascular events.[79–81] Although the biological mechanisms linking diet and cardiovascular disease are not completely understood, there are several intermediaries associated with diet and cardiovascular disease, including high body weight, high blood pressure, and uncontrolled lipids. With the Mediterranean diet, there is typically less obesity (and its other intermediaries, discussed previously), a decrease in adipokines, and a decrease in inflammatory cytokines, all contributing to fewer cardiovascular events.

Sedentary Behavior

Exercise can also have a favorable effect on improving cancer risk. Modest exercise has been associated with reduced incidence of prostate, breast, bladder, esophageal, kidney, and endometrial cancers.[82–85] Exercise seems to decrease not only primary incidence of cancer but also recurrence in cancer survivors. Sedentary women who begin exercising 150 minutes per week can decrease their risk of breast cancer recurrence by 6%.[86] Exercise has also been associated with a decrease in cancer mortality.[87,88] For each 15 minutes of exercise per day, cancer mortality decreases by 1%.[89] The cancer preventative effects also seem independent of weight. An individual with a healthy body weight who is inactive still has a higher risk for cancer compared with those who exercise.[90]

Exercise can have a favorable effect on cardiovascular profiles and heart failure.[91] Exercise can result in improvements in obesity, diabetes, and lipid profiles; a decrease in cardiovascular and cancer events with exercise can occur through these mechanisms (discussed previously). Through improvements in aerobic capacity, blood vessel capacitance, and vascular wall function, however, exercise can also improve cardiovascular disease.[92] Additionally, not all the benefits of exercise are related to weight management: as outlined in the INTERHEART Study, sedentary behavior, even in individuals with a healthy weight, results in an increase in cardiovascular mortality.[93] It seems the effects of exercise are dose related, with exercise of 150 minutes per week reducing the risk of cardiovascular events by 14%, with exercise of 200 minutes per week reducing the risk of cardiovascular events by 20%.[90,94,95]

Biologically, the effects of exercise on cancer and cardiovascular disease prevention are likely multifactorial. Some of these mechanisms overlap and have been described previously. For instance, exercise is often seen in conjunction with a healthier diet. Exercise decreases diabetes, hypertension, hyperlipidemia, and obesity. With physical activity, there is an overall decrease in adipose tissue. Thus the overall effect of exercise is a reduction in circulating sex and metabolic hormones, a decrease in insulin, decrease in leptin, and a decrease in inflammatory markers (CRP, tumor necrosis factor, and IL-6), several of which are known to be carcinogenic.[87] Additionally, the impacts of exercise on decreasing cancer mortality are likely related to better cardiac reserve and less cardiac toxicity of cancer treatment.

CARDIOVASCULAR DISEASE AND ONCOLOGIC DISEASES

Given the shared risk factors for cancer and cardiac disease, it is not surprising that many individuals with cancer also have cardiovascular disease.

Similarly, many individuals with cardiovascular disease also have a history of cancer. In a recent study on cancer survivors with a variety of cancers, 62% were overweight or obese, 55% had hypertension, and 21% had diabetes.[96] This study is consistent with many other published articles where survivors have higher rates of obesity, hyperglycemia, hyperlipidemia, and elevations in cardiac biomarkers, such as CRP.[97] In looking at childhood cancer survivors, compared with siblings without cancer, childhood cancer survivors were more likely to be on medications for hypertension, hyperlipidemia, and diabetes, even if their prior cancer treatment did not include chest radiation.[98]

Although some of the increased cardiac risk may be related to cancer treatments, such as chemotherapy and radiation, other studies suggest that patients with cancer likely have an elevated cardiac risk at the time of diagnosis, before receiving any chemotherapy or radiation. In a Dutch study, calcium artery scores were elevated in those with a new cancer diagnosis when compared with healthy controls in the Multi-Ethnic Study of Atherosclerosis (MESA) study.[99] In studies of prostate cancer patients in Canada, before starting androgen deprivation, individuals with prostate cancer had elevations in hypertension, hyperlipidemia, and glucose intolerance compared with population controls.[100] Additionally, the prostate cancer patients were also more likely to have metabolic syndrome compared with controls.[101] In summary, the findings of increased cardiac risk factors at the time of cancer diagnoses, compared with matched controls, provide further evidence for the shared biology underlying both cardiovascular disease and cancer.

Controlling cardiac risk factors may also improve cancer incidence and outcomes (Box 2). In the large European Prospective Investigation into Cancer and Nutrition (EPIC) study of 23,153 individuals ages 35 to 65 years, researchers examined whether those who adhered to lifestyle events of a BMI less than 30 kg/m^2, no tobacco use, exercise greater than 3.5 h/wk, and a healthy diet had improvements in chronic disease outcomes. After a mean follow-up of 7.8 years, adherence to all 4 lifestyles events compared with 0 lifestyle events resulted in decreases in chronic disease (adjusted HR 0.22), diabetes (adjusted HR 0.07), myocardial infarction (adjusted HR 0.19), stroke (adjusted HR 0.50), and cancer (adjusted HR 0.64).[102] Additionally, the Atherosclerosis Risk in Communities Study (ARIC) researchers examined the impact of 7 ideal cardiovascular health metrics (see Box 2) on individuals ages 45 to 64 years between 1987 to 2006. Adhering to 6 of the 7 health metrics resulted in a 51% lower incidence of cancer, after adjusting for age, gender, race, and ARIC study site.[103] Although these risk factors were picked to look at the reduction in cardiovascular events, they also resulted in a decrease in cancer risk.

CARDIAC RISK FACTORS AND CANCER OUTCOMES
Cardiac Medications and Cancer Outcomes

Several studies have examined the impact of cardiovascular medications on cancer outcomes and incidence. Antiglycemic agents as a whole have reported mixed results in cancer risk. Although small studies have suggested a possible increase in cancer risk with the use of insulin analogs,[104] a significant amount of data suggests metformin may actually reduce cancer risk.[105,106] Based on the hyperinsulinemia hypothesis discussed previously, biologically it seems feasible that antiglycemic agents are associated with a reduction in cancer. Mechanistically, metformin activates adenosine monophosphate-activated protein kinase in hepatocytes. This kinase is not only a regulator of lipids and glucose but also a tumor suppressor. Currently, there are ongoing studies looking at metformin and cancer in prostate cancer, colorectal cancer, breast cancer, nonsmall cell lung cancer,

bladder cancer, ovarian, and endometrial cancers (NCT02360618, NCT02115464, NCT02285855, NCT01340300, NCT02122185, NCT02065687, and NCT01243385).

Antihypertensives have mixed results in whether they may increase or decrease cancer risk. In animal models, furosemide and hydrochlorothiazide use results in a marginal increase in renal cell carcinoma and adrenal adenomatous growths.[107] A larger meta-analysis of studies in humans by Grossman and colleagues[60] also found an association between diuretics and renal cell carcinoma (odds ratio [OR] 1.55; 95% CI, 1.42–1.71). This risk has also been observed in individuals on diuretics for nonhypertensive reasons.[108] Other groups have examined the impact of β-blockers and angiotensin-converting enzyme (ACE) inhibitors on cancer. A review of 11 observational studies examining 113,048 individuals found a 6% decreased incidence of colon cancer in individuals on ACE inhibitors or angiotensin receptor blockers (ARBs).[109] Most other work has examined whether the use of ACE inhibitors, ARBs and β-blockers affect cancer outcomes.[110–112] In the Life After Cancer Epidemiology (LACE) cohort of breast cancer survivors, risk of breast cancer recurrence was slightly increased in women on ACE inhibitors (HR 1.56; 95% CI, 1.02–2.39) and decreased in those on β-blockers (HR 0.86; 95% CI, 0.57–1.32).[113] Another group examining 1449 patients found no difference in disease-free survival rates or overall survival rates in breast cancer survivors using ACEs or ARBs[110] but also found an improvement in responses with the use of β-blockers.[114] Given the mixed results from these studies and others, it is clear that further investigation needs to be performed to better understand the connection between ACE inhibitors, ARBs and β-blockers on cancer outcomes.

Inhibitors of hydroxymethylglutaryl coenzyme A reductase (HMGCR), otherwise known as statins, are well known to cause a reduction in cardiovascular mortality. Statins lead to a decrease in mevalonate and downstream regulators of cholesterol. Mevalonate and the downstream regulators of cholesterol can be critical to cancer growth and progression. In addition to their anti-inflammatory effects, statins likely lead to antitumor effects through this pathway and mechanism. These biological data have been confirmed in clinical studies.[115] Improved disease-free survivals have been demonstrated in breast cancer survivors and prostate cancer survivors taking statins.[116,117] Recently, a large study of more than 4000 veterans with multiple myeloma demonstrated a 12-month overall survival advantage in individuals with multiple myeloma on a statin.[118]

Similarly, in a large study by Nielsen and colleagues[119] of the Danish population with a cancer diagnosis between 1995 and 2007, there was a reduced cancer mortality among statin users compared with those who had never used statins in 13 different types of cancers (adjusted HR for death of any cause 0.82; 95% CI, 0.81–0.85).

Finally, the role of inflammatory drugs may also be associated with a decrease in many cancers. Aspirin use affects cyclooxygenase-dependent and cyclooxygenase-independent mechanisms; its use has been associated with a 24% risk reduction of primary colon cancer[120]; other studies suggest it is useful as a secondary preventative in colon cancer survivors. Additional ongoing clinical trials looking at the benefits of aspirin on breast cancer recurrence are being proposed by the Alliance for Clinical Trials in Oncology cancer clinical trial network.[121]

Controlling Cardiac Risk Factors May Actually Improve Cancer Outcomes

Risk factors for chemotherapy-related cardiac complications should be assessed in all patients diagnosed with cancer who are considered for cancer therapy, whether the administration of biologics, chemotherapy, or radiation therapy. Given that advancing age, prior cardiac dysfunction, coronary artery disease, hypertension, tobacco use, and obesity have been associated with an increased risk of anthracycline cardiac toxicity, it is recommended that all patients prescribed anthracyclines should be consulted about risk stratification and risk modification.[122] Given that a large number of other chemotherapies and targeted therapies can cause cardiac toxicity as well,[123] it is important to evaluate cardiac risk factors in all oncology patients. Hypertension has been linked as a risk factor for VEGF-induced hypertension[124] as well as trastuzumab cardiac toxicity.[125] Other models are being developed to look at risk factors for tyrosine kinase–induced cardiac toxicity.[126] Collaborative assessment by oncologists and cardiologists before the start of chemotherapy can lead to early identification of patients at risk as well as discussions about the utility and benefits of cardiac toxic medications as opposed to potential alternative therapies.[127] In some situations, as discussed previously, alternative noncardiac toxic chemotherapy regimens may be considered. A lower-intensity chemotherapy regimen, however, given out of concern for potential cardiac toxicity, may actually result in worsened cancer survival. In a large study of 17,000 individuals, management of these cardiac comorbidities, such as hypertension and diabetes, may actually improve cancer survival.[128,129] These data suggest a need for better collaboration between cardiologists and oncologists as part of not only primary prevention but also secondary prevention.

SUMMARY

There are many similar risk factors for both cancer and cardiovascular disease. There are substantial biological data to support the hypotheses that the pathogenesis of these 2 diseases overlaps. Exercise should be strongly encouraged and should continue to be a focus of ongoing research. The management of risk factors for cardiovascular disease and cancer, including tobacco use, a healthy diet, and normal weight, should be further addressed. Treatment of cardiac risk factors, including hypertension, hyperlipidemia, and diabetes, in cancer patients may actually improve overall outcomes not only in cancer patients on active therapy but also in cancer survivors. As a result, continued collaboration between oncology and cardiology is essential.

REFERENCES

1. Xu J, Murphy SL, Kochanek KD, et al. Deaths: final data for 2013. Natl Vital Stat Rep 2016;64(2):1–119.
2. DeVita VT, Lawrence TS, Rosenberg SA, editors. DeVita, Hellman and Rosenberg's cancer: principles and practice of oncology. 10th edition. Riverwoods (IL): Wolters Kluwer; 2014.
3. Libby P. Inflammation and cardiovascular disease mechanisms. Am J Clin Nutr 2006;83(2):456S–60S.
4. de Sanjose S, Quint WG, Alemany L, et al. Human papillomavirus genotype attribution in invasive cervical cancer: a retrospective cross-sectional worldwide study. Lancet Oncol 2010;11(11): 1048–56.
5. Huang JQ, Sridhar S, Chen Y, et al. Meta-analysis of the relationship between helicobacter pylori seropositivity and gastric cancer. Gastroenterology 1998;114(6):1169–79.
6. Thorley-Lawson DA, Gross A. Persistence of the epstein-barr virus and the origins of associated lymphomas. N Engl J Med 2004;350(13):1328–37.
7. Prabhu SR, Wilson DF. Evidence of epstein-barr virus association with head and neck cancers: a review. J Can Dent Assoc 2016;82:g2.
8. Zeineddine N, Khoury LE, Mosak J. Systemic sclerosis and malignancy: a review of current data. J Clin Med Res 2016;8(9):625–32.
9. Woodward J. Improving outcomes of refractory celiac disease - current and emerging treatment strategies. Clin Exp Gastroenterol 2016;9:225–36.

10. Kuper H, Adami HO, Trichopoulos D. Infections as a major preventable cause of human cancer. J Intern Med 2000;248(3):171–83.

11. Tarraga Lopez PJ, Albero JS, Rodriguez-Montes JA. Primary and secondary prevention of colorectal cancer. Clin Med Insights Gastroenterol 2014;7:33–46.

12. Coussens LM, Werb Z. Inflammation and cancer. Nature 2002;420(6917):860–7.

13. Tesfamariam B, Cohen RA. Free radicals mediate endothelial cell dysfunction caused by elevated glucose. Am J Physiol 1992;263(2 Pt 2):H321–6.

14. Stamler J, Wentworth D, Neaton JD. Is relationship between serum cholesterol and risk of premature death from coronary heart disease continuous and graded? findings in 356,222 primary screenees of the multiple risk factor intervention trial (MRFIT). JAMA 1986;256(20):2823–8.

15. Ridker PM, Koenig W, Fuster V. C-reactive protein and coronary heart disease. N Engl J Med 2004; 351(3):295–8 [author reply: 295–8].

16. Ridker PM, Rifai N, Rose L, et al. Comparison of C-reactive protein and low-density lipoprotein cholesterol levels in the prediction of first cardiovascular events. N Engl J Med 2002;347(20):1557–65.

17. Parrinello CM, Lutsey PL, Ballantyne CM, et al. Six-year change in high-sensitivity C-reactive protein and risk of diabetes, cardiovascular disease, and mortality. Am Heart J 2015;170(2):380–9.

18. Garcia M, Jemal A, Ward EM, et al. Global cancer facts and figures. Atlanta (GA): American Cancer Society; 2007.

19. Available at: http://www.cdc.gov/nchs/fastats/heart-disease.htm. Accessed September 1, 2016.

20. Giovannucci E, Harlan DM, Archer MC, et al. Diabetes and cancer: a consensus report. Diabetes Care 2010;33(7):1674–85.

21. Calle EE, Rodriguez C, Walker-Thurmond K, et al. Overweight, obesity, and mortality from cancer in a prospectively studied cohort of U.S. adults. N Engl J Med 2003;348(17):1625–38.

22. Calle EE, Thun MJ, Petrelli JM, et al. Body-mass index and mortality in a prospective cohort of U.S. adults. N Engl J Med 1999;341(15):1097–105.

23. Dobbins M, Decorby K, Choi BC. The association between obesity and cancer risk: a meta-analysis of observational studies from 1985 to 2011. ISRN Prev Med 2013;2013:680536.

24. Koene RJ, Prizment AE, Blaes A, et al. Shared risk factors in cardiovascular disease and cancer. Circulation 2016;133(11):1104–14.

25. Berrington de Gonzalez A, Hartge P, Cerhan JR, et al. Body-mass index and mortality among 1.46 million white adults. N Engl J Med 2010;363(23):2211–9.

26. Renehan AG, Tyson M, Egger M, et al. Body-mass index and incidence of cancer: a systematic review and meta-analysis of prospective observational studies. Lancet 2008;371(9612):569–78.

27. Tee MC, Cao Y, Warnock GL, et al. Effect of bariatric surgery on oncologic outcomes: a systematic review and meta-analysis. Surg Endosc 2013; 27(12):4449–56.

28. Sjostrom L, Narbro K, Sjostrom CD, et al. Effects of bariatric surgery on mortality in swedish obese subjects. N Engl J Med 2007;357(8):741–52.

29. Wilson PW, D'Agostino RB, Sullivan L, et al. Overweight and obesity as determinants of cardiovascular risk: the Framingham experience. Arch Intern Med 2002;162(16):1867–72.

30. Luft VC, Schmidt MI, Pankow JS, et al. Chronic inflammation role in the obesity-diabetes association: a case-cohort study. Diabetol Metab Syndr 2013;5(1):31.

31. Emanuela F, Grazia M, Marco de R, et al. Inflammation as a link between obesity and metabolic syndrome. J Nutr Metab 2012;2012:476380.

32. Vasan RS. Cardiac function and obesity. Heart 2003;89(10):1127–9.

33. Litwin SE. Cardiac remodeling in obesity: time for a new paradigm. JACC Cardiovasc Imaging 2010; 3(3):275–7.

34. Stocks T, Van Hemelrijck M, Manjer J, et al. Blood pressure and risk of cancer incidence and mortality in the metabolic syndrome and cancer project. Hypertension 2012;59(4):802–10.

35. Mendonca FM, de Sousa FR, Barbosa AL, et al. Metabolic syndrome and risk of cancer: which link? Metabolism 2015;64(2):182–9.

36. Despres JP. Body fat distribution and risk of cardiovascular disease: an update. Circulation 2012; 126(10):1301–13.

37. Gallagher EJ, LeRoith D. Epidemiology and molecular mechanisms tying obesity, diabetes, and the metabolic syndrome with cancer. Diabetes Care 2013;36(Suppl 2):S233–9.

38. Bjorge T, Stocks T, Lukanova A, et al. Metabolic syndrome and endometrial carcinoma. Am J Epidemiol 2010;171(8):892–902.

39. Borena W, Strohmaier S, Lukanova A, et al. Metabolic risk factors and primary liver cancer in a prospective study of 578,700 adults. Int J Cancer 2012;131(1):193–200.

40. Haggstrom C, Rapp K, Stocks T, et al. Metabolic factors associated with risk of renal cell carcinoma. PLoS One 2013;8(2):e57475.

41. Ankarfeldt MZ, Angquist L, Stocks T, et al. Body characteristics, [corrected] dietary protein and body weight regulation. Reconciling conflicting results from intervention and observational studies? PLoS One 2014;9(7):e101134.

42. Guo Y, Xu F, Lu T, et al. Interleukin-6 signaling pathway in targeted therapy for cancer. Cancer Treat Rev 2012;38(7):904–10.

43. Yao X, Huang J, Zhong H, et al. Targeting interleukin-6 in inflammatory autoimmune diseases and cancers. Pharmacol Ther 2014;141(2):125–39.

44. Martin SS, Qasim A, Reilly MP. Leptin resistance: a possible interface of inflammation and metabolism in obesity-related cardiovascular disease. J Am Coll Cardiol 2008;52(15):1201–10.

45. Chen C, Chang YC, Lan MS, et al. Corrigendum] leptin stimulates ovarian cancer cell growth and inhibits apoptosis by increasing cyclin D1 and mcl-1 expression via the activation of the MEK/ERK1/2 and PI3K/akt signaling pathways. Int J Oncol 2016;49(2):847.

46. Liu CL, Chang YC, Cheng SP, et al. The roles of serum leptin concentration and polymorphism in leptin receptor gene at codon 109 in breast cancer. Oncology 2007;72(1–2):75–81.

47. Satija A, Spiegelman D, Giovannucci E, et al. Type 2 diabetes and risk of cancer. BMJ 2015;350: g7707.

48. Tsilidis KK, Kasimis JC, Lopez DS, et al. Type 2 diabetes and cancer: umbrella review of meta-analyses of observational studies. BMJ 2015;350: g7607.

49. Denley A, Carroll JM, Brierley GV, et al. Differential activation of insulin receptor substrates 1 and 2 by insulin-like growth factor-activated insulin receptors. Mol Cell Biol 2007;27(10):3569–77.

50. Becker MA, Ibrahim YH, Oh AS, et al. Insulin receptor substrate adaptor proteins mediate prognostic gene expression profiles in breast cancer. PLoS One 2016;11(3):e0150564.

51. Clemmons DR. Modifying IGF1 activity: an approach to treat endocrine disorders, atherosclerosis and cancer. Nat Rev Drug Discov 2007;6(10): 821–33.

52. MacLeod DC, Strauss BH, de Jong M, et al. Proliferation and extracellular matrix synthesis of smooth muscle cells cultured from human coronary atherosclerotic and restenotic lesions. J Am Coll Cardiol 1994;23(1):59–65.

53. Giovannucci E. Insulin, insulin-like growth factors and colon cancer: a review of the evidence. J Nutr 2001;131(11 Suppl):3109S–20S.

54. Powell DR, Suwanichkul A, Cubbage ML, et al. Insulin inhibits transcription of the human gene for insulin-like growth factor-binding protein-1. J Biol Chem 1991;266(28):18868–76.

55. You L, Liu C, Tang H, et al. Advances in targeting insulin-like growth factor signaling pathway in cancer treatment. Curr Pharm Des 2014;20(17): 2899–911.

56. Carter BD, Abnet CC, Feskanich D, et al. Smoking and mortality–beyond established causes. N Engl J Med 2015;372(7):631–40.

57. Islami F, Torre LA, Jemal A. Global trends of lung cancer mortality and smoking prevalence. Transl Lung Cancer Res 2015;4(4):327–38.

58. Morris PB, Ference BA, Jahangir E, et al. Cardiovascular effects of exposure to cigarette smoke and electronic cigarettes: clinical perspectives from the prevention of cardiovascular disease section leadership council and early career councils of the american college of cardiology. J Am Coll Cardiol 2015;66(12):1378–91. http://dx.doi.org/10. 1016/j.jacc.2015.07.037.

59. Bangalore S, Kumar S, Kjeldsen SE, et al. Antihypertensive drugs and risk of cancer: network meta-analyses and trial sequential analyses of 324,168 participants from randomised trials. Lancet Oncol 2011;12(1):65–82.

60. Grossman E, Messerli FH, Goldbourt U. Carcinogenicity of antihypertensive therapy. Curr Hypertens Rep 2002;4(3):195–201.

61. Baik SK, Jo HS, Suk KT, et al. Inhibitory effect of angiotensin II receptor antagonist on the contraction and growth of hepatic stellate cells. Korean J Gastroenterol 2003;42(2):134–41.

62. Tseng TH, Hsu JD, Chu CY, et al. Promotion of colon carcinogenesis through increasing lipid peroxidation induced in rats by a high cholesterol diet. Cancer Lett 1996;100(1–2):81–7.

63. Swamy MV, Patlolla JM, Steele VE, et al. Chemoprevention of familial adenomatous polyposis by low doses of atorvastatin and celecoxib given individually and in combination to APCMin mice. Cancer Res 2006;66(14):7370–7.

64. Reddy BS. Dietary fat and its relationship to large bowel cancer. Cancer Res 1981;41(9 Pt 2):3700–5.

65. Nelson ER, Wardell SE, Jasper JS, et al. 27-hydroxycholesterol links hypercholesterolemia and breast cancer pathophysiology. Science 2013;342(6162): 1094–8.

66. Warner M, Gustafsson JA. On estrogen, cholesterol metabolism, and breast cancer. N Engl J Med 2014;370(6):572–3.

67. DuSell CD, Umetani M, Shaul PW, et al. 27-hydroxycholesterol is an endogenous selective estrogen receptor modulator. Mol Endocrinol 2008;22(1): 65–77.

68. Gonzalez CA, Jakszyn P, Pera G, et al. Meat intake and risk of stomach and esophageal adenocarcinoma within the european prospective investigation into cancer and nutrition (EPIC). J Natl Cancer Inst 2006;98(5):345–54.

69. Schwingshackl L, Hoffmann G. Adherence to mediterranean diet and risk of cancer: a systematic review and meta-analysis of observational studies. Int J Cancer 2014;135(8):1884–97.

70. Slattery ML, Potter JD, Sorenson AW. Age and risk factors for colon cancer (united states and australia): are there implications for understanding differences in case-control and cohort studies? Cancer Causes Control 1994;5(6):557–63.

71. Wang X, Ouyang Y, Liu J, et al. Fruit and vegetable consumption and mortality from all causes, cardiovascular disease, and cancer: systematic review

and dose-response meta-analysis of prospective cohort studies. BMJ 2014;349:g4490.

72. Buckland G, Agudo A, Lujan L, et al. Adherence to a mediterranean diet and risk of gastric adenocarcinoma within the european prospective investigation into cancer and nutrition (EPIC) cohort study. Am J Clin Nutr 2010;91(2):381–90.

73. Verberne L, Bach-Faig A, Buckland G, et al. Association between the mediterranean diet and cancer risk: a review of observational studies. Nutr Cancer 2010;62(7):860–70.

74. Baena Ruiz R, Salinas Hernandez P. Diet and cancer: risk factors and epidemiological evidence. Maturitas 2014;77(3):202–8.

75. Li Y, Hruby A, Bernstein AM, et al. Saturated fats compared with unsaturated fats and sources of carbohydrates in relation to risk of coronary heart disease: a prospective cohort study. J Am Coll Cardiol 2015;66(14):1538–48.

76. Wu H, Flint AJ, Qi Q, et al. Association between dietary whole grain intake and risk of mortality: two large prospective studies in US men and women. JAMA Intern Med 2015;175(3):373–84.

77. de Ferranti SD, de Boer IH, Fonseca V, et al. Type 1 diabetes mellitus and cardiovascular disease: a scientific statement from the American Heart Association and American Diabetes Association. Circulation 2014;130(13):1110–30.

78. Fox CS, Golden SH, Anderson C, et al. Update on prevention of cardiovascular disease in adults with type 2 diabetes mellitus in light of recent evidence: a scientific statement from the American Heart Association and the American diabetes Association. Circulation 2015;132(8):691–718.

79. Estruch R, Ros E, Salas-Salvado J, et al. Primary prevention of cardiovascular disease with a mediterranean diet. N Engl J Med 2013;368(14):1279–90.

80. de Lorgeril M, Renaud S, Mamelle N, et al. Mediterranean alpha-linolenic acid-rich diet in secondary prevention of coronary heart disease. Lancet 1994;343(8911):1454–9.

81. de Lorgeril M, Salen P. Wine ethanol, platelets, and mediterranean diet. Lancet 1999;353(9158):1067.

82. Johnson CB, Davis MK, Law A, et al. Shared risk factors for cardiovascular disease and cancer: implications for preventive health and clinical care in oncology patients. Can J Cardiol 2016;32(7):900–7.

83. Schmid D, Behrens G, Keimling M, et al. A systematic review and meta-analysis of physical activity and endometrial cancer risk. Eur J Epidemiol 2015;30(5):397–412.

84. Cao Y, Keum NN, Chan AT, et al. Television watching and risk of colorectal adenoma. Br J Cancer 2015;112(5):934–42.

85. Behrens G, Matthews CE, Moore SC, et al. The association between frequency of vigorous physical activity and hepatobiliary cancers in the NIH-AARP diet and health study. Eur J Epidemiol 2013;28(1):55–66.

86. Kodama S, Saito K, Tanaka S, et al. Cardiorespiratory fitness as a quantitative predictor of all-cause mortality and cardiovascular events in healthy men and women: a meta-analysis. JAMA 2009;301(19):2024–35.

87. Friedenreich CM. Physical activity and cancer: lessons learned from nutritional epidemiology. Nutr Rev 2001;59(11):349–57.

88. Friedenreich CM, Neilson HK, Woolcott CG, et al. Inflammatory marker changes in a yearlong randomized exercise intervention trial among postmenopausal women. Cancer Prev Res (Phila) 2012;5(1):98–108.

89. Wen CP, Wai JP, Tsai MK, et al. Minimum amount of physical activity for reduced mortality and extended life expectancy: a prospective cohort study. Lancet 2011;378(9798):1244–53.

90. Hu FB, Willett WC, Li T, et al. Adiposity as compared with physical activity in predicting mortality among women. N Engl J Med 2004;351(26):2694–703.

91. Pandey A, Garg S, Khunger M, et al. Dose-response relationship between physical activity and risk of heart failure: a meta-analysis. Circulation 2015;132(19):1786–94.

92. Pina IL, Apstein CS, Balady GJ, et al. Exercise and heart failure: a statement from the american heart association committee on exercise, rehabilitation, and prevention. Circulation 2003;107(8):1210–25.

93. Held C, Iqbal R, Lear SA, et al. Physical activity levels, ownership of goods promoting sedentary behaviour and risk of myocardial infarction: results of the INTERHEART study. Eur Heart J 2012;33(4):452–66.

94. Sui X, LaMonte MJ, Laditka JN, et al. Cardiorespiratory fitness and adiposity as mortality predictors in older adults. JAMA 2007;298(21):2507–16.

95. Li TY, Rana JS, Manson JE, et al. Obesity as compared with physical activity in predicting risk of coronary heart disease in women. Circulation 2006;113(4):499–506.

96. Weaver KE, Foraker RE, Alfano CM, et al. Cardiovascular risk factors among long-term survivors of breast, prostate, colorectal, and gynecologic cancers: a gap in survivorship care? J Cancer Surviv 2013;7(2):253–61.

97. Whitlock MC, Yeboah J, Burke GL, et al. Cancer and its association with the development of coronary artery calcification: an assessment from the multi-ethnic study of atherosclerosis. J Am Heart Assoc 2015;4(11) [pii:e002533].

98. Meacham LR, Chow EJ, Ness KK, et al. Cardiovascular risk factors in adult survivors of pediatric cancer–a report from the childhood cancer survivor

study. Cancer Epidemiol Biomarkers Prev 2010; 19(1):170–81.

99. Mast ME, Heijenbrok MW, Petoukhova AL, et al. Preradiotherapy calcium scores of the coronary arteries in a cohort of women with early-stage breast cancer: a comparison with a cohort of healthy women. Int J Radiat Oncol Biol Phys 2012;83(3): 853–8.

100. Davis MK, Rajala JL, Tyldesley S, et al. The prevalence of cardiac risk factors in men with localized prostate cancer undergoing androgen deprivation therapy in British Columbia, Canada. J Oncol 2015;2015:820403.

101. Morote J, Gomez-Caamano A, Alvarez-Ossorio JL, et al. The metabolic syndrome and its components in patients with prostate cancer on androgen deprivation therapy. J Urol 2015;193(6):1963–9.

102. Nothlings U, Ford ES, Kroger J, et al. Lifestyle factors and mortality among adults with diabetes: findings from the european prospective investigation into cancer and nutrition-potsdam study*. J Diabetes 2010;2(2):112–7.

103. Rasmussen-Torvik LJ, Shay CM, Abramson JG, et al. Ideal cardiovascular health is inversely associated with incident cancer: the atherosclerosis risk in communities study. Circulation 2013;127(12): 1270–5.

104. Grouven U, Hemkens LG, Bender R, et al. Risk of malignancies in patients with diabetes treated with human insulin or insulin analogues. Reply to Nagel JM, Mansmann U, Wegscheider K et al. [letter] and Simon D [letter]. Diabetologia 2010;53(1):209–11.

105. Pernicova I, Korbonits M. Metformin–mode of action and clinical implications for diabetes and cancer. Nat Rev Endocrinol 2014;10(3):143–56.

106. Johnson JA, Carstensen B, Witte D, et al. Diabetes and cancer (1): evaluating the temporal relationship between type 2 diabetes and cancer incidence. Diabetologia 2012;55(6):1607–18.

107. Lijinsky W, Reuber MD. Chronic carcinogenesis studies of acrolein and related compounds. Toxicol Ind Health 1987;3(3):337–45.

108. Chow WH, McLaughlin JK, Mandel JS, et al. Risk of renal cell cancer in relation to diuretics, antihypertensive drugs, and hypertension. Cancer Epidemiol Biomarkers Prev 1995;4(4):327–31.

109. Dai YN, Wang JH, Zhu JZ, et al. Angiotensin-converting enzyme inhibitors/angiotensin receptor blockers therapy and colorectal cancer: a systematic review and meta-analysis. Cancer Causes Control 2015;26(9):1245–55.

110. Chae YK, Brown EN, Lei X, et al. Use of ACE inhibitors and angiotensin receptor blockers and primary breast cancer outcomes. J Cancer 2013; 4(7):549–56.

111. Wang H, Liao Z, Zhuang Y, et al. Incidental receipt of cardiac medications and survival outcomes among patients with stage III non-small-cell lung cancer after definitive radiotherapy. Clin Lung Cancer 2015;16(2):128–36.

112. Song T, Choi CH, Kim MK, et al. The effect of angiotensin system inhibitors (angiotensin-converting enzyme inhibitors or angiotensin receptor blockers) on cancer recurrence and survival: a meta-analysis. Eur J Cancer Prev 2016;26(1): 78–85.

113. Ganz PA, Habel LA, Weltzien EK, et al. Examining the influence of beta blockers and ACE inhibitors on the risk for breast cancer recurrence: results from the LACE cohort. Breast Cancer Res Treat 2011;129(2):549–56.

114. Melhem-Bertrandt A, Chavez-Macgregor M, Lei X, et al. Beta-blocker use is associated with improved relapse-free survival in patients with triple-negative breast cancer. J Clin Oncol 2011;29(19):2645–52.

115. Ji Y, Rounds T, Crocker A, et al. The effect of atorvastatin on breast cancer biomarkers in high-risk women. Cancer Prev Res (Phila) 2016;9(5):379–84.

116. Dale KM, Coleman CI, Henyan NN, et al. Statins and cancer risk: a meta-analysis. JAMA 2006; 295(1):74–80.

117. Mucci LA, Stampfer MJ. Mounting evidence for prediagnostic use of statins in reducing risk of lethal prostate cancer. J Clin Oncol 2014;32(1):1–2.

118. Sanfilippo KM, Keller J, Gage BF, et al. Statins are associated with reduced mortality in multiple myeloma. J Clin Oncol 2016. [Epub ahead of print].

119. Nielsen SF, Nordestgaard BG, Bojesen SE. Statin use and reduced cancer-related mortality. N Engl J Med 2012;367(19):1792–802.

120. Rothwell PM, Wilson M, Elwin CE, et al. Long-term effect of aspirin on colorectal cancer incidence and mortality: 20-year follow-up of five randomised trials. Lancet 2010;376(9754):1741–50.

121. Available at: https://www.allianceforclinicaltrial sinoncology.org/main/public/standard.xhtml? path=/public/news-ABC-trial-Nov2015.

122. Accordino MK, Neugut AI, Hershman DL. Cardiac effects of anticancer therapy in the elderly. J Clin Oncol 2014;32(24):2654–61.

123. Yeh ET, Bickford CL. Cardiovascular complications of cancer therapy: incidence, pathogenesis, diagnosis, and management. J Am Coll Cardiol 2009; 53(24):2231–47.

124. Hamnvik OP, Choueiri TK, Turchin A, et al. Clinical risk factors for the development of hypertension in patients treated with inhibitors of the VEGF signaling pathway. Cancer 2015;121(2):311–9.

125. Ezaz G, Long JB, Gross CP, et al. Risk prediction model for heart failure and cardiomyopathy after adjuvant trastuzumab therapy for breast cancer. J Am Heart Assoc 2014;3(1):e000472.

126. Hurley PJ, Konety S, Cao Q, et al. Frequency and risk factors for tyrosine kinase inhibitor-associated

cardiotoxicity. J Clin Oncol 2016;34(Suppl) [abstract: 6596].

127. Lenihan DJ, Cardinale D, Cipolla CM. The compelling need for a cardiology and oncology partnership and the birth of the international CardiOncology society. Prog Cardiovasc Dis 2010;53(2):88–93.

128. Piccirillo J, Tierney R, Costas I, et al. Prognostic importance of comorbidity in a hospital-based cancer registry. JAMA 2004;291(20):2441–7.

129. Emerging Risk Factors Collaboration, Di Angelantonio E, Kaptoge S, Wormser D, et al. Association of cardiometabolic multimorbidity with mortality. JAMA 2015;314(1):52–60.

Alternative Biomarkers for Combined Biology

 CrossMark

Yong-Hyun Kim, MD[a,b], Jennifer Kirsop, BSc[c], Wai Hong Wilson Tang, MD[a,c,d],*

KEYWORDS

- Chemotherapy-related cardiac dysfunction • Heart failure • Malignancy • Biomarkers

KEY POINTS

- Chemotherapy-related cardiac dysfunction has been a problem as the development of effective antineoplastic agents has decreased mortality rates and increased the number of cancer survivors.
- To avoid chemotherapy-related cardiac dysfunction, early detection and timely discontinuation of cardiotoxic drugs has become a standard treatment strategy.
- Traditional biomarkers are commonly measured to detect early signs of chemotherapy-related cardiac dysfunction (CRCD), but their predictability in CRCD is inconsistent among studies.
- Alternative biomarkers have been investigated because of the need for more sensitive, accurate, and reliable biomarkers. Proteomics and genomics are under investigation in translational research and are potential reliable biomarkers.
- A combination of different methods may improve the accuracy in screening patients at high risk of CRCD.

INTRODUCTION

Chemotherapy-related cardiac dysfunction (CRCD) has challenged clinicians in choosing the best cardiotoxic agents such as anthracycline and several protein kinase inhibitors to treat cancers. Because the recommended total cumulative dose of doxorubicin (500–550 mg/m²) originated from statistical rather than pathophysiologic principles,[1] patients who may tolerate a higher dose of drug are deprived of the chance of appropriate treatment owing to this empirical dose limitation recommendation. Screening patients at risk of CRCD has mainly been dependent on the left ventricular ejection fraction (LVEF). Despite consensus statements from several groups,[2] there are multiple definitions for reduced LVEF. In fact, LVEF turned out to lack sensitivity to detect subclinical decline of ventricular function with chemotherapy treatment.[3,4] Therefore, endeavors have been made to find novel biomarkers capable of detecting early subclinical changes in various cardiovascular diseases.[5,6]

Over the decades, there have been many studies investigating the relationship between biomarkers and CRCD (Table 1). However, many of these studies are single-center observations and well-designed studies with good statistical power are rare. The majority of these studies involved clinically available biomarkers of myocardial necrosis (eg, cardiac troponin) or myocardial stress

Support: Dr W.H.W. Tang is supported by research grants from the National Institute of Health (R01HL103931).
Disclosure: None.
a Department of Cardiovascular Medicine, Kaufman Center for Heart Failure, Heart and Vascular Institute, Cleveland Clinic, Cleveland, OH, USA; b Cardiovascular Medicine, Korea University College of Medicine, Korea University Medical Center Ansan Hospital, 123 Jeokgeum-ro, Ansan-si 15355, Korea; c Department of Cellular and Molecular Medicine, Lerner Research Institute, Cleveland Clinic, Cleveland, OH, USA; d Center for Clinical Genomics, Cleveland Clinic, Cleveland, OH, USA
* Corresponding author. Heart and Vascular Institute, Cleveland Clinic, 9500 Euclid Avenue, Desk J3-4, Cleveland, OH 44195.
E-mail address: tangw@ccf.org

Table 1
Cardiac biomarker studies for chemotherapy related cardiac dysfunction

Author (Published Year)	Study Designs/ Duration of Observation	Biomarkers	Study Subjects	Results	Comments
No or very short interval from biomarker measurement to cardiac function evaluation					
Bauch et al,[91] 1992	Cross-sectional	ANP	16 pediatric patients.	ANP useful.	More cardiac events in patients with increased ANP.
Missov et al,[92] 1997	Cross-sectional	hs-TnI, CK-MB, myoglobin	30 patients with ANT vs 25 ANT-naïve patients vs 60 healthy controls.	cTnI useful.	Increased cTnI in only doxorubicin-treated patients. No ΔLVEF.
Nousiainen et al,[93] 1999	Cross-sectional	ANP, NTproANP, BNP	30 patients with lymphoma.	Not useful.	ΔNP was correlated with ΔLVEF. ΔNP was slower than ΔLVEF.
Hayakawa et al,[94] 2001	Cross-sectional	ANP, BNP	34 childhood cancer survivors vs healthy controls.	ANP, BNP useful.	ANP and BNP increased in patients and were correlated with LVEF.
Nousiainen et al,[95] 2002	Cross-sectional	ANP, NTproBNP, BNP	30 patients with lymphoma.	ANP, NTproBNP, BNP useful.	NP had no correlation with LV systolic function, but had correlation with LV diastolic function.
Poutanen et al,[96] 2003	Cross-sectional	NTproANP	39 childhood cancer survivors.	NTproANP useful.	NTproANP was correlated with cumulative ANT dose. No predictability suggested.

Kismet et al,[97] 2004	Cross-sectional	cTnT	24 patients with solid tumor.	cTnT Not useful.	No increase in cTnT during follow-up. No correlation between cTnT, cumulative dose of doxorobicin and cardiac functions.
Köseoğlu et al,[98] 2005	Cross-sectional	cTnI	22 pediatric patients with solid tumor.	cTnI not useful.	No correlation between cTnI, cumulative dose of doxorobicin and echocardiographic parameters.
Perik et al,[99] 2006	Cross-sectional	NTproBNP	15 patients with breast cancer.	NTproBNP useful.	Increased NTproBNP in patients with cardiotoxicity more than those without.
Aggarwal et al,[100] 2007	Cross-sectional	BNP	63 pediatric patients.	BNP useful.	BNP associated with LV dysfunction other than LVEF.
Jones et al,[101] 2007	Cross-sectional	BNP	26 postchemotherapy patients vs 10 matched controls.	BNP useful.	Increased BNP in patients. Correlation between BNP and LVEF.
Krawczuk-Rybak et al,[37] 2011	Cross-sectional	proBNP	44 pediatric patients with hematologic malignancies vs control groups.	BNP useful.	Increased proBNP in patients.

(continued on next page)

Table 1
(continued)

Author (Published Year)	Study Designs/ Duration of Observation	Biomarkers	Study Subjects	Results	Comments
D'Errico et al,[102] 2011	Cross-sectional	NTproBNP, cTnI	30 breast cancer patients with irradiation therapy vs 30 without irradiation therapy.	NTproBNP useful, cTnI not useful.	Increased NTproBNP in patient with radiation therapy.
Guler et al,[103] 2009	Cross-sectional	Total nitrite level	29 pediatric patients vs matched controls.	Nitrite level increased.	Increased nitrite level in patients.
Tragiannidis et al,[104] 2012	Cross-sectional	BNP	20 children with hematologic malignancies.	BNP useful.	Increased BNP and decreased LVEF after intensive chemotherapy.
Sherief et al,[105] 2012	Cross-sectional	cTnT, NTproBNP	50 acute leukemia survivors.	NTproBNP useful.	Increased NTproBNP in patients.
Pongprot et al,[7] 2012	Cross-sectional	NTproBNP, cTnT, CK-MB	30 pediatric patients.	NTproBNP useful.	Higher NTproBNP in LV dysfunction.
Mladosievicova et al,[106] 2012	Cross-sectional	NTproBNP	36 pediatric patients with ANT, 33 without ANT, 44 healthy controls.	NTproBNP useful.	Increased NTproBNP in patients with ANT exposure.
Arslan et al,[8] 2013	Cross-sectional	GDF-15, cTnI, myocardial strain	38 pediatric patients vs 32 matched controls.	GDF-15 useful. cTnI not useful.	Increased GDF-15 in patients.
Ylänen et al,[107] 2015	Cross-sectional	NTproBNP, cTnT, hs-cTnT, cTnI, cTnAAbs	76 childhood cancer survivors.	NTproBNP and cTnAAbs useful.	Increased NTproBNP and increased cTnAAbs in patients with cardiac dysfunction. No increase in hs-cTnT.

Study	Design/Interval	Biomarker	Patients	Conclusion	Findings
Pourier et al,[108] 2015	Cross-sectional	hs-cTnT, NTproBNP	64 childhood cancer survivors.	Hs-cTnT not useful.	No increase in hs-cTnT.
Şendur et al,[9] 2015	Cross-sectional	hs-CRP, NTproBNP	164 patients.	NTproBNP useful,	NTproBNP associated with LVEF loss.
van Boxtel et al,[109] 2015	Cross-sectional	NT-proBNP, TNF-α, galectin-3, IL-6, cTnI, ST2, sFlt-1	55 patients with breast cancer.	NTproBNP useful.	Correlation between ΔNTproBNP and ΔLVEF.
Oliveira-Carvalho et al,[80] 2015	Cross-sectional	cTnT, miR208a	59 breast cancer patients.	cTnT useful, miR208a not useful.	Increased cTnT, no increase in miR208.
Caram et al,[10] 2015	Cross-sectional	BNP, cTnT, NTproBNP, urine NTproBNP	269 breast cancer patients.	NTproBNP useful.	Correlation between NTproBNP and LV systolic dysfunction.
Short interval from biomarker measurement to cardiac function evaluation (< 3 mo)					
Kremer et al,[110] 2002	24 h	cTnT	38 pediatric patients.	cTnT not useful.	Measurement of cTnT within 24 h had low sensitivity for the identification of following cardiotoxicity.
Sandri et al,[111] 2003	72 h	cTnI	179 patients with solid or hematologic malignancies.	cTnI useful.	Increased cTnI predicted a decreased LVEF.
Specchia et al,[11] 2005	1 mo	cTnI, myoglobin, CPK, LDH	79 with hematologic malignancies.	cTnI useful.	ΔcTnI was correlated with ΔLVEF.
Polena et al,[112] 2005	48 h	cTnI	38 patients.	Not useful.	No change in cTnI, LVEF.
Kuittinen et al,[16] 2006	3 mo	NTproANP, NTproBNP	30 adults patients with NHL.	Probably not useful.	NP transiently increased but normalized within 3 mo.

(continued on next page)

Table 1
(continued)

Author (Published Year)	Study Designs/ Duration of Observation	Biomarkers	Study Subjects	Results	Comments
Mercuro et al,[17] 2007	7 d	BNP, cTnI, myoglobin, CK-MB, IL-6, glutathione peroxidase, ROS	16 patients with solid tumor.	ROS useful.	Level of ROS predicted reduction of myocardial strain (no reduction of LVEF).
Zver et al,[14] 2008	3 mo	cTnI, BNP, endothelin-1	30 patients with multiple myeloma.	BNP useful.	Increased BNP associated with LV diastolic dysfunction, no ΔLVEF.
Goel et al,[113] 2011	24 h	NTproBNP, cTnI	36 patients	Increased NTproBNP.	Increased NTproBNP in 39% of patients. No ΔLVEF.
Roziakova et al,[12] 2012	1 mo	NTproBNP, hs-cTnT	37 patients with hematologic malignancies.	NTproBNP, hs-cTnT useful.	Persistent increase in NTproBNP, hs-cTnT was associated with subsequent LV dysfunction.
Roziakova et al,[114] 2012	1–2 mo	NTproBNP, cTnT	21 patients with hematologic malignancies for hematopoietic stem cell transplantation.	NTproBNP, cTnT useful.	Increased NTproBNP, increased cTnT in treated patients.
Kittiwarawut et al,[15] 2013	3 mo	NTproBNP, cTnT, CK-MB	52 breast cancer patients.	NTproBNP useful.	Increased NTproBNP was associated with a subsequent decrease in LVEF.

Study	Time interval	Biomarker	Patients	Conclusion	Findings
Blaes et al,[13] 2015	1 mo	hs-cTnT, NTproBNP, cTnT, cTnI, CK-MB	18 breast or NHL patients.	hs-cTnT useful.	Baseline hs-cTnT before chemotherapy was associated with reduced LV systolic function 4 wk after chemotherapy.
Long interval from biomarker measurement to cardiac function evaluation (>3 mo)					
Lipshultz et al,[23] 1997	9 mo	cTnT	15 children with ALL.	cTnT useful.	Increased cTnT predicted LV dilatation and wall thinning after 9 mo.
Okumura et al,[32] 2000	7 mo	BNP, ANP	13 patients with acute leukemia.	BNP useful.	Increased BNP before development of subclinical or clinical HF.
Mathew et al,[115] 2001	9 mo	cTnI	15 pediatric patients.	Not useful.	No ΔcTnI, no ΔLVEF during follow-up.
Meinardi et al,[116] 2001	1 y	NTproANP and BNP	40 breast cancer patients.	NTproANP, BNP not useful.	NTproANP, BNP increased but no correlation between ΔNP and ΔLVEF.
Auner et al,[18] 2003	3–12 mo	cTnT	78 patients with hematologic malignancies.	cTnT useful.	Positive cTnT predicted delayed LV systolic dysfunction.
Kilickap et al,[33] 2005	4–6 mo	cTnT	41 patients.	cTnT useful.	Increased cTnT, but no ΔLVEF during follow-up. cTnT was correlated with LV diastolic dysfunction.

(continued on next page)

Table 1
(continued)

Author (Published Year)	Study Designs/ Duration of Observation	Biomarkers	Study Subjects	Results	Comments
Pichon et al,[26] 2005	2–3 y	BNP	12 breast cancer patients.	BNP useful.	Increased BNP in patients developing heart failure during follow-up. BNP was correlated with LVEF and cumulative dose of anthracycline.
Daugaard et al,[40] 2005	1 y	NTproANP, BNP	107 patients.	NTproANP, BNP not useful.	Correlation between NP and LVEF, but no correlation between ΔNP and ΔLVEF.
Ekstein et al,[117] 2007	4–6 mo	NTproBNP	23 pediatric patients vs 54 control.	Not useful.	Increased NTproBNP only after first cycle. No change in cardiac function.
Dodos et al,[38] 2008	6 mo	BNP, cTnT	100 patients.	Not useful.	No ΔBNP, No ΔcTnT during follow-up.
Horacek et al,[27] 2007	6 mo	NTproBNP, cTnT	26 patients with acute leukemia.	NTproBNP useful; cTnT not useful.	NTproBNP was correlated with LV systolic and diastolic dysfunction. cTnT did not increased during follow-up.
Horacek et al,[52] 2008	6 mo	Myoglobin, CK-MB, cTnT, cTnI, H-FABP, GPBB.	12 patients with acute leukemia.	GPBB useful	Increased GPBB in 16.7%, increased cTnI/cTnT in 8.3% of patients. No information on LV function.

Study	Time	Biomarker	Population	Conclusion	Comments
Lee et al,[118] 2008	6 mo to 2 y	BNP	86 patients with hematologic malignancies.	BNP useful.	Various cardiac events developed, but there was no LV dysfunction developed.
Feola et al,[28] 2011	2 y	cTnI, BNP	53 patients with breast cancer.	BNP useful, cTnI not useful.	Baseline BNP significantly associated with reduced LVEF at second year.
Cardinale et al,[19] 2010	34 mo	cTnI	251 patients with breast cancer.	cTnI useful.	Positive cTnI at baseline predicted reduced LVEF.
Horacek et al,[119] 2010	4–6 mo	GPBB, H-FABP, cTnT, cTnI, CK-MB, myoglobin	47 adults with acute leukemia.	GPBB useful.	Increased GPBB in 21.7%, cTnI/CTnT increased 8.3% of patients. No information on LV function.
Sawaya et al,[34] 2011	6 mo	NTproBNP, hs-cTnI	43 patients with breast cancers.	hs-cTnI useful, NTproBNP not useful.	hs-cTnI and longitudinal strain at 3 mo predicted cardiotoxicity at 6 mo.
Romano et al,[29] 2011	12 mo	NTproBNP	71 patients (no/transient increase in NTproBNP vs persistent increase in NTproBNP).	NTproBNP useful.	ΔNTproBNP predicted LV dysfunction at 3-, 6-, and 12-mo follow-up.
Morris et al,[59] 2011	18 mo	cTnI, CRP	95 patients with breast cancer.	cTnI not useful.	Increase in cTnI preceded decline in LVEF, but did not predict reduction of LVEF.

(continued on next page)

Table 1
(continued)

Author (Published Year)	Study Designs/ Duration of Observation	Biomarkers	Study Subjects	Results	Comments
Garrone et al,[56] 2012	40 mo	Hemoglobin, cTnI, BNP, catecholamines	50 patients with early breast cancer.	Hemoglobin useful.	ΔLVEF and Δhemoglobin predicted reduced LVEF or clinical heart failure at 40 mo.
Onitilo et al,[120] 2012	3–4 mo	BNP, hs-CRP, cTnI	54 patients with breast cancer.	hs-CRP useful, BNP and cTnI not useful.	hs-CRP predicted reduction of LVEF with high negative predictive value.
Sawaya et al,[20] 2012	15 mo	NTproBNP, ultrasensitive-cTnI, ST2	81 patients with breast cancer.	Ultrasensitive-cTnI useful, NTproBNP and ST2 not useful	hs-cTnI and longitudinal strain predicted reduced LVEF or clinical HF.
Mavinkurve-Groothuis et al,[35] 2013	1 y	NTproBNP, cTnT	60 pediatric patients with acute leukemia vs 60 age matched healthy controls.	NTproBNP, cTnT not useful.	NT proBNP, cTnT did not predict LV dysfunction evaluated by strain analysis (no Δ LV fractional shortening).
Ky et al,[21] 2014	15 mo	Ultrasensitive-cTnI, hs-CRP, NTproBNP, GDF-15, MPO, PlGF, sFlt-1, Galectin-3	78 patients with breast cancer.	Ultrasensitive-cTnI, MPO useful.	Increase in ultrasensitive-cTnI and increase in MPO associated with a subsequent decrease in LVEF or clinical HF.
Katsurada et al,[22] 2014	15 mo	hs-cTnT	19 patients with breast cancer.	hs-cTnT useful.	Increased hs-cTnT at 6 mo predicted ΔLVEF at 15 mo.

Study	Duration	Biomarkers	Population	Useful	Findings
Putt et al,[53] 2015	15 mo	hs-cTnI, hs-CRP, NT-proBNP, GDF-15, MPO, PlGF, sFlt-1, galectin-3	78 patients with breast cancer.	MPO, PlGF, GDF-15 useful.	Increased MPO, PlGF, GDF-15 was associated with cardiotoxicity at subsequent visits.
De Iuliis et al,[30] 2016	1 y	NTproBNP	100 patients with breast cancer.	NTproBNP useful.	Increase in NTproBNP before evident ΔLVEF.
Lenihan et al,[31] 2016	6–12 mo	cTnI, BNP	109 patients.	BNP useful.	Increased in BNP in patients with cardiac events.

Abbreviations: ALL, acute lymphocytic leukemia; ANP, atrial natriuretic peptide; ANT, anthracycline; BNP, B-type natriuretic peptide; CK-MB, creatinine kinase-MB type isoenzyme; CPK, creatine phosphokinase; cTnAAbs, cardiac troponin specific autoantibodies; cTnI, cardiac troponin I; cTnT, cardiac troponin T; GDF-15, growth differentiation factor-15; GPBB, glycogen phosphorylase BB; HF, heart failure; H-FABP, heart type fatty acid binding protein; hs-CRP, high sensitive C reactive protein; hs-TnI, highly sensitive troponin I; IL, interleukin; LDH, lactate dehydrogenase; LV, left ventricular; LVEF, left ventricular ejection fraction; miR208a, microRNA 208a; MPO, myoeloperoxidase; NHL, non-Hodgkin lymphoma; NP, natriuretic peptide; NTproANP, amino terminal pro-atrial natriuretic peptide; NTproBNP, Amino terminal pro B-type natriuretic peptide; PlGF, placental derived growth factor; ROS, reactive oxygen species; sFlt-1, soluble fms-like tyrosine kinase receptor 1; ST2, soluble form of interleukin-1 receptor; TNF-α, tumor necrosis factor-α.

(eg, natriuretic peptides). Studies have reported consistently an increase in cardiac troponin or natriuretic peptide in patients treated with anthracycline or anti–HER-2 monoclonal antibodies (see Table 1). Probably because of difficulties in follow-up, particularly in pediatric populations, these studies were designed as cross-sectional analyses where the biomarkers were supposed to predict development of cardiac dysfunction when there were significant correlations between changes of biomarkers level in serum and changes in cardiac function (ie, LVEF).[7–10] However, correlations between changes of serum biomarker levels and reduced cardiac function do not necessarily imply the ability of biomarkers to predict cardiac dysfunction, consistently to a lack in temporal causality.

There are other studies on the acute or subacute toxicity of anthracycline, with evaluations within a few days to months after administration of the agents, where the increase in troponin was assumed to predict reduced LVEF.[11–13] Increased natriuretic peptides in patients also seemed to predict development of CRCD,[14,15] but the natriuretic peptides would often normalize in subsequent cycles of chemotherapy.[16] Although the usefulness of cardiac troponin and natriuretic peptides in predicting cardiac dysfunction was proposed in short-term studies, the development of cardiac dysfunction was often judged based on the presence of left ventricular diastolic dysfunction or alteration of myocardial strain rather than the LVEF, because reductions in LVEF were not prominent in many short-term studies.[14,17] Oncologists' efforts to reduce the administration of cardiotoxic agents and subtle reductions in LVEF may be reasons many clinical studies failed to demonstrate predictability of the biomarkers.

In contrast, because normalization of both elevated biomarkers and cardiac function were frequently observed during short-term observation, longer observation studies were required. Despite still contradictory results, elevated cardiac troponin or natriuretic peptide seemed to predict the development of cardiac dysfunction or clinical heart failure during observation periods of more than three months after the completion of chemotherapy.[18–22] Increased cardiac troponin predicted cardiac remodeling, such as left ventricular dilatation and wall thinning, nine months after chemotherapy as well as functional deterioration.[23] In the largest study to date, Cardinale and colleagues showed that plasma cardiac troponin I (cTnI) measured at various time points was predictive of subsequent cardiotoxicity with high positive and negative predictive values in a study of 703 patients with diverse malignancies. In addition, patients with sustained elevation of cTnI had a greater reduction of left ventricular dysfunction than those whose cTnI levels normalized during follow-up. Death and symptomatic heart failure were more prevalent in patients with sustained elevation of cTnI as well.[19,24] High-sensitivity or ultrasensitive cardiac troponin assays drew attention in recent studies because they are known to detect as small an amount of myocardial necrosis as corresponding with 10 ng/L of cardiac troponin or less.[25] Ultrasensitive cTnI, along with the measurement of left ventricular systolic strain, predicted the development of CRCD in 81 patients who were treated with anthracycline followed by trastuzumab and taxanes where LVEF decreased from $64 \pm 5\%$ to $59 \pm 6\%$ ($P < .0001$) during 15 months of observation.[20]

The elevation of natriuretic peptides also preceded cardiac dysfunction and clinical heart failure and correlated with cumulative doses of anthracycline, suggesting predictability for development of CRCD.[26–31] In a Japanese study, natriuretic peptide, as detected by radionuclide angiography, increased before the development of clinical or subclinical heart failure. The authors suggested B-type natriuretic peptide (BNP) as a sensitive indicator of daunorubicin-induced cardiomyopathy.[32] However, because reduction of LVEF was not prominent in all of the long-term studies, other indicators of cardiac dysfunction such as left ventricular diastolic dysfunction or myocardial strain were adopted for endpoints like in the short-term observation studies discussed herein.[33–35]

CRITICISM AGAINST CARDIAC TROPONIN AND NATRIURETIC PEPTIDES

Several studies have raised questions about the usefulness of traditional biomarkers of cardiac dysfunction in predicting CRCD. Pavo and colleagues[36] evaluated amino-terminal proBNP (NT-proBNP), midregional proatrial natriuretic peptide, midregional proadrenomedullin, C-terminal pro–endothelin-1, copeptin, high-sensitivity cardiac troponin T (hs-cTnT), interleukin-6, high-sensitivity C-reactive protein (CRP), serum amyloid A, haptoglobin, and fibronectin in 555 patients with various malignancies and without evidence of cardiac disease. In the study, before antineoplastic chemotherapy, multiple vasoactive peptides and hs-cTnT were elevated and correlated significantly with systemic proinflammatory markers interleukin-6 and C-reactive protein. All of the biomarkers were elevated as the stage of the malignancy progressed. The presence of NT-proBNP, midregional proatrial natriuretic peptide, midregional proadrenomedullin, hs-cTnT, and copeptin were associated with all-cause mortality. The findings in the study may defy the traditional notion that increased troponin or natriuretic peptides are predictive of CRCD because the biomarkers were increased before chemotherapy. According to the results, higher troponin or natriuretic peptides seem to indicate that the patients in more severe status of malignancy and require more aggressive chemotherapy rather than discontinuation of chemotherapy.[36] Blaes and colleagues[13] also reported that patients with a reduced LVEF four weeks after the completion of chemotherapy had higher levels of hs-cTnT at baseline before chemotherapy, which suggests there are certain patients with latent cardiac dysfunction, which may be aggravated by chemotherapy more rapidly.

The majority of studies examined reported that natriuretic peptide levels are predictive of both short- and long-term cardiac dysfunction. Of note, serum natriuretic peptide increased during the early phase of chemotherapy and decreased gradually after the cessation of chemotherapy.[37] Furthermore, patients with persistently elevated natriuretic peptide seem more susceptible to future ventricular dysfunction.[29] However, because chemotherapy is usually accompanied by intravenous hydration during administration to reduce systemic toxicity, it is possible that the elevated natriuretic peptide might result from acute volume or pressure overload on the ventricles rather than cardiotoxicity by chemotherapy agents.[38] For example, in a placebo-controlled study by Reijers and Burggraaf,[39] when either trastuzumab or placebo in normal saline was infused into healthy volunteers, serum NT-proBNP was found to be elevated after 4 days in both groups. Another example comes from a study of patients with multiple myeloma who underwent chemotherapy containing cyclophosphamide.[14] The administration of cyclophosphamide is complicated frequently by hemorrhagic cystitis as well as cardiac injury and requires large amounts of hydration before and during treatment. In this study, serum BNP concentrations significantly increased, whereas cTnI was within normal range. Although there was no reduction in the LVEF, left ventricular diastolic dysfunction developed. Interestingly, functional mitral regurgitation developed in 40% of patients, suggesting overloaded intravascular volume, although the authors did not provide information on hydration or the weight change of enrolled patients.

In a study by Daugaard and colleagues,[40] natriuretic peptide showed significant correlation with LVEF when LVEF was less than 50% but no correlation when LVEF was 50% or greater. Changes in the serum natriuretic peptide level were not correlated with changes in the LVEF either. These results suggest that the release of natriuretic peptide does not increase without impaired cardiac dysfunction and, therefore, elevation of natriuretic peptide may follow reduced LVEF rather than precede it.[40] Conversely, because natriuretic peptides are usually measured during hospitalization, elevated natriuretic peptide may indicate latent left ventricular dysfunction that becomes prominent with hydration with or without chemotherapy.[41] Therefore, whether an elevated natriuretic peptide indicates toxicity of a chemotherapy agent per se rather than a latent cardiac dysfunction before chemotherapy that deteriorates into prominent cardiac dysfunction during chemotherapy must be clarified.

CANDIDATE ALTERNATIVE BIOMARKERS FOR CHEMOTHERAPY-RELATED CARDIAC DYSFUNCTION

With the usefulness of cardiac troponin and natriuretic peptides called into question, various other cardiac biomarkers validated for ischemic heart disease or heart failure have been investigated for usefulness in cardiooncology.[5] These potential biomarkers include peptides, hormones, and cytokines, and are representative of various potential mechanisms of cardiotoxicity (eg, oxidative stress, fibroblast proliferation or ischemia). For example, serum levels of myeloperoxidase (MPO), an enzyme produced by polymorphonuclear leukocytes with a proposed role in oxidative stress, were found to increase with worsening cardiac function and clinical outcomes,[42,43] whereas growth differentiation factor 15, which belongs to a superfamily of transforming growth factor-β cytokines and seems to be stimulated by oxidative stress, inflammation, or injury, was elevated in cancer survivors treated with anthracycline.[8,44] Other potential biomarkers involved in oxidative stress or inflammatory pathways include erythrocyte superoxide dismutase and resistin, which both increase in response to inflammatory stimuli.[45,46] Additional potential biomarkers representing fibroblast proliferation and cardiac hypertrophy include placental growth factor, soluble fms-like tyrosine kinase receptor 1, and galectin-3,[47–49] whereas glycogen phosphorylase BB was suggested as a potential biomarker in acute coronary syndrome because it is released during the early ischemic phase.[50–52]

In perhaps the most important study to date, Ky and colleagues[21] studied multiple biomarkers in

78 breast cancer patients who were treated with doxorubicin followed by trastuzumab. They investigated multiple biomarkers in patients with breast cancers, in which each biomarker represented a specific pathway of CRCD: cardiomyocyte injury (high-sensitivity cTnI), inflammation (high-sensitivity C-reactive protein and growth differentiation factor 15), neurohormonal activation (NT-proBNP), oxidative stress (MPO), antiangiogenesis and vascular remodeling (placental growth factor and soluble fms-like tyrosine kinase receptor 1), and fibrosis (galectin-3).[21] Among the evaluated biomarkers, hs-cTnI and MPO were associated with cardiotoxicity, whereas the others showed no association.[21,53] In particular, the interval increase in serum levels of the two biomarkers during the early phase after chemotherapy predicted cardiotoxicity. Combining troponin and MPO is proposed to produce better usefulness in predicting subsequent cardiotoxicity; the functional axis of the biomarkers was orthogonal.

However, in a conflicting study by Putt and colleagues,[53] growth differentiation factor 15 and placental growth factor, as well as MPO, did show significant association with cardiotoxicity at both the same visit and subsequent visits. Although the number of enrolled patients was relatively small, the study was designed to have enough power to detect significant hazards.[53] Interestingly, hs-cTnI and natriuretic peptides did not show significant association with cardiotoxicity, which the authors attributed to missing data.

Another potential biomarker of cardiotoxicity, ischemia-modified albumin (IMA), is produced when human serum albumin passes through ischemic tissue and undergoes modification at the N-terminus. The reactive oxygen species produced in ischemic tissue seem to play a role in this process.[54] Because IMA can be detected during the early stages of myocardial ischemia before apparent myocardial necrosis, it has been suggested as a biomarker of myocardial ischemia and, because oxidative stress is a leading mechanism of doxorubicin-induced cardiac injury, the ability of IMA to predict doxorubicin-induced cardiomyopathy was investigated. In a study with 152 breast cancer patients, an increase of IMA showed significant correlation with reduction in LVEF and had a greater area under the curve in receiver operator characteristic curves than those of cardiac troponin or creatinine kinase-MB type isoenzyme. Furthermore, combined measurement of IMA, troponin, and creatinine kinase-MB type isoenzyme had 92% sensitivity and 83% specificity for detection of cardiac injury at 12 months after chemotherapy.[55]

Finally, taking a different approach and moving away from biomarkers altogether, Garrone and colleagues[56] suggested that the degree of change in LVEF or rate of reduction in hemoglobin concentration held greater predictive value of further reduction of left ventricular systolic function than the measurement of one or two cardiac biomarkers such as cardiac troponin or natriuretic peptide. In a study of 50 early breast cancer patients with three years of follow-up, the reduction of LVEF to less than 53% or decreasing hemoglobin blood concentration greater than 0.33 g/dL per month during chemotherapy increased the odds of subsequent cardiotoxicity by 37.3 and 18.0, respectively, with a specificity of 93.3% and 80.0% and a sensitivity of 90.9% and 81.2%. The authors supposed the anthracycline had myelotoxicity to reduce hemoglobin concentration as well as cardiotoxicity. In any case, measuring and comparing the change in metabolomic parameters such as hemoglobin may shift the focus of investigation from biomarkers to inherent diathesis of individuals.[56]

UNDERREFINED STUDY DESIGNS MAY UNDERMINE CREDIBILITY IN PREVIOUS CARDIAC BIOMARKER STUDIES

In many studies dealing with CRCD, relatively low rates of adverse cardiac events, inadequate numbers, and high dropout rates resulted in diminished statistical power to prove usefulness of potential biomarkers. Notably, clinicians' efforts to reduce the administration of cardiotoxic agents to their patients might have helped to preserve cardiac function and potentially lead to statistically underpowered studies with inconsistent results. With current clinical guidelines somewhat conservative in defining CRCD (ie, reduction of LVEF > 10% or development of clinical heart failure),[2] investigators had difficulty in demonstrating the predictability of potential biomarkers.[57,58] Inconsistent timing of blood sampling among cohort studies or groups in a cohort might have also played a role in contradictory results in the biomarker studies. In particular, many chemotherapy protocols have changed to a 1-day hospital stay where frequent blood sampling for serial assessment of the biomarkers becomes implausible.[57]

In general principle, the usefulness of cardiac biomarkers in predicting cardiotoxicity must be demonstrated by their elevation in blood before a prominent reduction in LVEF during follow-up. However, many studies instead concluded that significant correlations among the blood levels of cardiac biomarkers, invasively or noninvasively measured left ventricular function, and cumulative anthracycline dose meant that the cardiac biomarkers were useful predictors of reduced cardiac function. However, correlations among the parameters at a certain time point do not guarantee the predictability of the biomarkers, only their correlation at the time point measured.[59] These interfering factors must be sorted out during study design to ensure that predictability can be discerned reliably.

PROTEOMICS/GENOMICS UNDER INVESTIGATION TO SEARCH FOR NOVEL BIOMARKERS

As another alternative to using cardiac troponin or natriuretic peptides, several authors have looked for biomarkers in the patient's genome or proteome. For example, quantifying the intercalation of anthracycline molecules into DNA to form doxorubicin–DNA adducts has been suggested as a potential preclinical marker of doxorubicin-induced myocardial injury. Depurination of deoxyguanine monophosphate and deoxyadenosine-5'-monophosphate occurs in parallel with increasing adriamycin concentration, enabling the quantification of the formed DNA adducts even at low doses of doxorubicin.[60] It is conceivable that analysis from more accessible tissue (eg, skeletal muscle lymph nodes) surrogating doxorubicin-exposed myocardium may make this diagnostic approach feasible in the near future, but its predictive value remains to be determined.

Drug-induced damage to organs can change circulating blood proteomes constantly, which may contain high amounts of previously undiscovered potential biomarkers. Detection of these low-molecular-weight peptide fragments may have specificity for the disease based on the unique microenvironment of damaged organs. As the most common analytical platform, serum proteomic pattern diagnostics can be used to produce a pattern of proteomic signatures. This method showed a 98.0% negative predictive value and a 69.4% positive predictive value in an animal study in which saline or doxorubicin with or without dexrazoane was administered. Rats administered with a weaker cardiotoxin, mitoxanthrone, were also classified as diseased, showing good classification accuracy of the method.[61] In contrast, because different drugs with different toxicities can induce similar metabolomic alterations, in studies of biomarkers based on metabolomics you must be able to distinguish between cardiotoxicity and other end-organ toxicities.[62] Meanwhile, S100A1, a member of the S100 protein family, is mainly expressed in cardiac muscle.

This protein is known to be a regulator of myocardial contractility by way of Ca^{2+}-induced Ca^{2+} release.[63] In rats treated with trastuzumab or lapatinib, serum cTnI was elevated, whereas the S100A1 level in serum was significantly reduced. Therefore, the authors suggested that measurement of S100A1 might be used as a detector of cardiotoxicity.[64]

Genomic biomarkers are a new area of exploration for the detection and prediction of cardiotoxicity. Toxicogenomic analysis was suggested as a potential tool to evaluate the toxicity mechanism of various chemicals and may be used to detect early pathology induced by the chemicals. This approach previously identified genes such as kidney injury molecule 1 (Kim1), lipocalin 2 (Lcn2), and secreted phosphoprotein 1 (Spp1) in rats, which are now acknowledged as promising genomic biomarkers of acute nephrotoxicity in humans.[65] Hearts from rats administered with cardiotoxic agents (including doxorubicin) upregulated expression of 36 genes that were related to inflammation and degeneration of myocardium. Contrary to cardiac troponin, which is normalized rapidly after the completion of chemotherapy, upregulated genes showed sustained elevation profiles that are advantageous to detect long-term cardiovascular complications at early stage toxicity screening. Intriguingly, 5 of 36 upregulated genes predicted cardiac dysfunction, even before the development of histopathologic changes with high specificity.[66] Todorova and colleagues[67] investigated genomic biomarkers from both hearts and peripheral blood cells from doxorubicin-exposed rats. Because obtaining cardiomyocytes from patients is not always possible, they hypothesized that genomic biomarkers from peripheral blood cells could surrogate for cardiomyocytes. They found 2411 genes are dysregulated both in heart and peripheral blood cells from doxorubicin-treated rats and suggested 188 molecules among the genes as potential biomarkers, which were known to be associated with decreased transcription and expression of RNA. Interestingly, the analysis of dysregulated genes expressed in both hearts and peripheral blood cells revealed the oxidative stress-related pathway is a main pathway in doxorubicin toxicity.[67] Doxorubicin seems to induce the premature senescence of cardiac progenitor cells and reduced regenerative capacity; consequentially, it provides a basis of doxorubicin-induced cardiomyopathy.[68] With cardiomyocytes treated with doxorubicin or other anthracyclines, dozens of unique protein features involving dysregulation of protein folding, translational regulation, and cytoskeleton regulation were overexpressed and suggested as potential biomarkers.[69–72] Similar to anthracycline, trastuzumab also upregulated or downregulated the expression of genes related to oxidative stress and apoptosis in mice.[73] However, generalization to clinical practice warrants much caution because very little about genomic biomarkers in this topic has been studied in human subjects.

MicroRNAs (miRNAs) are endogenous, 19 to 25 nucleotide-long, regulatory RNA molecules. Their functions were once thought to be limited to the developmental phase of some lower forms of life, but they are now acknowledged to play a role in posttranscriptional regulation of messenger RNAs in a diverse range of physiologic processes as well as in the developmental stage.[74] Four weekly administration of doxorubicin in rats revealed dysregulation of 25 miRNAs among 370 measurable miRNAs from excised rat hearts. Five of these dysregulated microRNAs (miR208b, miR215, miR216b, miR34c, and miR367) were thought to be potential cardiac biomarkers because they showed consistent dose-dependent alteration in amounts of administered doxorubicin. Interestingly, alteration of miRNAs occurred in the absence of histopathologic change, suggesting that miRNAs are the most sensitive of the cardiac biomarkers, indicating the earliest cardiac lesions are induced by doxorubicin. Another group of investigators evaluated 1179 unique miRNAs in mice. In this study, the number of differentially expressed miRNA increased as cumulative doses of doxorubicin increased. Among them, miR-34a, related to apoptosis signals, was upregulated at low cumulative doses of doxorubicin and suggested it was a potential biomarker.[75] Although the roles of upregulated miRNAs remain obscure, they can target certain messenger RNA transcriptions to mediate a homeostatic response to toxic stimulation by doxorubicin.[76] When cardiomyoctes from human pluripotent stems cells were treated with doxorubicin, dozens of miRNAs were differently expressed in the cells.[77] However, dysregulated miRNAs of interest still had discrepancies among the type of study, species of animals, and methods of administration of doxorubicin.[76,78,79] Disappointingly, when Oliveira-Cavalho and coworkers[80] investigated 59 patients with breast cancer who underwent a first round of chemotherapy with doxorubicin, cyclophosphamide, and paclitaxel, the level of miR208a in serum did not increase in all patients, although the cardiac troponin increased and LVEF decreased in patients with cardiotoxicity.[80]

NONBLOOD BIOMARKERS: COMBINING WITH NEW IMAGING MODALITIES

In part because of the controversial results from biomarker studies and in part because of the low sensitivity and specificity of LVEF in predicting CRCD, new imaging modalities have been examined to find a substitute for LVEF. In a systematic review of 1504 patients who underwent chemotherapy for cancers, a decrease in global longitudinal strain consistently detected early changes in ventricular function before a reduction in the LVEF. Longitudinal strain reduction between 9% and 19% using 2-dimensional speckle tracking methods or longitudinal strain rate reduction between 9% and 20% using tissue Doppler–based methods were observed during or immediately after chemotherapy in the absence of a reduction in LVEF. In 452 patients with known clinical cardiotoxicity, an early reduction of global longitudinal strain was associated with a subsequent reduction of the LVEF or the development of clinical heart failure.[81] Furthermore, a strain image-guided cardioprotective strategy seems to save medical costs significantly compared with a LVEF-guided strategy, justifying the routine evaluation of strain echocardiography for patients at high risk of CRCD.[82] However, because the degree of myocardial deformation varies depending on age, sex, pressure/volume load, and machine vendors, there is no universal agreement on normal strain, or strain rate values, that could guide preemptive treatment for CRCD. The absence of a consensus is a critical hindrance for strain imaging application in clinical practice.[83]

Novel scintigraphic methods were investigated to detect early functional change during doxorubicin administration. Nuclear cardiology technology may visualize tissue-level pathophysiology at an earlier stage when appropriate tracers are used. Sympathetic neuronal imaging with a wide variety of single photon emission computed tomography and PET tracers, In-111 antimyosin, which is a specific marker of myocyte injury and necrosis; Tc-99m annexin V, which visualized apoptosis and programmed cell death; fatty acid scintigraphy, which visualizes fatty acid retention in the lipid pool of the cytosol and can be impaired by cardiotoxic agents; and direct imaging of In-111 trastuzumab to study trastuzumab targeting of the myocardium have been considered.[84,85]

The induction of apoptosis is assumed as a mechanism of anthracycline-related cardiotoxicity. Caspase-3 may be an indicator of cardiomyocytes apoptosis because it is a catalytic enzyme functioning in the terminal step of apoptosis. When a synthesized caspase-3 substrate (tetrapeptidic caspase substrate labeled with flu-deoxyglucose F 18) tagged with a radioisotope was administered in mice treated with doxoru-bicin, increased uptake of the substrate repre-sented overexpression of caspase-3 activity, which was detected with microPET. It is possible to use CP18 with fludeoxyglucose F 18 as a biomarker of doxorubicin cardiotoxicity.[86]

Finally, cardiac MRI is a promising method to detect early change of CRCD. Serial cardiac MRI evaluation of both ventricles, using the latissimus dorsi muscle for the area of comparison, revealed myocardial edema before an apparent decrease of the LVEF in 46 patients. The LVEF decreased in 5% of patients at 4 months and in 26% of patients at 12 months, and the right ventricular ejection fraction decreased in 23% and 34% at the same points. During observation, NTproBNP did not in-crease and the hs-cTnT increased within normal range. Therefore, myocardial edema, evaluated by cardiac MRI, seems to be a useful method to detect early change in CRCD.[87] A decrease in the regional ventricular tissue velocity, which was evaluated with cardiac MRI, predicted a reduction of LVEF at 6 months of follow-up in patients treated with trastuzumab, whereas troponin and brain natriuretic peptide did not change.[88] The combined use of PET/MRI likely allows the acqui-sition of complimentary data on cardiac structure and function[89] and limits exposure to radiation.[90]

SUMMARY

Although the mechanism of CRCD requires further investigation, the combined use of traditional and novel antineoplastic agents has significantly reduced both morbidity and mortality of patients suffering from malignancies. Troponin and natri-uretic peptide, which are widely used biomarkers in the field of ischemic heart disease and heart fail-ure, have been evaluated for potential usefulness in the early detection of CRCD. Unfortunately, there are considerable controversies on their use-fulness because a significant number of studies failed to demonstrate the predictability of those biomarkers for short- and long-term cardiotoxicity, although many other studies succeeded in doing just that. Owing to an inconclusive usefulness of traditional biomarkers in cardiooncology, alterna-tive biomarkers have been investigated to replace traditional ones, including various peptides, hor-mones, cytokines, proteomics, microRNA, geno-mics, and various combinations thereof. Clearly, the endeavor to find alternative biomarkers in this field is not yet satisfactory and continued research will undoubtedly enlighten future directions of investigation.

REFERENCES

1. Friedman MA, Bozdech MJ, Billingham ME, et al. Doxorubicin cardiotoxicity. Serial endomyocardial biopsies and systolic time intervals. JAMA 1978; 240:1603–6.
2. Mousavi N, Tan TC, Ali M, et al. Echocardiographic parameters of left ventricular size and function as predictors of symptomatic heart failure in patients with a left ventricular ejection fraction of 50-59% treated with anthracyclines. Eur Heart J Cardiovasc Imaging 2015;16:977–84.
3. Swain SM, Whaley FS, Ewer MS. Congestive heart failure in patients treated with doxorubicin: a retro-spective analysis of three trials. Cancer 2003;97: 2869–79.
4. Jensen BV, Skovsgaard T, Nielsen SL. Functional monitoring of anthracycline cardiotoxicity: a pro-spective, blinded, long-term observational study of outcome in 120 patients. Ann Oncol 2002;13: 699–709.
5. Ky B, French B, Levy WC, et al. Multiple biomarkers for risk prediction in chronic heart failure. Circ Heart Fail 2012;5:183–90.
6. Zethelius B, Berglund L, Sundstrom J, et al. Use of multiple biomarkers to improve the prediction of death from cardiovascular causes. N Engl J Med 2008;358:2107–16.
7. Pongprot Y, Sittiwangkul R, Charoenkwan P, et al. Use of cardiac markers for monitoring of doxorubixin-induced cardiotoxicity in children with cancer. J Pediatr Hematol Oncol 2012;34:589–95.
8. Arslan D, Cihan T, Kose D, et al. Growth-differenti-ation factor-15 and tissue Doppler imaging in detection of asymptomatic anthracycline cardio-myopathy in childhood cancer survivors. Clin Bio-chem 2013;46:1239–43.
9. Sendur MA, Aksoy S, Yorgun H, et al. Comparison of the long term cardiac effects associated with 9 and 52 weeks of trastuzumab in her2-positive early breast cancer. Curr Med Res Opin 2015; 31:547–56.
10. Caram ME, Guo C, Leja M, et al. Doxorubicin-induced cardiac dysfunction in unselected patients with a history of early-stage breast cancer. Breast Cancer Res Treat 2015;152:163–72.
11. Specchia G, Buquicchio C, Pansini N, et al. Moni-toring of cardiac function on the basis of serum troponin I levels in patients with acute leukemia treated with anthracyclines. J Lab Clin Med 2005; 145:212–20.
12. Roziakova L, Bojtarova E, Mistrik M, et al. Serial measurements of cardiac biomarkers in patients after allogeneic hematopoietic stem cell transplan-tation. J Exp Clin Cancer Res 2012;31:13.
13. Blaes AH, Rehman A, Vock DM, et al. Utility of high-sensitivity cardiac troponin t in patients receiving

anthracycline chemotherapy. Vasc Health Risk Manag 2015;11:591–4.

14. Zver S, Zadnik V, Cernelc P, et al. Cardiac toxicity of high-dose cyclophosphamide and melphalan in patients with multiple myeloma treated with tandem autologous hematopoietic stem cell transplantation. Int J Hematol 2008;88:227–36.

15. Kittiwarawut A, Vorasettakarnkij Y, Tanasanvimon S, et al. Serum NT-proBNP in the early detection of doxorubicin-induced cardiac dysfunction. Asia Pac J Clin Oncol 2013;9:155–61.

16. Kuittinen T, Jantunen E, Vanninen E, et al. Cardiac effects within 3 months of beac high-dose therapy in non-Hodgkin's lymphoma patients undergoing autologous stem cell transplantation. Eur J Haematol 2006;77:120–7.

17. Mercuro G, Cadeddu C, Piras A, et al. Early epirubicin-induced myocardial dysfunction revealed by serial tissue Doppler echocardiography: correlation with inflammatory and oxidative stress markers. Oncologist 2007;12:1124–33.

18. Auner HW, Tinchon C, Linkesch W, et al. Prolonged monitoring of troponin t for the detection of anthracycline cardiotoxicity in adults with hematological malignancies. Ann Hematol 2003;82:218–22.

19. Cardinale D, Colombo A, Torrisi R, et al. Trastuzumab-induced cardiotoxicity: clinical and prognostic implications of troponin I evaluation. J Clin Oncol 2010;28:3910–6.

20. Sawaya H, Sebag IA, Plana JC, et al. Assessment of echocardiography and biomarkers for the extended prediction of cardiotoxicity in patients treated with anthracyclines, taxanes, and trastuzumab. Circ Cardiovasc Imaging 2012;5:596–603.

21. Ky B, Putt M, Sawaya H, et al. Early increases in multiple biomarkers predict subsequent cardiotoxicity in patients with breast cancer treated with doxorubicin, taxanes, and trastuzumab. J Am Coll Cardiol 2014;63:809–16.

22. Katsurada K, Ichida M, Sakuragi M, et al. High-sensitivity troponin t as a marker to predict cardiotoxicity in breast cancer patients with adjuvant trastuzumab therapy. Springerplus 2014;3:620.

23. Lipshultz SE, Rifai N, Sallan SE, et al. Predictive value of cardiac troponin t in pediatric patients at risk for myocardial injury. Circulation 1997;96:2641–8.

24. Cardinale D, Sandri MT, Colombo A, et al. Prognostic value of troponin I in cardiac risk stratification of cancer patients undergoing high-dose chemotherapy. Circulation 2004;109:2749–54.

25. Sherwood MW, Kristin Newby L. High-sensitivity troponin assays: evidence, indications, and reasonable use. J Am Heart Assoc 2014;3:e000403.

26. Pichon MF, Cvitkovic F, Hacene K, et al. Drug-induced cardiotoxicity studied by longitudinal B-type natriuretic peptide assays and radionuclide ventriculography. In Vivo 2005;19:567–76.

27. Horacek JM, Pudil R, Jebavy L, et al. Assessment of anthracycline-induced cardiotoxicity with biochemical markers. Exp Oncol 2007;29:309–13.

28. Feola M, Garrone O, Occelli M, et al. Cardiotoxicity after anthracycline chemotherapy in breast carcinoma: effects on left ventricular ejection fraction, troponin I and brain natriuretic peptide. Int J Cardiol 2011;148:194–8.

29. Romano S, Fratini S, Ricevuto E, et al. Serial measurements of NT-proBNP are predictive of not-high-dose anthracycline cardiotoxicity in breast cancer patients. Br J Cancer 2011;105:1663–8.

30. De Iuliis F, Salerno G, Taglieri L, et al. Serum biomarkers evaluation to predict chemotherapy-induced cardiotoxicity in breast cancer patients. Tumour Biol 2016;37:3379–87.

31. Lenihan DJ, Stevens PL, Massey M, et al. The utility of point-of-care biomarkers to detect cardiotoxicity during anthracycline chemotherapy: a feasibility study. J Card Fail 2016;22:433–8.

32. Okumura H, Iuchi K, Yoshida T, et al. Brain natriuretic peptide is a predictor of anthracycline-induced cardiotoxicity. Acta Haematol 2000;104:158–63.

33. Kilickap S, Barista I, Akgul E, et al. Ctnt can be a useful marker for early detection of anthracycline cardiotoxicity. Ann Oncol 2005;16:798–804.

34. Sawaya H, Sebag IA, Plana JC, et al. Early detection and prediction of cardiotoxicity in chemotherapy-treated patients. Am J Cardiol 2011;107:1375–80.

35. Mavinkurve-Groothuis AM, Marcus KA, Pourier M, et al. Myocardial 2d strain echocardiography and cardiac biomarkers in children during and shortly after anthracycline therapy for acute lymphoblastic leukaemia (ALL): a prospective study. Eur Heart J Cardiovasc Imaging 2013;14:562–9.

36. Pavo N, Raderer M, Hulsmann M, et al. Cardiovascular biomarkers in patients with cancer and their association with all-cause mortality. Heart 2015;101:1874–80.

37. Krawczuk-Rybak M, Dakowicz L, Hryniewicz A, et al. Cardiac function in survivors of acute lymphoblastic leukaemia and Hodgkin's lymphoma. J Paediatr Child Health 2011;47:455–9.

38. Dodos F, Halbsguth T, Erdmann E, et al. Usefulness of myocardial performance index and biochemical markers for early detection of anthracycline-induced cardiotoxicity in adults. Clin Res Cardiol 2008;97:318–26.

39. Reijers JA, Burggraaf J. Trastuzumab induces an immediate, transient volume increase in humans: a randomised placebo-controlled trial. EBioMedicine 2015;2:953–9.

40. Daugaard G, Lassen U, Bie P, et al. Natriuretic peptides in the monitoring of anthracycline

induced reduction in left ventricular ejection fraction. Eur J Heart Fail 2005;7:87–93.

41. Broeyer FJ, Osanto S, Ritsema van Eck HJ, et al. Evaluation of biomarkers for cardiotoxicity of anthracyclin-based chemotherapy. J Cancer Res Clin Oncol 2008;134:961–8.

42. Tang WH, Tong W, Troughton RW, et al. Prognostic value and echocardiographic determinants of plasma myeloperoxidase levels in chronic heart failure. J Am Coll Cardiol 2007;49:2364–70.

43. Tang WH, Brennan ML, Philip K, et al. Plasma myeloperoxidase levels in patients with chronic heart failure. Am J Cardiol 2006;98:796–9.

44. Wollert KC, Kempf T, Lagerqvist B, et al. Growth differentiation factor 15 for risk stratification and selection of an invasive treatment strategy in non ST-elevation acute coronary syndrome. Circulation 2007;116:1540–8.

45. Rohde LE, Bello-Klein A, Pereira RP, et al. Superoxide dismutase activity in adriamycin-induced cardiotoxicity in humans: a potential novel tool for risk stratification. J Card Fail 2005;11:220–6.

46. Schwartz DR, Briggs ER, Qatanani M, et al. Human resistin in chemotherapy-induced heart failure in humanized male mice and in women treated for breast cancer. Endocrinology 2013;154:4206–14.

47. Accornero F, van Berlo JH, Benard MJ, et al. Placental growth factor regulates cardiac adaptation and hypertrophy through a paracrine mechanism. Circ Res 2011;109:272–80.

48. Lenderink T, Heeschen C, Fichtlscherer S, et al. Elevated placental growth factor levels are associated with adverse outcomes at four-year follow-up in patients with acute coronary syndromes. J Am Coll Cardiol 2006;47:307–11.

49. Shah RV, Chen-Tournoux AA, Picard MH, et al. Galectin-3, cardiac structure and function, and long-term mortality in patients with acutely decompensated heart failure. Eur J Heart Fail 2010;12:826–32.

50. Horacek JM, Vasatova M, Pudil R, et al. Biomarkers for the early detection of anthracycline-induced cardiotoxicity: current status. Biomed Pap Med Fac Univ Palacky Olomouc Czech Repub 2014;158:511–7.

51. Horacek JM, Jebavy L, Vasatova M, et al. Glycogen phosphorylase bb as a potential marker of cardiac toxicity in patients treated with anthracyclines for acute leukemia. Bratisl Lek Listy 2013;114:708–10.

52. Horacek JM, Tichy M, Pudil R, et al. Multimarker approach to evaluation of cardiac toxicity during preparative regimen and hematopoietic cell transplantation. Neoplasma 2008;55:532–7.

53. Putt M, Hahn VS, Januzzi JL, et al. Longitudinal changes in multiple biomarkers are associated with cardiotoxicity in breast cancer patients treated

with doxorubicin, taxanes, and trastuzumab. Clin Chem 2015;61:1164–72.

54. Bar-Or D, Curtis G, Rao N, et al. Characterization of the co(2+) and ni(2+) binding amino-acid residues of the n-terminus of human albumin. An insight into the mechanism of a new assay for myocardial ischemia. Eur J Biochem 2001;268:42–7.

55. Ma Y, Kang W, Bao Y, et al. Clinical significance of ischemia-modified albumin in the diagnosis of doxorubicin-induced myocardial injury in breast cancer patients. PLoS One 2013;8:e79426.

56. Garrone O, Crosetto N, Lo Nigro C, et al. Prediction of anthracycline cardiotoxicity after chemotherapy by biomarkers kinetic analysis. Cardiovasc Toxicol 2012;12:135–42.

57. Stachowiak P, Kornacewicz-Jach Z, Safranow K. Prognostic role of troponin and natriuretic peptides as biomarkers for deterioration of left ventricular ejection fraction after chemotherapy. Arch Med Sci 2014;10:1007–18.

58. Bryant J, Picot J, Levitt G, et al. Cardioprotection against the toxic effects of anthracyclines given to children with cancer: a systematic review. Health Technol Assess 2007;11:iii, ix-x, 1–84.

59. Morris PG, Chen C, Steingart R, et al. Troponin I and C-reactive protein are commonly detected in patients with breast cancer treated with dose-dense chemotherapy incorporating trastuzumab and lapatinib. Clin Cancer Res 2011;17:3490–9.

60. Hahm S, Dresner HS, Podwall D, et al. DNA biomarkers antecede semiquantitative anthracycline cardiomyopathy. Cancer Invest 2003;21:53–67.

61. Petricoin EF, Rajapaske V, Herman EH, et al. Toxicoproteomics: serum proteomic pattern diagnostics for early detection of drug induced cardiac toxicities and cardioprotection. Toxicol Pathol 2004;32(Suppl 1):122–30.

62. Li Y, Ju L, Hou Z, et al. Screening, verification, and optimization of biomarkers for early prediction of cardiotoxicity based on metabolomics. J Proteome Res 2015;14:2437–45.

63. Donato R, Cannon BR, Sorci G, et al. Functions of s100 proteins. Curr Mol Med 2013;13:24–57.

64. Eryilmaz U, Demirci B, Aksun S, et al. S100a1 as a potential diagnostic biomarker for assessing cardiotoxicity and implications for the chemotherapy of certain cancers. PLoS One 2015;10:e0145418.

65. Wang EJ, Snyder RD, Fielden MR, et al. Validation of putative genomic biomarkers of nephrotoxicity in rats. Toxicology 2008;246:91–100.

66. Mori Y, Kondo C, Tonomura Y, et al. Identification of potential genomic biomarkers for early detection of chemically induced cardiotoxicity in rats. Toxicology 2010;271:36–44.

67. Todorova VK, Beggs ML, Delongchamp RR, et al. Transcriptome profiling of peripheral blood cells

identifies potential biomarkers for doxorubicin car-diotoxicity in a rat model. PLoS One 2012;7: e48398.

68. Piegari E, De Angelis A, Cappetta D, et al. Doxoru-bicin induces senescence and impairs function of human cardiac progenitor cells. Basic Res Cardiol 2013;108:334.

69. Bao GY, Wang HZ, Shang YJ, et al. Quantitative proteomic study identified cathepsin b associated with doxorubicin-induced damage in h9c2 cardio-myocytes. Biosci Trends 2012;6:283–7.

70. Lin ST, Chou HC, Chen YW, et al. Redox-proteomic analysis of doxorubicin-induced altered thiol activ-ity in cardiomyocytes. Mol Biosyst 2013;9:447–56.

71. Holmgren G, Synnergren J, Bogestal Y, et al. Iden-tification of novel biomarkers for doxorubicin-induced toxicity in human cardiomyocytes derived from pluripotent stem cells. Toxicology 2015;328: 102–11.

72. Chaudhari U, Nemade H, Wagh V, et al. Identifica-tion of genomic biomarkers for anthracycline-induced cardiotoxicity in human IPSC-derived car-diomyocytes: an in vitro repeated exposure toxicity approach for safety assessment. Arch Toxicol 2016;90(11):2763–77.

73. El Zarrad MK, Mukhopadhyay P, Mohan N, et al. Trastuzumab alters the expression of genes essen-tial for cardiac function and induces ultrastructural changes of cardiomyocytes in mice. PLoS One 2013;8:e79543.

74. Latronico MV, Condorelli G. MicroRNAs and car-diac pathology. Nat Rev Cardiol 2009;6:419–29.

75. Desai VG, C Kwekel J, Vijay V, et al. Early biomarkers of doxorubicin-induced heart injury in a mouse model. Toxicol Appl Pharmacol 2014;281:221–9.

76. Vacchi-Suzzi C, Bauer Y, Berridge BR, et al. Pertur-bation of microRNAs in rat heart during chronic doxorubicin treatment. PLoS One 2012;7:e40395.

77. Holmgren G, Synnergren J, Andersson CX, et al. MicroRNAs as potential biomarkers for doxorubicin-induced cardiotoxicity. Toxicol In Vitro 2016;34:26–34.

78. Horie T, Ono K, Nishi H, et al. Acute doxorubicin cardiotoxicity is associated with mir-146a-induced inhibition of the neuregulin-erbb pathway. Cardio-vasc Res 2010;87:656–64.

79. Xu C, Lu Y, Pan Z, et al. The muscle-specific micro-rnas mir-1 and mir-133 produce opposing effects on apoptosis by targeting hsp60, hsp70 and caspase-9 in cardiomyocytes. J Cell Sci 2007; 120:3045–52.

80. Oliveira-Carvalho V, Ferreira LR, Bocchi EA. Circu-lating mir-208a fails as a biomarker of doxorubicin-induced cardiotoxicity in breast cancer patients. J Appl Toxicol 2015;35:1071–2.

81. Thavendiranathan P, Poulin F, Lim KD, et al. Use of myocardial strain imaging by echocardiography for the early detection of cardiotoxicity in patients dur-ing and after cancer chemotherapy: a systematic review. J Am Coll Cardiol 2014;63:2751–68.

82. Nolan MT, Plana JC, Thavendiranathan P, et al. Cost-effectiveness of strain-targeted cardioprotec-tion for prevention of chemotherapy-induced cardi-otoxicity. Int J Cardiol 2016;212:336–45.

83. Lang RM, Badano LP, Mor-Avi V, et al. Recommen-dations for cardiac chamber quantification by echocardiography in adults: an update from the American Society of Echocardiography and the Eu-ropean Association of Cardiovascular Imaging. J Am Soc Echocardiogr 2015;28:1–39.e14.

84. Schwartz RG, Jain D, Storozynsky E. Traditional and novel methods to assess and prevent chemotherapy-related cardiac dysfunction nonin-vasively. J Nucl Cardiol 2013;20:443–64.

85. de Geus-Oei LF, Mavinkurve-Groothuis AM, Bellersen L, et al. Scintigraphic techniques for early detection of cancer treatment-induced cardiotoxic-ity. J Nucl Med Technol 2013;41:170–81.

86. Su H, Gorodny N, Gomez LF, et al. Noninvasive molecular imaging of apoptosis in a mouse model of anthracycline-induced cardiotoxicity. Circ Cardi-ovasc Imaging 2015;8:e001952.

87. Grover S, Leong DP, Chakrabarty A, et al. Left and right ventricular effects of anthracycline and trastu-zumab chemotherapy: a prospective study using novel cardiac imaging and biochemical markers. Int J Cardiol 2013;168:5465–7.

88. Fallah-Rad N, Walker JR, Wassef A, et al. The utility of cardiac biomarkers, tissue velocity and strain imag-ing, and cardiac magnetic resonance imaging in pre-dicting early left ventricular dysfunction in patients with human epidermal growth factor receptor ii-positive breast cancer treated with adjuvant trastuzu-mab therapy. J Am Coll Cardiol 2011;57:2263–70.

89. Hahn VS, Lenihan DJ, Ky B. Cancer therapy-induced cardiotoxicity: basic mechanisms and po-tential cardioprotective therapies. J Am Heart As-soc 2014;3:e000665.

90. Catana C, Guimaraes AR, Rosen BR. PET and MR imaging: the odd couple or a match made in heav-en? J Nucl Med 2013;54:815–24.

91. Bauch M, Ester A, Kimura B, et al. Atrial natriuretic peptide as a marker for doxorubicin-induced cardi-otoxic effects. Cancer 1992;69:1492–7.

92. Missov E, Calzolari C, Davy JM, et al. Cardiac troponin I in patients with hematologic malig-nancies. Coron Artery Dis 1997;8:537–41.

93. Nousiainen T, Jantunen E, Vanninen E, et al. Natri-uretic peptides as markers of cardiotoxicity during doxorubicin treatment for non-Hodgkin's lym-phoma. Eur J Haematol 1999;62:135–41.

94. Hayakawa H, Komada Y, Hirayama M, et al. Plasma levels of natriuretic peptides in relation to doxorubicin-induced cardiotoxicity and cardiac

function in children with cancer. Med Pediatr Oncol 2001;37:4–9.

95. Nousiainen T, Vanninen E, Jantunen E, et al. Natriuretic peptides during the development of doxorubicin-induced left ventricular diastolic dysfunction. J Intern Med 2002;251:228–34.

96. Poutanen T, Tikanoja T, Riikonen P, et al. Long-term prospective follow-up study of cardiac function after cardiotoxic therapy for malignancy in children. J Clin Oncol 2003;21:2349–56.

97. Kismet E, Varan A, Ayabakan C, et al. Serum troponin t levels and echocardiographic evaluation in children treated with doxorubicin. Pediatr Blood Cancer 2004;42:220–4.

98. Köseoğlu V, Berberoglu S, Karademir S, et al. Cardiac troponin I: is it a marker to detect cardiotoxicity in children treated with doxorubicin? Turk J Pediatr 2005;47:17–22.

99. Perik PJ, Lub-De Hooge MN, Gietema JA, et al. Indium-111-labeled trastuzumab scintigraphy in patients with human epidermal growth factor receptor 2-positive metastatic breast cancer. J Clin Oncol 2006;24:2276–82.

100. Aggarwal S, Pettersen MD, Bhambhani K, et al. B-type natriuretic peptide as a marker for cardiac dysfunction in anthracycline-treated children. Pediatr Blood Cancer 2007;49:812–6.

101. Jones LW, Haykowsky M, Peddle CJ, et al. Cardiovascular risk profile of patients with her2/neu-positive breast cancer treated with anthracycline-taxane-containing adjuvant chemotherapy and/or trastuzumab. Cancer Epidemiol Biomarkers Prev 2007;16:1026–31.

102. D'Errico MP, Grimaldi L, Petruzzelli MF, et al. N-terminal pro-B-type natriuretic peptide plasma levels as a potential biomarker for cardiac damage after radiotherapy in patients with left-sided breast cancer. Int J Radiat Oncol Biol Phys 2011;82:e239–46.

103. Guler M, Yilmaz T, Ozercan I, et al. The inhibitory effects of trastuzumab on corneal neovascularization. Am J Ophthalmol 2009;147:703–8.e2.

104. Tragiannidis A, Dokos C, Tsotoulidou V, et al. Brain natriuretic peptide as a cardiotoxicity biomarker in children with hematological malignancies. Minerva Pediatr 2012;64:307–12.

105. Sherief LM, Kamal AG, Khalek EA, et al. Biomarkers and early detection of late onset anthracycline-induced cardiotoxicity in children. Hematology 2012;17:151–6.

106. Mladosievicova B, Urbanova D, Radvanska E, et al. Role of NY-proBNP in detection of myocardial damage in childhood leukemia survivors treated with and without anthracyclines. J Exp Clin Cancer Res 2012;31:86.

107. Ylänen K, Poutanen T, Savukoski T, et al. Cardiac biomarkers indicate a need for sensitive cardiac imaging among long-term childhood cancer survivors exposed to anthracyclines. Acta Paediatr 2015;104:313–9.

108. Pourier MS, Kapusta L, van Gennip A, et al. Values of high sensitive troponin t in long-term survivors of childhood cancer treated with anthracyclines. Clin Chim Acta 2015;441:29–32.

109. van Boxtel W, Bulten BF, Mavinkurve-Groothuis AM, et al. New biomarkers for early detection of cardiotoxicity after treatment with docetaxel, doxorubicin and cyclophosphamide. Biomarkers 2015;20:143–8.

110. Kremer LC, Bastiaansen BA, Offringa M, et al. Troponin t in the first 24 hours after the administration of chemotherapy and the detection of myocardial damage in children. Eur J Cancer 2002;38:686–9.

111. Sandri MT, Cardinale D, Zorzino L, et al. Minor increases in plasma troponin I predict decreased left ventricular ejection fraction after high-dose chemotherapy. Clin Chem 2003;49:248–52.

112. Polena S, Shikara M, Naik S, et al. Troponin I as a marker of doxorubicin induced cardiotoxicity. Proc West Pharmacol Soc 2005;48:142–4.

113. Goel S, Simes RJ, Beith JM. Exploratory analysis of cardiac biomarkers in women with normal cardiac function receiving trastuzumab for breast cancer. Asia Pac J Clin Oncol 2011;7:276–80.

114. Roziakova L, Bojtarova E, Mistrik M, et al. Abnormal cardiomarkers in leukemia patients treated with allogeneic hematopoietic stem cell transplantation. Bratisl Lek Listy 2012;113:159–62.

115. Mathew P, Suarez W, Kip K, et al. Is there a potential role for serum cardiac troponin I as a marker for myocardial dysfunction in pediatric patients receiving anthracycline-based therapy? A pilot study. Cancer Invest 2001;19:352–9.

116. Meinardi MT, van Veldhuisen DJ, Gietema JA, et al. Prospective evaluation of early cardiac damage induced by epirubicin-containing adjuvant chemotherapy and locoregional radiotherapy in breast cancer patients. J Clin Oncol 2001;19:2746–53.

117. Ekstein S, Nir A, Rein AJ, et al. N-terminal-proB-type natriuretic peptide as a marker for acute anthracycline cardiotoxicity in children. J Pediatr Hematol Oncol 2007;29:440–4.

118. Lee HS, Son CB, Shin SH, et al. Clinical correlation between brain natriuretic peptide and anthracyclin-induced cardiac toxicity. Cancer Res Treat 2008;40:121–6.

119. Horacek JM, Vasatova M, Tichy M, et al. The use of cardiac biomarkers in detection of cardiotoxicity associated with conventional and high-dose chemotherapy for acute leukemia. Exp Oncol 2010;32:97–9.

120. Onitilo AA, Engel JM, Stankowski RV, et al. High-sensitivity c-reactive protein (hs-CRP) as a biomarker for trastuzumab-induced cardiotoxicity in her2-positive early-stage breast cancer: a pilot study. Breast Cancer Res Treat 2012;134:291–8.

Cardio-oncology
The Role of Big Data

Anant Mandawat, MD[a], Andrew E. Williams, PhD[b], Sanjeev A. Francis, MD[c],*

KEYWORDS

- Big data • Cardio-oncology • Pharmacovigilant

KEY POINTS

- Despite its challenges, a "big data" approach offers a unique opportunity within the field of cardio-oncology.
- A pharmacovigilant approach using large data sets can help characterize cardiovascular toxicities of the rapidly expanding armamentarium of targeted therapies.
- Creating a broad coalition of data sharing can provide insights into the incidence of cardiotoxicity and stimulate research into the underlying mechanisms.
- Population health necessitates the use of big data and can help inform public health interventions to prevent both cancer and cardiovascular disease.
- As a relatively new discipline, Cardio-Oncology is poised to take advantage of big data.

Big data is like teenage sex; everyone talks about it, nobody really knows how to do it, everyone thinks everyone else is doing it, so everyone claims they are doing it.[1]
—Dan Ariely, Duke University Professor of Behavior Economics

Patients with cancer are living longer due to improvements in treatment.[2] As cancer survivors live longer, they are at risk of complications of heart disease in part due to effects of cardiotoxicity from chemotherapy and radiotherapy. Cardio-oncology is the discipline that focuses on the intersection of cancer and cardiovascular disease.[3] A major facet of this intersection is chemotherapy-related or radiotherapy-related heart disease.[2,4] Cancer therapy may result in damage to the heart from a direct toxic effect of the therapy or indirectly by worsening cardiac risk factors like hypertension.[2] However, at present, there is variation in screening and treatment practices.[5] For a relatively young discipline like cardio-oncology, research and

discovery are essential for growth and understanding. In particular, there is a call to study the direct and indirect effects of chemotherapy and radiation on heart function. This call includes strategies for primary and second prevention, identification of surrogate markers, guidelines for screening, and risk prediction models.[2,6] More information on the early and late effects of systemic treatments and mechanisms of injury is needed. The focus of this review is to describe the potential of big data to achieve these goals in cardio-oncology.

Cardio-oncology is an exciting new field primed for the application of big data. In 2015, President Barack Obama announced the Precision Medicine Initiative, and in 2016, Vice-President Joe Biden declared the Cancer Moonshot, which will allocate more than $1 billion in advancing patient level care and oncology. Importantly, these initiatives will direct significant resources that could be used toward the collection and application of big data in cardiology and oncology.[7,8] Research in

a Division of Cardiovascular Medicine, Duke University School of Medicine, 2301 Erwin Road, Durham, NC 27710, USA; b Division of Health Services Research, Center for Outcomes Research and Evaluation, Maine Medical Center Research Institute, 509 Forest Avenue, Suite 200, Portland, MW 04101, USA; c Division of Cardiovascular Medicine, Maine Medical Center, 22 Bramhall Street, Portland, ME 04102, USA
* Corresponding author.
E-mail address: SFrancis@mmc.org

Heart Failure Clin 13 (2017) 403–408
http://dx.doi.org/10.1016/j.hfc.2016.12.010
1551-7136/17/© 2016 Elsevier Inc. All rights reserved.

cardio-oncology is a unique opportunity for both clinical and research collaboration between the cardiology and oncology.[9]

Big data has been an elusive term to define, as characterized in Prof Dan Ariely's opening quote.

It is estimated that there is 2.3 trillion gigabytes of data created each day. As of 2011, the global size of data is health care is estimated to be 161 billion gigabytes (IBM).[10] A framework for defining big data has been developed using the 4 "V's": volume, variety, veracity, and velocity (IBM). Importantly, big data is not just about large amounts of data; rather, it is characterized by data heterogeneity, validity, and its high speed of new inputs. Big data in health care includes insurance claims data, public health data, electronic health records, genomic data, mobile health data, and social health data. The goal of big data is to leverage information from such sources to meaningfully inform patients, physicians, and researchers. Examples can be found in the priorities of the new Cancer Moonshot Task Force to support data sharing, analytical collaborations, and public-private partnerships between the Veterans Administration and IBM Watson.[8]

The European Organization for Research and Treatment of Cancer has advocated for a systematic collection of data in cardio-oncology.[2] Perhaps more than any other discipline within cardiology, cardio-oncology would benefit from leveraging multiple sources of data. Statistically, the absolute event rate of chemotherapy-induced cardiomyopathy may be relatively low depending on the specific drug and patient population being studied[11] (rate of cardiac events between 1.3 [control] and 4.0% [trastuzumab arm] at 7 years follow-up of 1830 patients). Big data presents an opportunity to detect relatively low-frequency events that nonetheless can have significant clinical impact. Aleman and colleagues[2] support an international registry for cardio-oncology. Unlike acute coronary syndrome, cardio-oncology is a relatively young discipline in which new fundamental pathophysiology and phenotypes continue to be understood, and whose identification and surveillance will require large amounts of data. In addition, chemotherapy-induced cardiomyopathy is a complex interaction between a patient's demographics, genetics, comorbidities, medications, laboratory tests, imaging, and functional status, requiring integration of multiple data sources, including electronic health records and genomics, for research on risk assessment and treatment.

The current infrastructure in cardio-oncology is limited. Recent initiatives are designed to streamline development of new cancer therapeutics at an accelerated rate.[8] However, cancer therapeutics receives approval based on randomized clinical trials with cardiac events prone to variable ascertainment and adjudication. In addition, patients enrolled in randomized trials may represent the "healthier" patients with cancer who are younger with a lower incidence of cardiovascular disease or risk. The incidence of cardiotoxicity observed in clinical trials may not be an accurate reflection of the risk in typical clinical practice.

There are several examples of using big data within cardiology. Patel and colleagues[12] used data from CathPCI, a registry part of the American College of Cardiology National Cardiovascular Data Registry, to analyze almost 400,000 patients from 663 hospitals undergoing elective coronary angiography. They showed that almost two-thirds of patients undergoing the procedure had nonobstructive disease, encouraging the need for better risk stratification before angiography. Speaking to the power of big data, the CathPCI registry from its inception in 1998 to 2013 contained data on more than 12 million records from 1577 participating US centers.[13] This year, the *International Journal of Medical Journal Editors* released a proposal advocating for release of deidentified data within 6 months of trial publication.[14] Recent high-profile editorials have supported this push for transparency and open data access of clinical trial data,[15–17] an important source of data for toxicities of new cancer therapeutics.

Chen and colleagues[18] and Ezaz and colleagues[19] are 2 examples of using big data in cardio-oncology. Both studies used the Surveillance, Epidemiology, and End Results–Medicare data. Chen and colleagues[18] calculated incidence rates of heart failure or cardiomyopathy over 3 years in 45,000 women aged 67 to 94 with breast cancer who received anthracycline, trastuzumab, a combination of both, or neither. It leveraged big data to elucidate incidence rates that otherwise would be difficult to assess due to low event rates. Ezaz and colleagues[19] analyzed data on 1664 women with breast cancer receiving adjuvant trastuzumab and created a risk score for the development of heart failure and cardiomyopathy. Unlike other disciplines that have to use existing tools, which at times are outdated, cardio-oncology has the luxury to design its own research infrastructure from the ground up.

Cardio-oncology would benefit from several initiatives that could contribute to the big data research mission. First, a clinically meaningful and consistent definition of cardio-toxicity is needed. The most adopted definition is the Cardiac Review and Evaluation Committee of trastuzumab-associated cardiotoxicity definition of either a reduction of left ventricular ejection fraction (LVEF) of 5% or greater to less than 55% with symptoms of heart failure or an asymptomatic reduction of LVEF 10% or greater to less than 55%. An expert consensus statement from the American Society of Echocardiography and the European Society of Cardiovascular Imaging defined cardiotoxicity as a decline of greater than 10% to an LVEF less than 53%. In addition, it is the first guideline to include a change in strain as criteria for subclinical left ventricular dysfunction. Nevertheless, studies have shown that there can be an interreader variability of 10% when assessing an ejection fraction by transthoracic echocardiography.[20] Although sensitive, an asymptomatic reduction of LVEF of 10% may not be very clinically useful and result in false positives that could confound clinically meaningful endpoints. Alternatively, a change in strain is often used as an early marker of cardiotoxicity, although it is unclear if this should be included as part of the definition of chemotherapy-induced cardiomyopathy. For research that ultimately impacts patient care, a clinically useful definition is essential. Second, chemotherapy-related or radiotherapy-related heart disease needs International Classification of Disease (ICD) diagnosis codes for rapid incorporation into administrative sources of big data like Medicare and the Healthcare Cost and Utilization Project as well as local electronic health records. Such data sets will be useful for following demographics and trends in incidence of disease. Third, a national cardio-oncology registry funded by a private-public partnership is needed. Similar to the America College of Cardiology's National Cardiovascular Data Registry, a registry is needed that can pool data across multiple institutions and collect granular variables like stage of cancer, receptor status, chemotherapy dose, and strain patterns that are lacking in administrative datasets. A registry is important in collecting "real world" data as clinical trials often comprise a more selected population.[4] Such a registry could also be a unique basic science opportunity to understand common molecular mechanisms shared by the heart and cancer (eg, cell proliferation, adhesion, and apoptosis) from the use of cancer therapeutics, ultimately using these similar pathways for cardiovascular drug development.[9] The elucidation of the cardiac effects of the HER2 pathway has led to research into a new class of medications for heart failure and has aptly been termed "bench to bedside back to bench" research.[9,21]

Although early efforts in understanding cardiotoxicity have been focused on traditional cancer therapies, such as anthracyclines and chest radiotherapy, the advent of targeted pathway inhibitors has ushered in a revolution in cancer chemotherapy. First-in-class drugs such as Imatinib and Trastuzumab changed the paradigm for cancer therapy. Tyrosine-kinase inhibitors (TKIs) and immunomodulatory therapies are rapidly being introduced into the market offering new treatment options and hope for many patients with cancer. The length of time before a cancer is approved by the US Food and Drug Administration (FDA) has also decreased, with some drugs bypassing the standard phase 1-2-3 trial structure.[22,23]

The rapid entry of drugs into the market necessitates a greater role for after-marketing surveillance and pharmacovigilance to determine the potential for cardiotoxicity. To date, pharmacovigilance analyses have simply used big data from administrative claims or electronic health records to correlate cancer therapy exposure with subsequent incident heart disease. Big data also holds the promise of a more advanced approach that complements correlational pharmacovigilance analyses by using knowledge of drug mechanisms to clarify the importance of potential signals of cardiotoxic risk, which may not have been suggested by preclinical trials. A systems pharmacology approach could do this by suggesting whether a potential signal has a known pharmacologic basis. With sufficient development, such an approach might also be able to predict characteristic phenotypes that should be anticipated in surveillance efforts.

These ideas and the challenges in implementing them were recently presented to the Observational Health Data Sciences[24] and Informatics group by Dr Darrell Abernethy of the FDA's Office of Clinical Pharmacology.[25] Initial efforts involved collaboration with data mining vendors that linked pharmacovigilance data such as the FDA's Adverse Event Reporting (FAERS) database to sources of information on drug chemistry or drug targets. That has evolved recently to a more integrated approach that starts with either a drug molecule or, in the case of large molecules, the drug on- and off-target, and tries to map that through the biological system to the clinical phenotype of an adverse drug reaction. The current focus is on mapping TKI through their known biological mechanisms to the clinical phenotype of impaired left ventricular function or cardiomyopathy.[26] The positive and negative controls in this research would be between TKIs that do have a clear link to cardiac toxicity versus TKIs that do not. The goal would be to clearly characterize the targets and pharmacology of TKIs in each group. When complete, this approach is intended to be a model for predicting other drug-outcome relationships.

This work is in the infrastructure-building phase. One methodologic hurdle is the lack of an overarching ontology of adverse events that enables effective integration of the diverse data streams required for these analyses. Data types may include gene expression array, RNA sequencing, histopathologic data, animal toxicologic data, and human clinical phenotypes. The overarching ontology will define the relational terms between separate ontologies for each of these different data types.

Another important methodologic challenge is posed by the requirement that big data analyses use data that are incomplete. Typical systems analyses use ordinary differential equations to determine relationships of interest among nodes and edges in a network defined the relational terms in an overarching ontology. Big data does not meet the completeness for this analytical approach, so alternative analytical methods that are robust when dealing with incomplete data are needed.

Beyond the organization and analysis of the data, there are challenges to finding and developing the data on drug mechanisms. Improved collaboration between the pharmaceutical industry, academic institutions, individual investigators, and health care systems may allow the level of data sharing necessary to achieve this lofty goal. Indeed, the National Cancer Institute has developed the Experimental Therapeutics Clinical Trials Network, which among its goals includes improved collaboration among the various stakeholders as well as an integration of molecular, pharmacologic, and clinical data.[27]

Another important challenge is finding big data sources that meet the analytical requirements for clinical phenotyping. Adequate phenotypic characterization requires data from clinical assessments (office encounters, case report forms), laboratory data, and imaging data. Adjudication of clinical endpoints can be challenging when relying on billing data or ICD-10 coding. Data in the National Cancer Institute's Cancer Clinical Trials program that contain Common Terminology Criteria for Adverse Events descriptors of cardiac function and cardiovascular activity are also inadequate. Data from pharmaceutical companies are considerably richer and better able to characterize phenotypes, although it is still unclear whether they will be sufficient to meet the analytical needs of the approach envisioned by the FDA. Two FDA-sponsored big data sources FAERS and Sentinel are attempts to broaden the data-sharing coalition. The FDA Sentinel program includes a broad group, including large insurers, health care systems, and academic institutions.[28] Networks such as PCORnet[29] and OHDSI[24] may represent significant untapped sources of data and informatics expertise needed to characterize and analyze clinical phenotypes. PCORnet is an initiative of the Patient Centered Outcomes Research Institute, the aim of which is to leverage large health data sets and partnerships with patient organizations to facilitate patient-centered research. Assembling these broad coalitions is an important step in the creation of robust, meaningful data sets (Fig. 1). The computational approaches necessary to work with these data sets continue to evolve and will be a critical aspect of generating meaningful conclusions from such large data sets.

In addition to the cardiotoxicity from cancer therapies, there is growing evidence suggesting

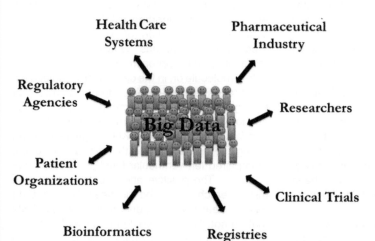

Fig. 1. A broad coalition of stakeholders is necessary to generate robust and complete data sets that can lead to meaningful conclusions.

a shared biology between cancer and cardiovascular disease. Epidemiologic evidence reveals common risk factors, such as smoking, obesity, and diabetes. Cancer and cardiovascular disease share some common cellular processes, including inflammation and oxidative stress.[30] Data from the ARIC study suggest that if patients adhere to the 7 ideal cardiovascular health metrics the incidence of cancer was lower.[31] Additional research is necessary to identify the link between cancer and cardiovascular disease. A big data approach may better characterize the complex interplay between genetic factors, lifestyle, and environmental factors. Analysis of population level health data may ultimately lead to targeted interventions to help prevent both cancer and cardiovascular disease.

Despite the challenges outlined above, a "big data" approach offers a unique opportunity within the field of Cardio-Oncology. A pharmacovigilant approach using large data sets can help characterize cardiovascular toxicities of the rapidly expanding armamentarium of targeted therapies. Creating a broad coalition of data sharing can provide insights into the incidence of cardiotoxicity and stimulate research into the underlying mechanisms. Population health necessitates the use of big data and can help inform public health interventions to prevent both cancer and cardiovascular disease. As a relatively new discipline, Cardio-Oncology is poised to take advantage of big data.

REFERENCES

1. Pathak J. Big data tools and methods for computational medicine. Big data course for computational medicine. Presented at the NIH's Big Data Course for Computation Medicine. Weil Cornell Medical Center, New York, July 11, 2016.

2. Aleman BM, Moser EC, Nuver J, et al. Cardiovascular disease after cancer therapy. EJC Suppl 2014; 12:18–28.

3. Francis SA, Asnani A, Neilan T, et al. Optimizing cardio-oncology programs for cancer patients. Future Oncol 2015;11(14):2011–5.

4. Francis SA, Cheng S, Arteaga CL, et al. Heart failure and breast cancer therapies: moving towards personalized risk assessment. J Am Heart Assoc 2014;3:e000780.

5. Khouri MG, Douglas PS, Mackey JR, et al. Cancer therapy-induced cardiac toxicity in early breast cancer: addressing the unresolved issues. Circulation 2012;126:2749–63.

6. Bhave M, Shah AN, Akhter N, et al. An update on the risk prediction and prevention of anticancer therapy-induced cardiotoxicity. Curr Opin Oncol 2014;26: 590–9.

7. Office of the Press Secretary, The White House. Fact Sheet: President Obama's Precision Medicine Initiative. 2015. Available at: www.whitehouse.gov. Accessed September 4, 2016.

8. Office of the Press Secretary, The White House. Fact Sheet: At Cancer Moonshot Summit, Vice President Biden announces new actions to accelerate progress towards ending cancer as we know it. 2016. Available at: www.whitehouse.gov. Accessed September 4, 2016.

9. Bellinger AM, Arteaga CL, Force T, et al. Cardio-oncology: how new targeted cancer therapies and precision medicine can inform cardiovascular discovery. Circulation 2015;132:2248–58.

10. IBM Big Data and Analytics Hub. The Four V's of Big Data. Available at http://www.ibmbigdatahub.com/infographic/four-vs-big-data. Accessed August 27, 2016.

11. Romond EH, Jeong JH, Rastogi P, et al. Seven-year follow-up assessment of cardiac function in NSABP B-31, a randomized trial comparing doxorubicin and cyclophosphamide followed by paclitaxel (ACP) with ACP plus trastuzumab as adjuvant therapy for patients with node-positive, human epidermal growth factor receptor 2-positive breast cancer. J Clin Oncol 2012;30:3792–9.

12. Patel MR, Peterson ED, Dai D, et al. Low diagnostic yield of elective coronary angiography. N Engl J Med 2010;362:886–95.

13. Moussa I, Hermann A, Messenger JC, et al. The NCDR CathPCI Registry: a US national perspective on care and outcomes for percutaneous coronary intervention. Heart 2013;99:297–303.

14. Taichman DB, Backus J, Baethge C, et al. Sharing clinical trial data: a proposal from the International Committee of Medical Journal Editors sharing clinical trial data. Ann Intern Med 2016; 164:505–6.

15. Academic Research Organization Consortium for Continuing Evaluation of Scientific S-C, Patel MR, Armstrong PW, Bhatt DL, et al. Sharing data from cardiovascular clinical trials–a proposal. N Engl J Med 2016;375:407–9.

16. Krumholz HM, Waldstreicher J. The Yale Open Data Access (YODA) Project–a mechanism for data Sharing. N Engl J Med 2016;375:403–5.

17. Navar A, Pencina MJ, Rymer JA, et al. USe of open access platforms for clinical trial data. JAMA 2016; 315:1283–4.

18. Chen J, Long JB, Hurria A, et al. Incidence of heart failure or cardiomyopathy after adjuvant trastuzumab therapy for breast cancer. J Am Coll Cardiol 2012;60:2504–12.

19. Ezaz G, Long JB, Gross CP, et al. Risk prediction model for heart failure and cardiomyopathy after adjuvant trastuzumab therapy for breast cancer. J Am Heart Assoc 2014;3:e000472.

20. Thavendiranathan P, Grant AD, Negishi T, et al. Reproducibility of echocardiographic techniques for sequential assessment of left ventricular ejection fraction and volumes: application to patients undergoing cancer chemotherapy. J Am Coll Cardiol 2013;61(1):77–84.

21. De Keulenaer GW, Doggen K, Lemmens K. The vulnerability of the heart as a pluricellular paracrine organ: lessons from unexpected triggers of heart failure in targeted ErbB2 anticancer therapy. Circ Res 2010;106:35–46.

22. Chabner BA. Early accelerated approval for highly targeted cancer drugs. N Engl J Med 2011; 364(12):1087–9.

23. Chabner BA. While we're at it, let's whack the FDA. Oncologist 2016;21(3):259–60.

24. Available at: http://www.ohdsi.org. Accessed September 11, 2016.

25. Bai JP, Abernethy DR. Systems pharmacology to predict drug toxicity: integration across levels of biological organization. Annu Rev Pharmacol Toxicol 2013;53:451–73.

26. Sarntivijai S, Zhang S, Jagannathan DG, et al. Linking MedDRA(®)-coded clinical phenotypes to biological mechanisms by the ontology of adverse events: a pilot study on tyrosine kinase inhibitors. Drug Saf 2016;39(7):697–707.

27. Available at: https://ctep.cancer.gov/initiativesPrograms/etctn.htm. Accessed September 11, 2016.

28. Available at: http://www.fda.gov/Safety/FDAsSentinelInitiative/ucm149340.htm. Accessed September 11, 2016.

29. Available at: http://www.pcornet.org. Accessed September 11, 2016.

30. Koene RJ, Prizment AE, Blaes A, et al. Shared risk factors in cardiovascular disease and cancer. Circulation 2016;133(11):1104–14.

31. Rasmussen-Torvik LJ, Shay CM, Abramson JG, et al. Ideal cardiovascular health is inversely associated with incident cancer: the Atherosclerosis Risk In Communities study. Circulation 2013;127(12):1270–5.

Current Concepts of Cardiac Amyloidosis
Diagnosis, Clinical Management, and the Need for Collaboration

Alexandra J. Ritts, MD[a], Robert F. Cornell, MD, MS[b],
Kris Swiger, MD[c], Jai Singh, MD[c], Stacey Goodman, MD[b],
Daniel J. Lenihan, MD, FACC[d],*

KEYWORDS

- Cardiac amyloidosis • Multiple myeloma • TTR • Cardiotoxicity • Proteasome inhibitors
- Immunomodulatory drugs

KEY POINTS

- Cardiac amyloidosis is a complex and vexing clinical condition that requires a high degree of suspicion for the diagnosis with a substantial amount of discipline to discern the extent of disease and the best available therapy.
- There is a complex interplay between multiple organ systems, and the clinical presentation may involve a myriad of confusing clinical symptoms.
- The diagnosis of cardiac amyloidosis can be confirmed with a combination of physical findings, cardiac biomarkers, noninvasive testing, and, if necessary, myocardial biopsy. Genetic testing is critical to establish the type of amyloidosis.
- The treatment of cardiac amyloidosis is determined by the type, either amyloid light-chain or transthyretin, or less likely, a very rare inherited amyloidosis.
- The future for drug development in the treatment of cardiac amyloidosis is bright, and the need for earlier diagnosis is imperative.

INTRODUCTION

Patients with cardiac amyloidosis commonly develop diastolic and systolic dysfunction, progressive heart failure (HF), arrhythmias, and symptoms of orthostatic hypotension. Amyloidosis is a rare group of diseases characterized by the extracellular deposition of misfolded precursor proteins in a beta-pleated sheet conformation that renders the proteinaceous material an insoluble fibril. Systemic deposition of these amyloid fibrils results in organ damage and dysfunction, with affected tissue demonstrating a characteristic apple-green birefringence under polarized light when stained with Congo red.[1] The nature of the organ dysfunction depends on the organ affected and the

[a] Department of Internal Medicine, Vanderbilt University School of Medicine, 1215 21st Avenue South, Suite 5209, Nashville, TN 37232, USA; [b] Division of Hematology and Oncology, Department of Internal Medicine, Vanderbilt University School of Medicine, 1215 21st Avenue South, Suite 5209, Nashville, TN 37232, USA; [c] Division of Cardiovascular Medicine, Department of Internal Medicine, Vanderbilt University School of Medicine, 1215 21st Avenue South, Suite 5209, Nashville, TN 37232, USA; [d] Division of Cardiovascular Medicine, Department of Internal Medicine, Vanderbilt University Medical Center, 1215 21st Avenue South, Suite 5209, Nashville, TN 37232, USA
* Corresponding author.
E-mail address: daniel.lenihan@vanderbilt.edu

Heart Failure Clin 13 (2017) 409–416
http://dx.doi.org/10.1016/j.hfc.2016.12.003
1551-7136/17/© 2016 Elsevier Inc. All rights reserved.

intensity of protein deposition. This review focuses on cardiac dysfunction but includes other organs and the manner in which that dysfunction may impact the cardiovascular system.

In order to have a solid basic understanding of cardiac amyloidosis, it is important to recognize that there are multiple sources of amyloid fibrils that can deposit in cardiac tissue. The 2 most common types of amyloidosis affecting the heart include light chain (AL) amyloidosis and transthyretin (TTR) amyloidosis (subcategorized into mutant [TTRm] and wild-type [TTRwt]), although other rarer systemic amyloid processes have been described that can affect the heart.[2] Given the tendency for amyloidosis to have systemic involvement, a diagnosis of cardiac amyloidosis should be strongly considered in patients presenting with HF who also have findings indicating other typical organ system dysfunction seen with systemic amyloidosis. Because protein deposition can be diffuse, the patterns of involvement can be myriad, and a clinician needs to be aware of the possible connections in order to detect the disease at the earliest possible moment. Commonly involved organ systems that may be affected by amyloidosis include the kidney, gastrointestinal tract, liver, pulmonary, soft tissue, and nervous system.

DIAGNOSIS

There are multiple classifications of the type of systemic amyloidosis that must be considered. The 2 most common, constituting more than 90% of all cardiac-related amyloidosis, are AL and TTR amyloidosis.

Amyloid Light-Chain Amyloidosis

AL amyloidosis is the most common systemic amyloidosis type in the United States with approximately 4500 new cases diagnosed yearly.[3] The disease is the result of an abnormal population of bone marrow plasma cells producing an improperly folded light chain protein (of either kappa or lambda type) that deposits systemically. It is mainly a disease of older individuals, frequently diagnosed in patients between ages 50 to 80, although cases have been reported at younger ages. Men are more commonly affected than women, representing approximately two-thirds of all cases.[3]

Cardiac involvement is estimated in more than 50% of patients diagnosed with AL amyloidosis and has been identified as the greatest predictor of poor prognosis.[4] Notably, AL amyloidosis is commonly associated with multiple myeloma, a plasma cell dyscrasia that frequently presents with hypercalcemia, renal insufficiency, anemia, and bony lytic lesions. Median life expectancy in patients with AL amyloidosis has been previously estimated to be approximately 1 year (0.75 years after HF onset), but this estimate has increased in recent years with the advent of new therapies and routine use of autologous hematopoietic stem cell transplantation in treatment.[4,5]

Transthyretin Amyloidosis

In TTR amyloidosis, the liver produces TTR (prealbumin), a protein that has an intrinsic potential and tendency to misfold and deposit in tissues, causing organ tissue damage and dysfunction. The generation and deposition of amyloid in this disease can be either the result of a TTRm or a gradual deposition of TTR protein over time that mimics a process of early aging, and an absence of a known transthyretin gene mutation, referred to as TTRwt. The most common TTRm gene mutations have been described to be a valine to isoleucine substitution at position 122 (Val122Ile), a valine to methionine substitution at position 30 (Val30Met), and threonine to alanine substitution at position 60 (Thr60Ala), although at least 34 mutations have been reported in the United States, and more than 100 worldwide.[6–8]

In general, in the United States, wild-type disease (TTRwt) is more commonly diagnosed in patients that are older and of African descent, whereas patients with a common mutation in TTR-m (Val122Ile) are more likely to be younger, white, and female.[6] Median survival for patients with either type of TTR amyloidosis is typically longer than patients with AL amyloidosis.[9,10]

SIGNS AND SYMPTOMS

Initial signs of cardiac amyloidosis can be subtle, with patients commonly noting symptoms of fatigue and weakness. As the disease advances, amyloid deposition throughout the heart frequently results in progressive mechanical cardiac dysfunction. The classic triad of HF symptoms (fatigue, shortness of breath, and edema) become evident and can raise suspicion for a diagnosis of cardiac amyloidosis (Box 1).

Amyloid deposition in the ventricles and atrium can result in biventricular wall thickening without dilation and subsequently increased atrial pressure, resulting in profound atrial dilation and atrial wall thickening.[11] These structural changes certainly are not detected until late in the process, and the development of important diastolic filling impairment will likely precede obvious structural changes. As the deposition persists, ultimately systolic left ventricular (LV) dysfunction ensues and the hemodynamic and functional impairment becomes recalcitrant. A common presentation is a patient with classical HF symptoms, including dyspnea, orthopnea, paroxysmal nocturnal dyspnea, and lower extremity edema, but left ventricular (LV) systolic function is normal. It is imperative that amyloidosis is considered when a patient presents with symptomatic HF and abnormal cardiac biomarker testing, regardless of the left ventricular ejection fraction (LVEF). This principle is especially true when there is evidence of early structural change on imaging, such as mild left ventricular hypertrophy (LVH) or biatrial enlargement in a patient who has diastolic HF without a history of hypertension. A major clinical tipoff that amyloidosis is a possibility is when those patients have orthostasis upon presentation or if their baseline blood pressure is relatively hypotensive, because most patients with diastolic dysfunction would be expected to be hypertensive. Angina is not uncommon in patients with cardiac amyloidosis and

thought to be frequently secondary to amyloid deposition in small coronary arteries and infrequently coronary artery disease.[12,13] Other symptoms that may be indicators of a systemic amyloidosis condition include jaw claudication, difficulty swallowing, diarrhea, symptoms of peripheral neuropathy, and substantial weight change (either gain or loss). Deposition of amyloid in the heart can also lead to conduction system dysfunction, with arrhythmias and sudden death. Patients will frequently present with complaints of lightheadedness, palpitations, and syncope. In addition to affecting the conduction system, both AL and TTR amyloidosis can substantially affect the nervous system, resulting in peripheral neuropathy that frequently results in orthostatic hypotension and autonomic dysfunction that becomes a very difficult constellation of conditions to manage especially when HF is a prominent component. In TTR in particular, the pattern of fibril deposition most often occurs in the heart, kidney, and nerves. Common signs and symptoms experienced by these patients other than HF include rhythm disturbances, extremity tingling, and palpitations.[14–16] It should be noted that a personal history of carpal tunnel is a frequent historical event in both TTRm and TTRwt patients and can be a clue to diagnosis (see Box 1).[14]

CLINICAL EVALUATION

Screening for cardiac amyloidosis should be considered in all patients with unexplained HF but especially those with normal LVEF upon presentation (Figs. 1–6). Minimal evaluation should include an electrocardiogram (ECG), which can be notable for characteristic amyloid infiltration patterns of low-voltage or "pseudoinfarct" patterns in patients without a history of coronary disease (Box 2). Initial cardiac laboratory evaluation should consist of measurement of N-terminal pro-brain natriuretic peptide (NT-pro BNP) and troponin T, if available, because these 2 markers have been shown to be

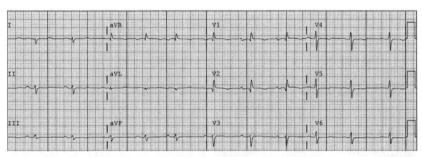

Fig. 1. There is a classic low voltage in all leads, and there is also a suggestion of an anterior infarction in a patient with normal LV function and no evidence of a regional wall motion abnormality due to ischemic heart disease (this is a pseudoinfarction pattern).

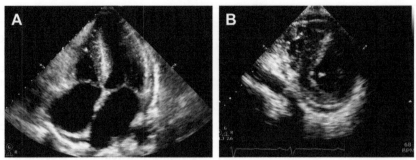

Fig. 2. Echocardiography is an initial test that may indicate cardiac amyloidosis. (*A*) Apical 4-chamber view showing typical concentric biventricular hypertrophy with biatrial enlargement. In the absence of a long history of hypertension or renal failure, one must consider an infiltrative process with this constellation of findings. (*B*) Parasternal short-axis view showing a "D"-shaped septum indicating right ventricular volume overload and a small pericardial effusion sometimes seen with cardiac amyloidosis.

First Image   Null of Myocardium   Null of Blood Pool   Last Image

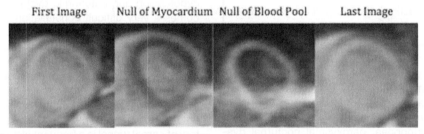

Fig. 3. Cardiac MRI short-axis views of inversion time (TI) scout images that show the myocardium nulls before the blood pool, indicating extensive expansion of the myocardial interstitium.

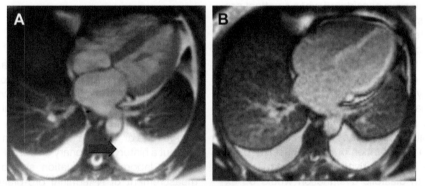

Fig. 4. (*A, B*) Cardiac MRI 4-chamber long-axis views obtained before (*A*) and after (*B*) gadolinium administration confirm dense, circumferential, near transmural late gadolinium enhancement of the entire left ventricle. There is no apparent right ventricular or atrial enhancement. Bilateral pleural effusions are evident by this imaging (*arrow*).

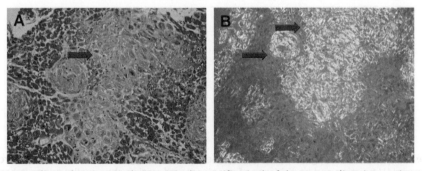

Fig. 5. (*A*) Hematoxylin and eosin stain (×66 original magnification) of the myocardium in a patient with cardiac amyloidosis. The architecture of the myocyte is destroyed by protein infiltration (*arrow*). (*B*) Apple-green birefringence with polarized light is diffusely evident on this biopsy sample (*arrows*).

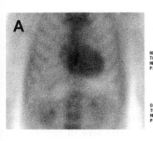

HEART
TOTAL 145.237
MEAN 117.696
PIXELS 1234

CONTRALATERAL
TOTAL 82.555
MEAN 66.846
PIXELS 1235

Fig. 6. (A) Technetium pyrophosphate scanning showing intense cardiac uptake. (B) The ratio of cardiac uptake compared with lung uptake is higher than 50%, consistent with transthyretin-related cardiac amyloidosis.

sensitive for detection of cardiac abnormalities as well as staging of disease severity and prognosis in patients with AL amyloidosis.[17] There are modified staging systems using BNP and troponin I, so these cardiac biomarkers are alternative options especially in TTR-related amyloidosis.[18] Additional blood testing is needed to establish the extent of systemic disease in the case of AL amyloidosis, such as serum free light chains, calcium, and creatinine, but a more complete list is not necessary to confirm cardiac involvement. There is a suggestion that a novel biomarker, hepatocyte growth factor (HGF), may allow an earlier diagnosis of cardiac amyloid, but these data are preliminary.[19] A transthoracic echocardiogram should be obtained, with attention to whether characteristic findings of amyloid are present, such as LVH, diastolic filling impairment, and an "apical sparing" abnormal strain pattern that may be characteristic of cardiac amyloid.[20] Cardiac MRI is frequently obtained if the estimated glomerular filtration rate is acceptable to allow the use of gadolinium contrast to evaluate for hyperenhancement.[21] For the diagnosis of TTR-related cardiac amyloidosis, a technetium pyrophosphate scan can be diagnostic, potentially precluding the need for cardiac biopsy.[22,23] In situations where the diagnosis of amyloidosis has not been confirmed with alternative biopsy locations, and the patient is persistently symptomatic, a

myocardial biopsy is necessary. These procedures are generally quite safe when done with experienced operators, and the pathologic staining is best done at institutions that are adept at those techniques. Additional genetic screening that examines the commonly identified mutations associated with amyloid should be performed in most, if not all, cases of cardiac amyloidosis because both AL and TTR closely mimic each other.[6,24,25]

STAGING

Cardiac staging systems, such as the Mayo criteria, have been generated that correlate the cardiac involvement of AL amyloidosis to the NT-pro BNP and serum troponin T.[17,26] These values have been used to risk stratify patients to different treatments (eg, stem-cell transplant or chemotherapy), follow response to therapy, and generate median survival rates. Hematologic response to treatment evaluates the difference of involved and uninvolved immunoglobulin free light chain values. However, organ-specific responses, including potential cardiac response, do not always correlate to hematologic response to treatment. The modified Mayo staging reflects the prognostic addition of free light chain level to pre-existing cardiac criteria.[17] HF severity as defined by ejection fraction decreases 10% or greater or New York Heart Association class decreases of 2 or more has also been added to the updated cardiac staging and treatment response criteria.[27] There is a new staging system proposed for TTR cardiac amyloidosis that uses similar criteria.[28]

MEDICAL THERAPY FOR CARDIAC AMYLOIDOSIS
Not Amyloid Specific

The treatment of HF encountered with cardiac amyloidosis is usually different than the standard treatment used for typical systolic HF. In many cases, these patients have diastolic HF, and thus, there is a paucity of guideline-directed optimal medical therapy in this setting alone. More importantly, it is commonplace that they have prominent orthostasis and hypotension that

---

Box 2
Typical testing that is potentially useful in detecting cardiac amyloidosis

ECG

Cardiac biomarkers (BNP, NT-pro BNP, troponin I, troponin T)

Echocardiography, particularly strain imaging

Technetium pyrophosphate scan

Cardiac MRI

Cardiac biopsy

Genetic screening for common mutations

Novel biomarkers (HGF)

limits any tolerance of vasodilator-based therapy. In fact, there is some evidence that beta-blocker–based therapy, a cornerstone of therapy for systolic dysfunction, may be harmful in the setting of cardiac amyloidosis.[29] In addition, digoxin has also been associated with a higher risk of adverse events and is generally not used in this setting. As a result, diuretics are a mainstay of treatment, and typically, a combination of loop diuretics (eg, furosemide or bumetanide) and potassium-sparing diuretics (eg, spironolactone) works well together to maintain adequate volume and potassium balance (Box 3). There is a substantial need to use electrical therapy in patients with cardiac amyloidosis, and this may include a pacemaker, implantable cardio-defibrillator, or perhaps atrial ablation techniques to name a few important tools.[30]

Amyloid Specific

The treatment of cardiac amyloidosis specifically is highly dependent on whether the cause is AL or TTR. Other more rare conditions, such as hereditary fibrinogen A alpha-chain–type amyloidosis, would be managed individually, and a definitive treatment may involve transplantation of an involved organ. For this section, the focus is on current or developing medical therapy for cardiac amyloidosis. The current treatment of AL amyloidosis, which includes cardiac involvement, uses typical therapy for multiple myeloma. Bortezomib

and other proteasome inhibitors, cyclophosphamide, immunomodulatory agents (such as revlimid and pomalidomide), and dexamethasone, form a set of chemotherapy regimens that have shown initial promise for extending the length and enhancing the quality of life in patients with AL cardiac amyloidosis.[31] There is an antibody for light chain amyloidotic protein that is currently under clinical trials for efficacy. The role of autologous stem cell transplantation is currently under investigation and certainly plays a role in consolidating contemporary therapy for AL amyloidosis.[32–34] The treatment of TTR cardiac amyloidosis is also rapidly developing in the last 5 years.[35] There are ongoing trials looking at protein-stabilizing medications, like tafamidis, to prevent the deposition of amyloidotic proteins into tissues. There are RNA silencer therapies intended to shut off the production of TTR from the liver in order to reduce or eliminate amyloidotic protein production.[36] Diflunisal, a nonsteroidal medication, may stabilize the protein and may be useful in the reduction of neuropathy.[37] There is some evidence that TTR degradation and extraction can be enhanced by using doxycycline to disrupt fibril formation if used with bile salts.[36]

Transplantation

The role of transplantation is quite complex in the case of amyloidosis. Stem cell transplantation is an important component in the treatment of AL cardiac amyloidosis as mentioned previously. Solid organ transplantation may be a critical component of managing the other organs affected. In terms of the use of cardiac transplantation as an adjunct for the treatment of amyloidosis, this is not a common occurrence, but in selected patients it is lifesaving therapy.[38]

SUMMARY

Cardiac amyloidosis is a complex and vexing clinical condition that requires a high degree of suspicion for the diagnosis with a substantial amount of discipline to discern the extent of disease and the best available therapy. There is a complex interplay between multiple organ systems, and the clinical presentation may involve a myriad of confusing clinical symptoms. The diagnosis of cardiac amyloidosis can be confirmed with a combination of physical findings, cardiac biomarkers, noninvasive testing, and, if necessary, myocardial biopsy. Genetic testing is critical to establish the type of amyloidosis. The treatment of cardiac amyloidosis is determined by the type, either AL or TTR, or less likely a very rare inherited amyloidosis. For AL amyloid, the current

---

Box 3
Summary of medical treatment options in cardiac amyloidosis

Nonamyloid specific

    Diuretics (loop and potassium sparing)

    Sodium restriction

    Avoiding nephrotoxic treatments

Amyloid specific

AL

    Bortezomib-based treatment with dexamethasone

    Immunomodulatory agents (revlimid, pomalidomide)

    Cyclophosphamide

    Dexamethasone

    Doxycycline

TTR

    Diflunisal

    Tafamidis

treatment with combination chemotherapy and possibly an autologous stem cell transplant forms the contemporary treatment paradigm. Specific treatments for TTR cardiac amyloidosis are currently under development and include protein stabilizers, protein silencers, and strategies intended to enhance degradation. The future for drug development in the treatment of cardiac amyloidosis is bright, and the need for earlier diagnosis is imperative.

REFERENCES

1. Merlini G, Bellotti V. Molecular mechanisms of amyloidosis. N Engl J Med 2003;349:583–96.
2. Wechalekar AD, Gillmore JD, Hawkins PN. Systemic amyloidosis. Lancet 2016;387:2641–54.
3. Gertz MA, Dispenzieri A, Sher T. Pathophysiology and treatment of cardiac amyloidosis. Nat Rev Cardiol 2015;12:91–102.
4. Gertz MA. Immunoglobulin light chain amyloidosis: 2016 update on diagnosis, prognosis, and treatment. Am J Hematol 2016;91:947–56.
5. Falk RH, Alexander KM, Liao R, et al. AL (light-chain) cardiac amyloidosis: a review of diagnosis and therapy. J Am Coll Cardiol 2016;68:1323–41.
6. Maurer MS, Hanna M, Grogan M, et al. Genotype and phenotype of transthyretin cardiac amyloidosis: THAOS (Transthyretin Amyloid Outcome Survey). J Am Coll Cardiol 2016;68:161–72.
7. Zhen DB, Swiecicki PL, Zeldenrust SR, et al. Frequencies and geographic distributions of genetic mutations in transthyretin- and non-transthyretin-related familial amyloidosis. Clin Genet 2015;88: 396–400.
8. Plante-Bordeneuve V, Said G. Familial amyloid polyneuropathy. Lancet Neurol 2011;10:1086–97.
9. Ruberg FL, Maurer MS, Judge DP, et al. Prospective evaluation of the morbidity and mortality of wild-type and V122I mutant transthyretin amyloid cardiomyopathy: the Transthyretin Amyloidosis Cardiac Study (TRACS). Am Heart J 2012;164:222–8.e1.
10. Ruberg FL, Berk JL. Transthyretin (TTR) cardiac amyloidosis. Circulation 2012;126:1286–300.
11. Falk RH, Quarta CC, Dorbala S. How to image cardiac amyloidosis. Circ Cardiovasc Imaging 2014;7: 552–62.
12. Quarta CC, Solomon SD, Uraizee I, et al. Left ventricular structure and function in transthyretin-related versus light-chain cardiac amyloidosis. Circulation 2014;129:1840–9.
13. Dorbala S, Vangala D, Bruyere J Jr, et al. Coronary microvascular dysfunction is related to abnormalities in myocardial structure and function in cardiac amyloidosis. JACC Heart Fail 2014;2:358–67.
14. Falk RH. Cardiac amyloidosis: a treatable disease, often overlooked. Circulation 2011;124:1079–85.
15. Gonzalez-Lopez E, Gallego-Delgado M, Guzzo-Merello G, et al. Wild-type transthyretin amyloidosis as a cause of heart failure with preserved ejection fraction. Eur Heart J 2015;36:2585–94.
16. Mohammed SF, Mirzoyev SA, Edwards WD, et al. Left ventricular amyloid deposition in patients with heart failure and preserved ejection fraction. JACC Heart Fail 2014;2:113–22.
17. Kumar S, Dispenzieri A, Lacy MQ, et al. Revised prognostic staging system for light chain amyloidosis incorporating cardiac biomarkers and serum free light chain measurements. J Clin Oncol 2012; 30:989–95.
18. Damy T, Maurer MS, Rapezzi C, et al. Clinical, ECG and echocardiographic clues to the diagnosis of TTR-related cardiomyopathy. Open Heart 2016;3: e000289.
19. Swiger KJ, Friedman EA, Brittain EL, et al. Plasma hepatocyte growth factor is a novel marker of AL cardiac amyloidosis. Amyloid 2016;23:1–7.
20. Senapati A, Sperry BW, Grodin JL, et al. Prognostic implication of relative regional strain ratio in cardiac amyloidosis. Heart 2016;102:748–54.
21. Boynton SJ, Geske JB, Dispenzieri A, et al. LGE provides incremental prognostic information over serum biomarkers in AL cardiac amyloidosis. JACC Cardiovasc Imaging 2016;9:680–6.
22. Gillmore JD, Maurer MS, Falk RH, et al. Nonbiopsy diagnosis of cardiac transthyretin amyloidosis. Circulation 2016;133:2404–12.
23. Castano A, Haq M, Narotsky DL, et al. Multicenter study of planar technetium 99m pyrophosphate cardiac imaging: predicting survival for patients with ATTR cardiac amyloidosis. JAMA Cardiol 2016;1: 880–9.
24. Kristen AV, Brokbals E, Aus dem Siepen F, et al. Cardiac amyloid load: a prognostic and predictive biomarker in patients with light-chain amyloidosis. J Am Coll Cardiol 2016;68:13–24.
25. Swiecicki PL, Zhen DB, Mauermann ML, et al. Hereditary ATTR amyloidosis: a single-institution experience with 266 patients. Amyloid 2015;22:123–31.
26. Dispenzieri A, Gertz MA, Kyle RA, et al. Serum cardiac troponins and N-terminal pro-brain natriuretic peptide: a staging system for primary systemic amyloidosis. J Clin Oncol 2004;22:3751–7.
27. Palladini G, Hegenbart U, Milani P, et al. A staging system for renal outcome and early markers of renal response to chemotherapy in AL amyloidosis. Blood 2014;124:2325–32.
28. Grogan M, Scott CG, Kyle RA, et al. Natural history of wild-type transthyretin cardiac amyloidosis and risk stratification using a novel staging system. J Am Coll Cardiol 2016;68:1014–20.
29. Selvanayagam JB, Hawkins PN, Paul B, et al. Evaluation and management of the cardiac amyloidosis. J Am Coll Cardiol 2007;50:2101–10.

30. Tan NY, Mohsin Y, Hodge DO, et al. Catheter ablation for atrial arrhythmias in patients with cardiac amyloidosis. J Cardiovasc Electrophysiol 2016;27: 1167–73.

31. Sperry BW, Ikram A, Hachamovitch R, et al. Efficacy of chemotherapy for light-chain amyloidosis in patients presenting with symptomatic heart failure. J Am Coll Cardiol 2016;67:2941–8.

32. Sher T, Dispenzieri A, Gertz MA. Evolution of hematopoietic cell transplantation for immunoglobulin light chain amyloidosis. Biol Blood Marrow Transpl 2016;22:796–801.

33. Warsame R, Bang SM, Kumar SK, et al. Outcomes and treatments of patients with immunoglobulin light chain amyloidosis who progress or relapse postautologous stem cell transplant. Eur J Haematol 2014;92:485–90.

34. D'Souza A, Dispenzieri A, Wirk B, et al. Improved outcomes after autologous hematopoietic cell transplantation for light chain amyloidosis: a center for International Blood and Marrow Transplant Research Study. J Clin Oncol 2015;33:3741–9.

35. Gertz MA, Benson MD, Dyck PJ, et al. Diagnosis, prognosis, and therapy of transthyretin amyloidosis. J Am Coll Cardiol 2015;66:2451–66.

36. Brunjes DL, Castano A, Clemons A, et al. Transthyretin cardiac amyloidosis in older Americans. J Card Fail 2016;22(12):996–1003.

37. Berk JL, Suhr OB, Obici L, et al. Repurposing diflunisal for familial amyloid polyneuropathy: a randomized clinical trial. JAMA 2013;310:2658–67.

38. Davis MK, Kale P, Liedtke M, et al. Outcomes after heart transplantation for amyloid cardiomyopathy in the modern era. Am J Transplant 2015;15:650–8.

Printed and bound by CPI Group (UK) Ltd, Croydon, CR0 4YY

03/10/2024

01040298-0011